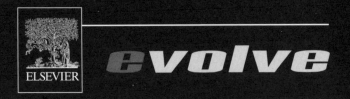

ELSEVIER

To access your Student Resources, visit the Web address below:

http://evolve.elsevier.com/

- **WebLinks**

  An exciting resource that lets you link to hundreds of websites carefully chosen to supplement the content of the textbook. The WebLinks are regularly updated, with new ones added as they develop.

JOINT RANGE of MOTION
and
MUSCLE LENGTH TESTING

JOINT RANGE of MOTION
and
MUSCLE LENGTH TESTING

· ·

NANCY BERRYMAN REESE, PhD, PT
Associate Professor
Department of Physical Therapy
University of Central Arkansas
Conway, Arkansas

Adjunct Assistant Professor
Department of Anatomy
University of Arkansas for Medical Sciences
Little Rock, Arkansas

WILLIAM D. BANDY, PhD, PT, SCS, ATC
Professor
Department of Physical Therapy
University of Central Arkansas
Conway, Arkansas

Photographer: Michael Morris, FBCA
University of Arkansas for Medical Sciences
Little Rock, Arkansas

SAUNDERS
An Imprint of Elsevier

SAUNDERS
An Imprint of Elsevier

The Curtis Center
Independence Square West
Philadelphia, Pennsylvania 19106

Library of Congress Cataloging-in-Publication Data

Reese, Nancy Berryman.
    Joint range of motion and muscle length testing/Nancy Berryman Reese, William D. Bandy.

       p.   cm.

    ISBN-13: 978-0-7216-8942-5   ISBN-10: 0-7216-8942-6

    1. Joints—Range of motion—Measurement. 2. Muscles—Measurement. 3. Physical therapy.
I. Bandy, William D.   II. Title.
    [DNLM: 1. Range of Motion, Articular. 2. Muscles—physiology.   WE 103 R329j 2002]

RC932 .R435 2002

612.795—dc21   2001020321

Editor-in-chief: Andrew M. Allen
Developmental Editor: Rachael Zipperlen
Manuscript Editor: Jeffrey L. Scheib
Production Manager: Guy Barber
Illustration Specialist: Robert F. Quinn
Page layout: Lynn Foulk

JOINT RANGE OF MOTION AND MUSCLE LENGTH TESTING

ISBN-13: 978-0-7216-8942-5

ISBN-10: 0-7216-8942-6

Printed in the United States of America.

Last digit is the print number: 9   8   7   6   5   4   3

· ·

To our parents, Steve and Geneva Berryman and Dick and Betty Bandy, whose love and guidance have sustained us throughout our lives.

"My son, keep your father's commands and do not forsake your mother's teaching. Bind them upon your heart forever; fasten them around your neck. When you walk, they will guide you; when you sleep, they will watch over you; when you awake, they will speak to you. For these commands are a lamp, this teaching is a light," Prov. 6:20–23a (NIV)

PREFACE

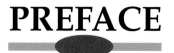

In writing *Joint Range of Motion and Muscle Length Testing*, we had two primary goals. The first was to create a highly organized, easy-to-follow text that contained comprehensive techniques for measuring joint range of motion and muscle length of the spine and extremities. Our second goal was to provide the most accurate, up-to-date information possible on norms for range of motion in all age groups and on reliability and validity of the techniques included in the text.

We believe that *Joint Range of Motion and Muscle Length Testing* fulfills both of our established goals. A comprehensive set of techniques is included that details measurement of both joint range of motion and muscle length of the spine and extremities using the goniometer, the inclinometer, and the tape measure. In fact, we believe that this text provides the most complete information available to date on measurement of muscle length of the upper and lower extremities and on measurement of range of motion of the spine. Every effort was made to provide a combination of instructions, illustrations, and layout for each technique that would allow the reader to easily follow and comprehend the intent of the authors. We hope our readers find that such is the case.

Fulfillment of our second goal was more difficult than we had at first imagined. The community of health care providers who measure range of motion of patients has relied for far too long on norms of range of motion that have little or no scientific basis. We sought to update those poorly based norms with norms derived from population-based studies of normal range of motion. Unfortunately, a comprehensive review of the literature revealed a paucity of studies with samples of sufficient size and randomness to allow the data to be generalized to the population. However, we were able, in some cases, to provide updated norms for range of motion based on values obtained in the literature. A more detailed explanation of our literature review and its findings is located in Appendix C. Additionally, comprehensive information regarding studies that have focused on reliability or validity of

techniques of measuring joint range of motion and muscle length is found in Chapters 7, 10, and 15.

Overall, *Joint Range of Motion and Muscle Length Testing* is divided into four sections. Section I provides the background needed for the reader to better understand and utilize the information in Sections II through IV. Chapter 1 differentiates joint range of motion from muscle length testing, includes a history of measurement techniques, and then introduces the basic concepts of measurement. Chapter 2 also provides background information, but deals with the clinical relevance of information related to joint range of motion and muscle length. This chapter presents information on changes in range of motion and muscle length that occur with age, differences between men and women, as well as differences due to culture and occupation. In addition, Chapter 2 provides basic, but important, information regarding reliability and validity of measurement, in general.

The majority of chapters in Sections II through IV are related to the specific techniques used to measure joint range of motion and muscle length. We have attempted to describe each technique in a similar manner for the ease of use of the reader. Additionally, each section also contains one chapter devoted to the reliability and validity of the specific measurement techniques introduced in that section.

The chapters in Section II are devoted to measurement of the upper extremity. Chapters 3 through 5 describe the actual techniques for the measurement of joint range of motion of the upper extremity. Chapter 6 describes techniques for the measurement of muscle length. Finally, Chapter 7 presents information on the reliability and validity of the upper extremity techniques described in Chapters 3 through 6.

The three chapters in Section III provide information on the measurement of range of motion of the spine. Chapter 8 describes techniques for measurement of the lumbar and thoracic spine, and Chapter 9 is related to the cervical spine and temporomandibular joint. The reader should note that these chapters are organized by motion and not by measurement device. For example, all techniques for measuring cervical flexion (tape measure, inclinometer, CROM) are presented together in Chapter 8. In Chapter 10, information about the reliability and validity of measurement techniques of the spine is presented.

Section IV is organized in a similar manner to Section II, with Chapters 11 through 13 describing techniques related to measurement of joint range of motion of the lower extremity, and Chapter 14 presenting information on muscle length tests for the lower extremity. In Chapter 15, the reader is presented with information on reliability and validity of the methods described in Chapters 11 through 14.

Finally, the Appendices provide related information for performing an examination of an individual's range of motion and muscle length. Appendices A and B include information on capsular patterns that may affect joint range of motion and sample forms for recording range of motion and muscle length testing. Within Appendix C are found tables of traditionally accepted norms for joint range of motion, revised range of motion tables based on a comprehensive critique of the available literature, and data to support changes in range of motion norms. A complete set of tables summarizing all reviewed studies which examined range of motion of the spine and extremities can be found at www.wbsaunders.com/SIMON/Reese/joint/.

Mastery of techniques used to measure joint range of motion and muscle length can be achieved only through repeated practice. The reader is highly encouraged to practice initially on individuals with full range of motion in a supervised setting. Once the novice feels comfortable with the techniques, practice should occur on patients with impairments in range of motion and muscle length, again under close supervision. With repeated practice, the novice should quickly become proficient in the measurement of joint range of motion and muscle length using the techniques described in this text.

NANCY BERRYMAN REESE
WILLIAM D. BANDY

ACKNOWLEDGMENTS

Writing a book is never an easy task, and doing so with a co-author presents its own set of challenges. So, before we thank the long list of all those who supported us in completing this book, first we must thank each other. We each would like to thank the other for all the exhausting work, dedication, and attention to detail that went into the creation of *Joint Range of Motion and Muscle Length Testing*. We are grateful for mutual patience, for forgiveness when patience gave way to heated discussions or worse, and for the encouragement that each of us gave to the other to strive to perform at a higher level. Most importantly, we are thankful for a strong and abiding friendship which saw us through this project and will sustain us in those to come.

Throughout the creation and writing of this book, we have had incredible support from the editorial staff at W.B. Saunders. Our sincere thanks go to our editor, Andrew Allen, whose encouragement led us to undertake this task, and to Rachael Zipperlen, our developmental editor, who gently kept us focused and provided us with invaluable help and support. During preparation of the figures, we had the incredible opportunity to work again with Michael Morris, FBCA, who did all the beautiful photography for the text. He is a consummate professional, and having each had the experience of working with him on two books, we can't imagine ever using another photographer. Research, secretarial support, and proofing was provided by our brilliant graduate assistants, Danyelle Lusby, Stacey Ihler, Jenny Hood, Amanda Whitehead, and Vicki Readnour, to whom we are forever grateful. We would be still in the process of writing without their able assistance. Models for the photographs in this text included physical therapy students Rachel Ladin, Trigg Ross, Michael Adkins, Rachel Cloud, Blake Wagner, and Brooke Bridges as well as Jamie Bandy and Brandon Chandler. Sherry Holmes served as the model for the examiner in many of the photographs. We appreciate the patience and hard work of all the models, especially when the studio got cold and their muscles got fatigued from long sessions of posing for the camera.

Our most important thanks go to those who provided us with emotional support during the completion of this project. We both have been blessed for many years to work for a creative and supportive chairperson, Dr. Venita Lovelace-Chandler, and with a talented and dedicated group of faculty in the Department of Physical Therapy at the University of Central Arkansas. We are continuously grateful for their support and encouragement and for their tolerance of missed deadlines in the name of "the book." Finally, our largest debt of gratitude goes to our families: to Nancy's husband David and daughters Elizabeth and Nicole, and to Bill's wife Beth and daughters Melissa and Jamie. The love, support, and tolerance that they have shown us through all these years is cherished more than any of them can know. We are truly humbled that God has blessed us with such wonderful families.

NANCY BERRYMAN REESE
WILLIAM D. BANDY

CONTENTS

S E C T I O N

1

INTRODUCTION

MEASUREMENT of RANGE of MOTION and MUSCLE LENGTH: BACKGROUND, HISTORY, and BASIC PRINCIPLES

Historically, early reports of the procedures for the examination of range of motion (ROM) suggested using visual approximation.[23] In fact, as late as the 1960s, the initial edition (1965) of a text for measuring joint range of motion published by the American Academy of Orthopaedic Surgeons (AAOS)[2] suggested that visual estimation is as good as, or better than, goniometric measurement. This opinion was shared by Rowe,[81] who suggested that visual estimation was especially important when bony landmarks were difficult to see or to palpate. However, none of these authors provide any objective data to support their claims.

More recently, Watkins et al.[94] reported that reliability of the measurement of knee flexion was greater when using a goniometer than when using visual estimation. Additionally, two studies in which the lead author was Youdas[101, 102] reported that the use of instruments to examine the ankle and the cervical spine resulted in more accurate measurements than did visual estimates. Given that research has indicated that objective measurement is more accurate than visual examination for the measurement of joint range of motion, and that scientists, the government, and the public demand improved outcomes of patient intervention, accurate and standardized measurements are of utmost importance.

The purpose of Chapter 1 is to lay the groundwork for standardized measurement of range of motion and muscle length. To this end, the chapter defines the difference between joint range of motion and muscle length as well as presents basic but important information on kinematics (including the definitions of arthrokinematics and osteokinematics). Additionally, background information and history of a variety of measurement techniques, related both to joint range of motion and to muscle length testing, are provided. Finally, suggested procedures for standardized measurement are presented. After reading Chapter 1, the reader will have gained general information on the measurement of range of motion and muscle length, which serves as the basis for performance of the more specific measurement techniques presented in subsequent chapters.

JOINT RANGE OF MOTION VS. MUSCLE LENGTH

Joint range of motion is an integral part of human movement. In order for an individual to move efficiently and with minimal effort, full range of motion across the joints is imperative. In addition, appropriate range of motion allows the joints to adapt more easily to stresses imposed on the body, as well as decreasing the potential for injury. Full range of motion across a joint is dependent on two components: joint range of motion and muscle length.[103]

Joint range of motion is the motion available at any single joint and is influenced by the associated bony structure and the physiologic characteristics of the connective tissue surrounding the joint. Important connective tissue that limits joint range of motion includes ligaments and joint capsule.[37]

Muscle length refers to the ability of the muscle surrounding the joint to lengthen, allowing one joint or a series of joints to move through the available range of motion. The terms *muscle length* and *flexibility* are often used synonymously to describe the ability of muscle to be lengthened to the end of the range of motion. In this book, the term *muscle length* is used to refer to the end of the range of the muscle across the joint.[103]

According to Kendall et al.,[57] "For muscles that pass over *one joint* only, the range of motion and range of muscle length will measure the same. . . . For muscles that pass over *two or more* joints, the normal range of muscle length will be less than the total range of motion of the joints over which the muscle passes." Therefore, if the goal is to measure joint range of motion of a joint in which a two-joint muscle is involved, the second joint should be placed in a shortened position. If the goal is to measure muscle length, the muscle should be placed in an elongated position across all joints affected, and a measurement should be taken.[57]

An example to illustrate the difference between range of motion and range of muscle length is the measurement of knee flexion. In order to measure knee flexion joint motion, the hip should be flexed (the patient is supine) to put the rectus femoris muscle in a shortened position, and to allow full joint motion at the knee (illustrated in Chapter 12, Figs. 12–1 through 12–4). In order to measure muscle length of the rectus femoris muscle (a two-joint muscle), the patient is placed in the prone position, which extends the hip and lengthens the rectus femoris muscle (described in Chapter 14, Figs. 14–13 through 14–15).

KINEMATICS

Soderberg[91] defines *kinematics* as "the description of motion without regard to forces." In other words, kinematics describes human movement and ignores the cause of the motion (for example, forces, momentum, energy). This description of motion may include movement of the center of gravity of the body or movement of the extremities, or it may include motion specific to one joint. Kinematics can be subcategorized into specific movements, referred to as *arthrokinematics* and *osteokinematics*. To more fully understand kinematics as it relates to measurement of range of joint motion and muscle length, clarification of the terms arthrokinematics and osteokinematics is necessary.

In addition, an understanding of anything that can affect normal kinematic range of motion is important, especially the concept of the capsular pattern. Information related to the capsular pattern is presented in Appendix A.

ARTHROKINEMATICS

Arthrokinematics refers to the actual movements of the joint surfaces in relation to one another. In addition to the movement of the lever arm of the bone during range of motion activities, the articulating ends of the bone roll and slide (or glide) on each other. Roll is a rotary motion that occurs when new points on one joint surface come in contact with new points on a second joint surface. Slide is a translatory motion and occurs when one joint surface glides across a second surface so that the same point on one surface is continually in contact with new points on the second surface.[52] Although arthrokinematic motion is vital to normal range of motion, this textbook does not address the measurement or grading of this type of motion.

OSTEOKINEMATICS

The quality and degree of motion actually observed in the bony lever arm is called osteokinematic motion. Osteokinematic motion is the movement of the whole bone resulting from rolling and sliding (arthrokinematics) between the articulating surfaces that compose the joint measured.[37] For example, when raising the arm overhead, the bony lever arm (the humerus) moving overhead is the osteokinematic motion. But in order for this motion to occur, the head of the humerus must roll and slide on the glenoid fossa (arthrokinematic motion). In most cases, osteokinematic motion is the actual motion that is measured and is the focus of this textbook.

Osteokinematic description of movement follows a generalized system based on definitions of planes of movement around axes of rotation. For effective discussion of planes of motion and axes of movement, a reference point is required, a point referred to as the anatomical position. This reference point (anatomical position) is defined as "standing erect with the head, toes, and palms of the hands facing forward and with the fingers extended."[90] When measuring the range of motion at a joint, the starting position is typically the anatomical position. Figures 1–1 through 1–4 all show the model standing in the anatomical position.

Osteokinematic movement may be described as occurring in one of three imaginary planes of the body arranged perpendicular to each other, with the axes of each plane intersecting the center of gravity of the body. These imaginary planes are referred to as the cardinal planes of the body. It should be emphasized that human motion is not limited to movement in these cardinal planes, but that this system of planes of movement around axes of rotation provides a simple method for describing range of motion and muscle length.[90]

Sagittal Plane

The sagittal plane is a vertical plane that divides the body into right and left sides (Fig. 1–1). Photographically, this is a side view. Joint movement in the sagittal plane occurs around a line perpendicular to the plane that is referred to as the medial-lateral axis. The osteokinematic motions that occur in the

Sagittal plane

Medial-lateral axis

sagittal plane are flexion and extension (Fig. 1–2).[90] *Gray's Anatomy* defines flexion as occurring "when the angle between two bones is decreased."[22] In other words, during flexion, the two bony levers move around the joint axis so that the two levers approach each other. Flexion at the ankle is given a special term, with the approximation of the foot and the leg in the sagittal plane being referred to as dorsiflexion.

Extension is the opposite of flexion. It occurs when the two bony levers move away from each other and is defined as "the act of straightening a

Fig. 1–2. Osteokinematic motions; note that model is standing in anatomical position.

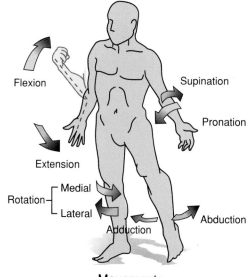

Flexion

Supination

Pronation

Extension

Rotation — Medial / Lateral

Abduction

Adduction

Movements

limb," which "occurs when the angle between the bones is increased."[22] Hyperextension is defined as extension beyond the normal anatomical range of motion. Plantarflexion of the foot at the ankle in the sagittal plane is the opposite of dorsiflexion.

Frontal Plane

The frontal (or coronal) plane is a vertical plane that divides the body into anterior (ventral, or front) and posterior (dorsal, or back) halves (Fig. 1–3). Photographically, this is a front view. Joint movement in the frontal plane occurs around a line perpendicular to the plane that is referred to as the anterior-posterior axis. The osteokinematic motions that occur in the frontal plane are abduction, adduction, and lateral flexion of the spine (see Fig. 1–2).[90]

Abduction is defined as occurring "when a limb is moved away from the midsagittal plane or when the fingers or toes are moved away from the median longitudinal axis of the hand or foot."[90] Abduction of the wrist is often referred to as radial deviation. The median longitudinal axis of the hand is the third metacarpal, and for the foot this axis is the second metatarsal. An exception to this definition is abduction that takes place at the carpometacarpal (CMC) joint of the thumb, which is defined as "that action by which the thumb is elevated anterior to the palm."[22] Therefore, abduction at the CMC joint actually takes place in the sagittal plane.

Adduction is the opposite of abduction and "occurs when a limb is moved toward, or beyond the midsagittal plane or when the fingers or toes are moved toward the median longitudinal axis of the hand or foot."[22] Adduction of the wrist is often referred to as ulnar deviation. At the CMC joint of the thumb, adduction is moving the thumb posteriorly toward the palm (sagittal plane movement).

Fig. 1–3. Frontal plane; note that model is standing in anatomical position.

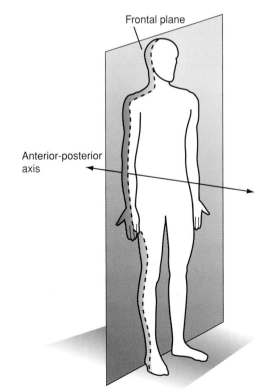

Frontal plane

Anterior-posterior axis

Transverse Plane

The transverse plane is a horizontal plane that divides the body into upper (superior, or cranial) and lower (inferior, or caudal) halves (Fig. 1–4). Photographically, this is a view from the top of the head. Joint movement in the transverse plane occurs around a line perpendicular to the plane (a line running from cranial to caudal) that is referred to as the longitudinal (or long) axis. The osteokinematic motions that occur in the transverse plane are medial rotation, lateral rotation, pronation, and supination (see Fig. 1–2).[90]

Rotation "is a form of movement in which a bone moves around a central axis without undergoing any other displacement."[22] Medial (or internal) rotation refers to rotation toward the body's midline, and lateral (or external) rotation refers to rotation away from the body's midline. Pronation is defined as medial rotation of the forearm and occurs when the segment is turned in a way that causes the palm of the hand to face posteriorly (in relation to anatomical position). Supination is lateral rotation of the forearm and occurs when the segment is turned so that the palm of the hand faces anteriorly (related to anatomical position).

Special Case: Oblique Axis at the Foot and Ankle

Motions occurring at the talocrural, subtalar, and midtarsal joints do not take place around the previously described cardinal axes. Contemporary explanations describe motion at these joints as occurring around oblique axes that lie at angles to all three cardinal planes.[29, 79] These so-called triplanar axes run in an anteromedial-to-posterolateral direction and allow motion in all three planes simultaneously (Fig. 1–5). The motions thus produced have been termed pronation (a combination of dorsiflexion, abduction, and eversion) and supination (a combination of plantarflexion, adduction, and inversion).[27, 79]

Fig. 1–4. Transverse plane; note the model is standing in anatomical position.

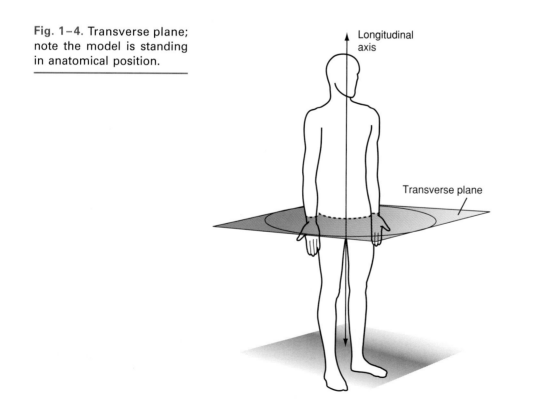

Longitudinal axis

Transverse plane

Fig. 1–5. Oblique axis of foot and ankle.

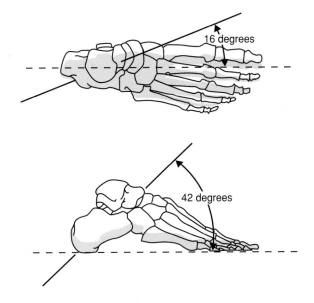

16 degrees

42 degrees

HISTORY OF INSTRUMENTS TO MEASURE RANGE OF MOTION AND MUSCLE LENGTH

UNIVERSAL GONIOMETER

The inspiration for the universal goniometer appears to have been devices used to measure range of motion that were developed in France early in the 1900s.[88] Initial publications describing the use of goniometers are apparently contained in the French medical literature, and descriptions of goniometric use did not appear in the American or British literature until the second decade of the 20th century.[38, 41] With the advent of each of the World Wars came an increased interest in, and use of, the goniometer.[66] Although many variations and specialized designs of the goniometer have been developed over the years,[13, 20, 41, 71, 80, 86, 93, 98, 100] today's universal goniometer remains little changed from the instrument described by Clark[19] in 1920.

Measurement Techniques

While reliable goniometers were available for measuring joint range of motion early in the 20th century, examiners did not agree on the correct procedures for performing goniometric measurements. In 1920, Clark[19] attempted to alleviate this problem by providing some standards for examining and recording joint range of motion using the universal goniometer. He described a standardized starting position for measurement that was identical to the anatomical position currently used, with the exception of the position of the ankle, which Clark[19] described as fully extended (plantarflexed). Additionally, Clark[19] provided values for the normal range of motion of joints of the spine and extremities, although the source and method of measurement on which these values were based were not stated. However, no description of techniques for patient positioning and goniometer placement was included in Clark's[19] recommendations.

Numerous other individuals and groups have proposed methods for measuring and recording joint range of motion using the universal goniometer.*

---

* See references 2, 3, 15, 21, 29, 66, 72, 77, 80, 86, 96.

The most widely accepted techniques appear to be those published by the American Academy of Orthopaedic Surgeons,[2, 44] which were based on work done by Cave and Roberts.[15] These techniques, which are cited more than the techniques of any other group in studies involving measurement of range of motion, were developed by a committee of the American Academy of Orthopaedic Surgeons in the early 1960s. The pamphlet containing the original techniques was sent to members of the American Academy of Orthopaedic Surgeons in 1961, and subsequently to orthopaedic societies in Australia, Great Britain, Canada, New Zealand, and South Africa. Following multiple revisions, the techniques were published in booklet form by the American Academy of Orthopaedic Surgeons[2] in 1965, with the approval of orthopaedic societies in all countries to which the original pamphlet was sent. The most recent version of the AAOS techniques was published by Greene and Heckman in 1994.[44]

While the AAOS techniques[44] provide illustrations to aid in the measurement of range of motion, specific landmarks for alignment of the goniometer during measurement are not provided. Instructions consist primarily of line drawings of a subject in what is termed the "zero starting position," with limits of normal range of motion indicated in some but not all cases. These norms are based, for the most part, on studies of adults, with small sample sizes and no accompanying reliability data. The reliability of techniques used to measure joint motion also is not discussed.

Efforts have been made, and continue to be made, to refine the techniques of goniometry used to measure range of motion of the joints. Several groups of investigators have examined the reliability of currently used techniques (see Chapters 7, 10, and 15), and, in some cases, recommendations have been made as to preferred techniques for measuring a particular joint motion, based on reliability studies. However, the most reliable techniques for measuring motion at the majority of joints in the body are yet to be determined, and much additional work remains to be done in this area.

Methods of Documentation

Currently, the most widely accepted method of recording range of motion information is based on a system of measurement known as the 0–180 system. This system defines the anatomical position as the 0-degree starting position of all joints except the forearm, which is fully supinated. Thus, neutral extension at each joint is recorded as 0 degrees, and, as the joint flexes, motion progresses toward 180 degrees. The 0–180 system, which was first described by Silver[86] in 1923, has been endorsed by the AAOS[44] and the American Medical Association (AMA),[3] as well as in the physical therapy literature.[66] Descriptions of how to document range of motion using the 0–180 method are provided later in this chapter.

Other measurement systems have been used as a basis for the recording of range of motion, but these methods are rarely used today. In 1920, Clark[19] described a system for recording range of motion based on the idea that neutral extension at each joint is recorded as 180 degrees, movement toward flexion approaches 0 degrees, and movement toward extension past neutral also approaches 0 degrees.[19] According to this 180–0 system, the shoulder position that would be indicated as 145 degrees flexion according to the 0–180 system, would be designated as 35 degrees flexion according to the 180–0 system. A second system that has been used in the past but is not in common use today is based on a full 360-degree circle, in which the 0-degree position of each joint is full flexion, neutral extension is recorded as 180 degrees, and motions toward extension past neutral approach 360 degrees.[68, 97]

OTHER MEASUREMENT DEVICES

While the universal goniometer remains the most widely used instrument in the measurement of joint motion, limitations in the application of this device to some joints have led to the development of specialized devices for measuring joint motion. Most of these devices are designed to measure motion at only one, or at most a few, joints, although some are capable of more wide-spread application. Examples of highly specialized devices for measuring joint range of motion include the Therabite, for measuring motion of the temporomandibular joint (see Figs. 9–67 and 9–68 for a description of its use), and specialized devices for measuring motion of the shoulder,[1, 80] forearm,[4, 20, 26, 50] wrist,[26, 50] hand,[31, 47, 71] hip,[34, 46, 80] knee,[34] and foot and ankle.[5, 12, 28, 65, 69, 78]

Some of the more specialized devices for measuring joint range of motion are adaptable for measuring motion at several joints. Examples of such devices include the inclinometer (also called the bubble goniometer, pendulum goniometer, and gravity goniometer) and the electrogoniometer, as well as various types of radiographic, photographic, and video recording equipment. Of these specialized devices, the inclinometer is probably the most widely used, because of its portability and relatively low cost.

Inclinometer

In the early 1930s, Fox and van Breeman[39] reported measuring range of motion using an instrument called the pendulum goniometer, which consisted of a circular scale "to the center of which is attached a weighted pointer at one end so that it remains vertical while the scale rotates around it." Early studies reported using a pendulum goniometer to measure range of motion of the upper and lower extremities.[42, 48, 66]

In 1955, Leighton[60] introduced a similar instrument, referred to as the "Leighton flexometer," consisting of a 360-degree dial and a weighted pointer mounted in a case. The dial and pointer operated freely, with movement being controlled by gravity. The device was strapped to the segment being measured, the dial was locked at the extreme of motion, and the arc of movement was registered by the pointer. Leighton's[60] study was one of the first to use the device to attempt to provide normative data on range of motion and muscle length in 30 joints of the extremities and trunk in a group of 16-year-old males. More recently, Ekstrand et al.[30] used a modification of the Leighton flexometer in the measurement of range of motion of the hip, knee, and ankle.

Schenker[85] introduced the fluid goniometer (bubble goniometer) in 1956. The fluid goniometer contains a 360-degree scale with a fluid-filled circular tube containing a small air bubble. Strapping the device to the segment being measured and moving the segment causes the scale to rotate while the bubble remains stationary, thereby indicating the range of motion in the scale. The fluid goniometer has been used to measure the shoulder,[18] knee,[76] elbow,[73] ankle,[65] and cervical spine.[8]

Loebl[61] was the first to use the term *inclinometer* to describe the wide range of measuring instruments that rely on the principle of gravity. In general, these instruments are calibrated or referenced on the basis of gravity, with a starting zero position that is indicated by a fluid level or, more commonly, a weighted needle. Today, the term *inclinometer* includes devices labeled for how the instrument works (gravity goniometer, bubble goniometer) as well as for the manufacturer that developed the measurement tool (Myrin goniometer, Rangiometer, CROM, BROM).[59]

Electrogoniometer

Electrogoniometers, which convert angular motion of the joint into an electric signal, first appeared in the 1950s.[55] The basic principle of this type of gonionmeter has been modified to produce a variety of styles of electrogoniometer that are currently in use. Some electrogoniometers are designed to measure motion at a single joint, such as the elbow[67] or the hip,[32] whereas others are designed to measure motion at a variety of joints.[4, 17, 43, 70] Designs range from fairly cumbersome devices to more compact, portable systems. Although many electrogoniometers are capable of measuring motion in several planes simultaneously, the cost of these devices and the skill required for application have caused electrogoniometers to be used primarily in research applications.

Photography and Video Recording Equipment

Still photography has been used to measure joint range of motion for decades[99, 104] and remains in use today.[10, 35] Although still photography has been reported to be more accurate than standard methods of goniometry in measuring range of motion of the elbow joint,[35] measuring range of motion using still photography requires more time and effort than is practical in a normal clinical situation. Video recording techniques also have been used to measure joint range of motion.[10, 16, 56, 83] While many motion analysis systems are commercially available, the examination of joint range of motion using video recording equipment, such as motion analysis systems, remains generally confined to the research arena because of the prohibitive cost and decreased portability of such equipment.

Radiographic Equipment

The gold standard against which all other techniques of measuring joint range of motion are compared is radiographic measurement of joint motion. Radiographic techniques have been used to study the amount and type of motion occurring at various joints, as well as to examine the validity of goniometry.[6, 33, 62–64, 75, 92, 95] However, the routine use of radiographic techniques for the measurement of joint motion is not recommended because of the health risks of repeated exposure to radiation and because of the high costs involved.

MEASUREMENT METHODS OF MUSCLE LENGTH

A review of the literature indicates that muscle length is measured using primarily two methods. The first method uses the traditional *composite tests*, which consist of measuring movement across more than one muscle or more than one joint.[49] Frequently used composite tests include the sit-and-reach test (Fig. 1–6), Apley's scratch test (Fig. 1–7), the shoulder-lift test (Fig. 1–8), and the fingertip-to-floor test (Fig. 1–9). The second method is *direct measurement* of muscle length, in which excursion between adjacent segments of one joint is involved.[53]

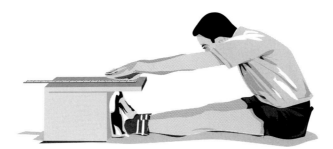

Fig. 1–6. Sit and reach test: Composite muscle length test for lower extremity.

COMPOSITE METHOD

Examination of muscle length originated in the physical education literature and can be traced back to the 1940s, when a large number of veterans returned from World War II with limited movement capabilities.[7] Following World War II, great emphasis was placed on physical fitness testing, with *flexibility* being one component that was measured. In 1941, Cureton[24] published a "14-Item Motor Fitness Test" that contained four measures of flexibility. These flexibility measurements consisted of composite tests involving flexion and extension of the entire length of the body.

Interest in the importance of examining muscle length was heightened when Kraus[58] reported that a lack of flexibility and strength were major factors in the high incidence of back pain in the United States. Testing by Kraus,[58] using strength testing and composite flexibility tests, indicated that American children were minimally fit and significantly less fit than European children, leading to the further increase in use of fitness testing. Fleischman[36] used six fitness tests to perform a factor analytic study that concluded that flexibility was "one of the important parts of overall fitness."

In the 1970s, the American Alliance for Health, Physical Education, Recreation, and Dance (AAHPERD) built on the work of these fitness pioneers and developed language to describe *health-related physical fitness*. Health-related physical fitness consists of qualities that "have been formed to contribute to one's general health by reducing the risk of cardiovascular disease,

Fig. 1–7. Apley's scratch test: Composite muscle length test for upper extremity. (From Magee DJ: Orthopedic Physical Assessment, 3rd ed. Philadelphia, WB Saunders, 1997, with permission.)

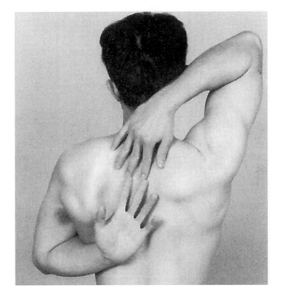

Fig. 1–8. Shoulder lift test: Composite muscle length test for upper extremity.

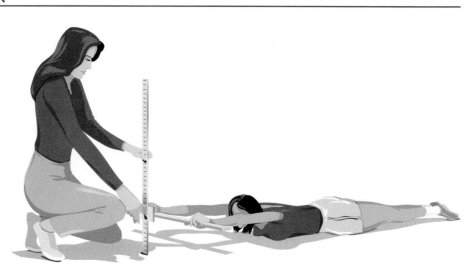

problems associated with obesity, and chronic back problems."[7] Health-related fitness consists of five categories that should be examined: aerobic endurance, muscular endurance, muscular strength, body composition, and flexibility. The AAHPERD developed a standardized health-related fitness test battery, referred to as the "Physical Best Assessment Program." Included in this program is the composite flexibility test referred to as the sit-and-reach test (described later in this text in Chapter 8).[7]

DIRECT MEASUREMENT

Flexibility is not only one of the five specific components of health-related physical fitness defined by the AAHPERD, but research indicates that flexibility is highly specific to each muscle involved. It does not exist as a general characteristic, but is specific to the joint and muscle in question.[11, 49, 53]

Fig. 1–9. Fingertip-to-floor test: Composite muscle length test for lumbar spine.

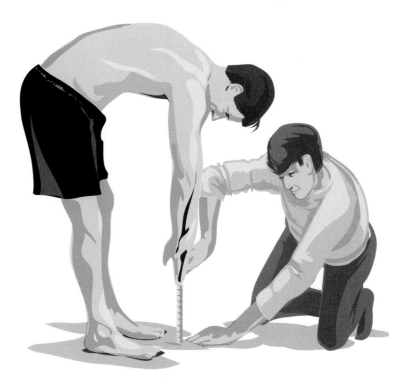

This research has shown that it is possible to have ideal muscle length in one muscle crossing a joint and poor flexibility at another joint in the body. Harris[49] suggested that "there is no evidence that flexibility exists as a single general characteristic of the human body. Thus, no one composite test can give a satisfactory index of the flexibility characteristics of an individual."

Hubley-Kozey[53] suggested that composite tests do not provide accurate measurements of flexibility because these tests are combinations of movements across several joints and involve several muscles. The author continues by indicating that composite tests are of questionable accuracy, owing to difficulty in determining which muscles actually are being examined and to the complexity of the movement. In conclusion, Hubley-Kozey[53] suggests that composite tests "serve as gross approximations for flexibility, at best."

Based on the information provided by authors such as Harris[49] and Hubley-Kozey,[53] composite measurement does not appear to be the appropriate measurement technique for muscle length. Therefore, in this text every effort is made to provide only direct measurement of flexibility in the description of the techniques for upper (Chapter 6) and lower (Chapter 14) extremity muscle length testing.

PROCEDURES FOR MEASUREMENT

INSTRUMENTATION

Three primary types of instruments will be employed in the measurement of range of motion and muscle length in this text. These instruments include the universal goniometer and the variations of this measurement tool, the inclinometer and its variations, and linear forms of measurement such as the tape measure. A description of each type of instrument and exercises that will help the student become familiar with each instrument are presented in this section.

Universal Goniometer

The universal goniometer is produced in a variety of forms and sizes (Fig. 1–10). Most commonly, the universal goniometer is made of either metal or clear plastic and consists of a central protractor portion on which are mounted two arms of varying lengths. The protractor portion of the

Fig. 1–10. Various styles and sizes of universal goniometers.

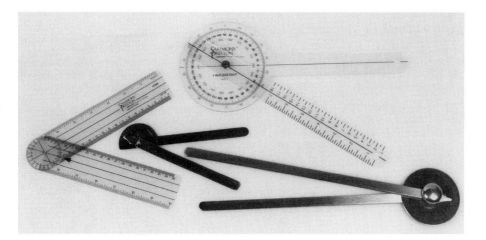

Fig. 1–11. Plastic universal goniometer with full circle protractor. Stationary arm, moving arm, and axis are labeled. Scale of goniometer marked in increments of one degree.

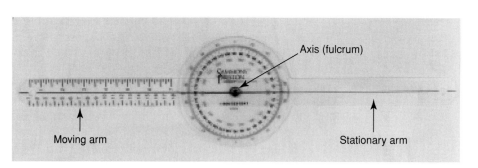

Moving arm

Axis (fulcrum)

Stationary arm

goniometer may be either a full circle or a half circle, both of which are calibrated in degrees. Although the scales of some goniometers are marked in gradations of 2.5 or 5 degrees, for optimal accuracy the scale should be marked at 1-degree intervals. Many goniometers are marked with a line that runs from the 0-degree to the 180-degree mark on the protractor. This line represents the base line of the protractor and serves as a reference point for measurements. One of the two arms of the goniometer is an extension of the protractor (the stationary arm), while the other arm is riveted to, and can move independently of, the protractor (the moving arm) (Fig. 1–11). The central rivet, which attaches the moving arm to the protractor, functions as the axis, or fulcrum, of the goniometer.

If the goniometer is made of metal, the end of the moving arm that is in contact with the protractor (the proximal end) should either be tapered to a point on its end or contain a cutout so that the degree indicators on the protractor scale can be viewed (see Fig. 1–10). This concern is not present with a plastic goniometer, since the scale can be easily viewed through the plastic arm. The arms of a plastic goniometer generally are calibrated along their length in centimeters or inches, for convenience when linear measurements are needed. Additionally, a prominent line extends from the axis of the goniometer down the midline of each arm, providing a landmark on the goniometer that can be maintained in line with bony landmarks on the body during goniometric measurements (see Fig. 1–11).

Many modifications of the basic design for the universal goniometer exist. One of the most common, and one that is used in this text, is the finger goniometer. The finger goniometer is basically a scaled-down version of the universal goniometer, with some modifications so that it fits the finger joints more precisely (Fig. 1–12). The finger goniometer is designed to be used over the dorsum of the finger joints, and many styles have broad arms that lie flat against the dorsal surfaces of the metacarpals or phalanges when the

Fig. 1–12. Two styles of finger goniometers.

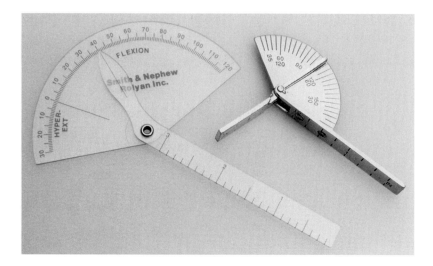

goniometer is in place. Some styles of finger goniometer are limited as to the amount of extension that can be measured because of a physical block built into the goniometer at 30 degrees of extension.

Further Exploration: Familiarization with the Universal Goniometer

The activities in Box 1–1 are designed to help the reader become familiar with a goniometer and attain proficiency in manipulating the device and reading the scale correctly. Select a goniometer and locate the parts and features listed in Box 1–1. Make sure several different styles of goniometers are examined and the features of each are compared.

BOX 1–1. FEATURES OF THE GONIOMETER (See Fig. 1–11)

Protractor
1. Is the protractor a half or a full circle?
2. Is the protractor marked in 1-, 2.5-, or 5-degree increments?
3. Is there a single scale marked on the protractor, or is more than one scale present?
4. If more than one scale is present, are the scales marked in the same direction, or in opposite directions?
5. Locate the base line of the protractor (line extending between the 0-degree mark and the 180-degree mark). The base line is the reference from which measurements are made.

Stationary arm (see Fig. 1–11)
1. Locate the line that extends from the protractor of the goniometer down the midline of the stationary arm. This is an extension of the protractor's base line.
2. Are there markings along the length of the stationary arm? If so, are the markings in centimeters or in inches?

Moving arm (see Fig. 1–11)
1. If the goniometer is metal, is a tapered end or cutout present on the proximal end of the moving arm?
2. If the goniometer is plastic, is the length of the arm marked in centimeters or in inches?
3. Locate the prominent line along the midline of the arm.
4. Holding the goniometer so that the stationary arm is in your right hand and the moving arm is in your left hand, move the moving arm to different positions and read the scale of the goniometer. The reading is taken at the point where the midline of the proximal end of the free arm crosses the scale of the protractor.
5. If more than one scale is present on the protractor, move the moving arm and read first one and then the other scale. Note how the scales relate to each other.
6. Position the moving arm at your estimation of various angles (e.g., 45 degrees, 60 degrees, 90 degrees), and then read the scale of the goniometer, and see how close your estimate was. If more than one scale is present on the goniometer, note the reading from each scale and examine the relationship between the two scales.
7. Reverse the goniometer so that the stationary arm is in your left hand and the moving arm is in your right hand. Repeat steps 4, 5, and 6 while holding the goniometer in this position. Note any differences in which scale must be read.

Inclinometer

An inclinometer consists of a circular, fluid-filled disk with a bubble or weighted needle that indicates the number of degrees on the scale of a protractor. The majority of inclinometers are calibrated or referenced to gravity, analogous to the principle related to the level used by a carpenter. Since gravity does not change, using gravity as a reference point means that the starting position of the inclinometer can be consistently identified and repeated.

Inclinometers are available in two types: mechanical and electronic. The least expensive of the two is the mechanical, with most inclinometers today consisting of a protractor and a weighted gravity-pendulum indicator that remains in the vertical position to indicate degrees on the protractor (Fig. 1–13).

A second type of mechanical inclinometer is the fluid-level inclinometer, which indicates degrees by the alignment of the meniscus (bubble) of the fluid to the protractor. Although used in the past, the fluid-level goniometer is not used frequently today; most clinicians who use inclinometers choose to use the weighted gravity-pendulum device.

Electronic inclinometers are more expensive, may have to be connected to computers with special programs and software, and must frequently be calibrated against some horizontal surface between measurements. Given that the mechanical inclinometer is easy to use, inexpensive, and fairly well represented in research in the literature, this textbook only presents information related to the mechanical inclinometer.

The inclinometer can be held against the patient during a variety of movements, or the device can be mounted on a frame. Examples of mounting the inclinometer onto a plastic frame include the cervical range of motion (CROM) device and the back range of motion (BROM) device (both manufactured by Performance Attainment Associates, Roseville, Minnesota).

CROM

The CROM device consists of a plastic frame that is placed over the subject's head, aligned on the bridge of the nose and on the ears, and secured to the

Fig. 1–13. Freestanding inclinometer.

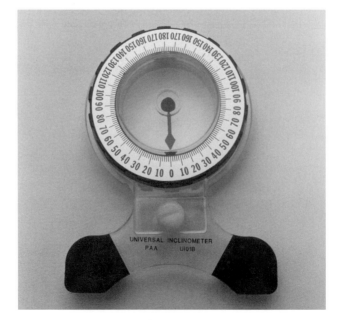

Fig. 1–14. CROM; note inclinometers mounted vertically in frontal plane (to measure lateral flexion), vertically in the sagittal plane (to measure flexion and extension), and in the horizontal plane on top of the head (to measure rotation).

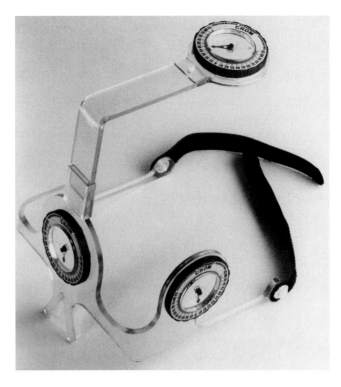

back of the head with straps made of Velcro (Fig. 1–14). Cervical flexion and extension are measured by an inclinometer mounted on the side of the headpiece. An inclinometer mounted on the front of the headpiece is used to measure lateral flexion. Both inclinometers work by force of gravity. To measure cervical rotation, a compass inclinometer is attached to the top of the headpiece in the transverse plane and operated in conjunction with a magnetic yoke. The yoke consists of two padded bars, mounted on the shoulders, that contain magnetic poles.

BROM

The BROM device consists of two plastic frames, which are secured to the lumbar spine of the subject by two elastic straps. One frame consists of an L-shaped slide arm that is free to move within a notch of the fixed base unit during flexion and extension; range of motion is read from a protractor scale (Fig. 1–15). The second frame has two measurement devices attached to it (Fig. 1–16). One attachment is a vertically mounted gravity-dependent inclinometer, which measures lateral flexion. The second attachment is a horizontally mounted compass to measure rotation. During the measurement of trunk rotation, the device requires a magnetic yoke to be secured to the pelvis.

Further Exploration: Familiarization with the Inclinometer

The activities in Box 1–2 are designed to help the reader become familiar with an inclinometer and attain proficiency in manipulating the device and reading the scale correctly. Make sure several different styles of inclinometers are examined and the features of each are compared. Compare various free-standing inclinometers to the inclinometers mounted on the CROM and the BROM.

Fig. 1–15. Apparatus for measuring flexion and extension using BROM.

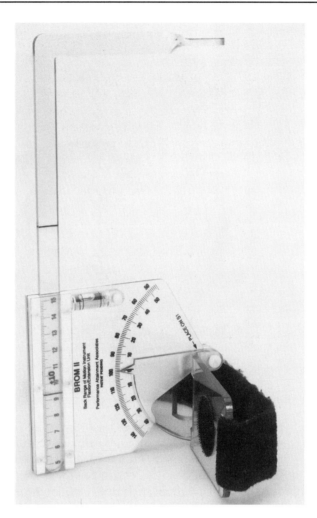

Tape Measure

One of the simplest procedures for measuring range of motion and muscle length is the tape measure (or ruler) (Fig. 1–17). Tape measures can be made of cloth or metal. They can possess a centimeter scale, an inch scale, or both. The tape measure is easy to use and readily available in most clinics. One

Fig. 1–16. Apparatus for measuring lateral flexion and rotation using BROM; note inclinometers mounted vertically (to measure lateral flexion) and horizontally (to measure rotation).

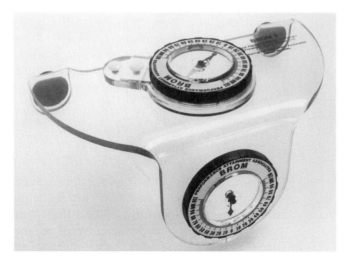

BOX 1–2. FEATURES OF THE INCLINOMETER

1. Is the free-standing inclinometer fixed to a base that is a straight-edge, or is it fixed to a two-point contact base? Can you speculate on the advantage of one base over the other?
2. Is the protractor on the inclinometer immobile, or does it rotate, allowing you to set the zero point?
3. Is the scale of the protractor marked in 1-, 2.5-, or 5-degree increments?
4. Does the scale of the protractor have a 0-to-360–degree scale running in a full circle, or does it have a 0-to-180–degree scale running in the clockwise direction and another 0-to-180–degree scale running in the counter-clockwise direction?
5. Is the scale of the protractor indicated by a weighted pointer, by a floating bubble, or by both?
6. Holding the inclinometer vertically in your hand with 0 degrees at the bottom and 180 degrees at the top, tip the inclinometer in a clockwise direction. What happens to the indicator (weighted pointer or bubble)? Read the scale of the inclinometer. Try turning the inclinometer in a counter-clockwise direction. What happens? Read the scale of the inclinometer.
7. Place the inclinometer horizontally on a flat surface such as a table. Turn the inclinometer in a clockwise direction. What happens to the indicator (weighted pointer or bubble)? Keeping the inclinometer on the flat surface, turn the inclinometer in a counter-clockwise direction. What happens?

---

negative aspect related to the use of the tape measure is that most systems of rating range of motion and muscle length impairment rely on measurements in degrees.

Further Exploration: Familiarization with the Tape Measure

The activities in Box 1–3 are designed to help the reader become familiar with a simple tape measure and attain proficiency in manipulating the device and reading the scale correctly. Make sure several different styles of tape measures are examined and the features of each are compared.

Fig. 1–17. Tools for linear measurement: Ruler, tape measure, Therabite.

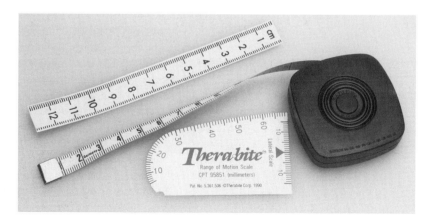

BOX 1–3. FEATURES OF THE TAPE MEASURE

1. Is the tape measure cloth or metal?
2. Does the tape measure retract into a receptacle, or is the tape measure free-standing?
3. Is the tape measure marked in centimeters on one side and inches on the other?
4. Is the zero point at the very tip of the tape measure, or is the zero point indented from the tip of the tape measure?
5. For practice: From a sitting position, cross one leg over the other. Palpate the following anatomical landmarks on your own crossed leg: medial malleolus and tibial tubercle. Using a tape measure, measure the distance between these two landmarks three times, removing the tape measure between each measurement. Did you get the exact same measurement each time? Be honest!

TECHNIQUES FOR MEASURING RANGE OF MOTION AND MUSCLE LENGTH

Regardless of the instrument being used, the individual employing the instrument must become skilled in the use of the measurement tool. Once a level of comfort in handling and reading a measurement device has been attained, the user must become skillful in using the instrument to measure joint range of motion and muscle length. Skill in the use of any measurement device comes only after much repeated practice. Practice in using an instrument should continue until the user has established a high level of intra-rater reliability (more detailed information on reliability is presented in Chapter 2). That is, repeated measurements taken by the same person on the same subject should be identical or within a small margin of error. Since techniques of measurement differ from joint to joint, each examiner should practice the techniques until all measurements can be performed in a reliable manner.

Many of the steps involved in measuring joint range of motion and muscle length are the same, no matter which joint is being measured. These steps provide the basic framework for measurement, and are outlined in Table 1–1 and expounded in this section. How the basic steps are applied at each joint, such as which landmarks are used for alignment of the instrument or what patient positioning is used, differs from joint to joint. The use of standardized techniques is critical for accurate measurement of joint range of motion and muscle length. Without standardized techniques, range of motion and muscle length measurements are likely to be unreliable and, thus, of questionable validity.[40, 84] The specific techniques for measuring range of motion at each joint are provided in Chapters 3 through 5 for the upper extremity, Chapters 8 and 9 for the spine and the temporomandibular joint, and Chapters 11 through 13 for the lower extremity. The specific techniques for measuring muscle length are presented in Chapters 6 and 14.

Preparation for Measurement

Prior to measuring a patient's range of motion or muscle length, the examiner should determine whether the measurement of active range of motion or passive range of motion is most appropriate. Active range of motion (AROM), which occurs when a patient moves a joint actively through its available range of motion, and passive range of motion (PROM), which occurs when the examiner moves the patient's joint through the available range of motion, both may be used to examine the amount of motion available at a given joint. Although in many cases the examiner will be interested in how much AROM the patient possesses, sometimes PROM may be the motion of interest. For example, a patient with supraspinatus tendinitis may be unwilling to abduct the shoulder more than 75 degrees because of pain, so AROM would be limited to 0–75 degrees. To ensure that the patient is not developing adhesive capsulitis of the shoulder, the examiner also may wish to measure the amount of passive shoulder abduction present. In some instances the examiner has no choice but to measure PROM, as the patient is unable or unwilling to perform AROM. Such cases include measuring range of motion in infants, young children, and in any patient who lacks the motor control to perform active movement at the joint in question. In its *Guides to the Evaluation of Permanent Impairment*, the American Medical Association[3] recommends the measurement and comparison of both AROM and PROM in the evaluation process.

Active and passive range of motion may differ widely for a given joint in an individual, particularly if muscle weakness, pain, or related pathologies are present. Studies that have compared AROM and PROM in subjects without pathology have reported that PROM is greater than AROM for most joints.[14, 45, 46, 54, 89] In many cases, the increase in PROM over AROM is significant. However, PROM is not greater than AROM at all joints. For example, measurements of ankle dorsiflexion range of motion tend to be higher when the patient actively dorsiflexes the ankle than when passive motion alone is measured.[10, 74] Because of the variability that exists between AROM and PROM even in pathology-free individuals, care should be taken to document the type of range of motion (AROM or PROM) measured in each patient.

Instructing the Patient

Patients should be provided with thorough instructions prior to performing any examination technique, including taking range of motion and muscle length measurements. Measurement of range of motion and muscle length,

Table 1–1. PROCEDURES FOR MEASURING JOINT RANGE OF MOTION AND MUSCLE LENGTH

1. Determine the type of measurement to be performed (AROM or PROM).
2. Explain the purpose of the procedure to the patient.
3. Position the patient in the preferred patient position for the measurement.
4. Stabilize the proximal joint segment.
5. Instruct the patient in the specific motion that will be measured while moving the patient's distal joint segment passively through the ROM. Determine the patient's end-feel at the end of the PROM.
6. Return the patient's distal joint segment to the starting position.
7. Palpate bony landmarks for measurement device alignment.
8. Align the measurement device with the appropriate bony landmarks.
9. Read the scale of the measurement device and note the reading.
10. Have the patient move actively, or move the patient passively, through the available ROM.
11. Repalpate the bony landmarks and readjust the alignment of the measurement device as necessary.
12. Read the scale of the measurement device and note the reading.
13. Record the patient's ROM. The record should include, at a minimum:
    a. Patient's name and identifying information
    b. Date measurement was taken
    c. Identification of person taking measurement
    d. Type of motion measured (AROM or PROM) and device used
    e. Any alteration from preferred patient position
    f. Readings taken from measurement device at beginning and end of ROM.

AROM; active range of motion; PROM, passive of motion; ROM, range of motion.

particularly active motion, requires the full cooperation of the patient. As the patient's understanding of the procedure increases, so does the likelihood that the patient will provide his or her best effort during the process.

Before beginning the procedure, describe to the patient exactly what will be taking place and why the measurement must be performed. Show the patient the measurement tool, and explain, in layperson's terms, its purpose and how it will be used. Instruct the patient in the position he or she is to assume, again using layperson's terms and avoiding terms such as *supine* or *prone*. Detailed explanations of every step of the procedure should not be provided initially, as this will only confuse the patient. A brief, general explanation is best at this point, and further explanations may be given once the procedure is in progress. An example of initial patient instructions is as follows:

> "Ms. Haynes, I need to measure how much you can move your knee. This information will tell me how much progress you are making since your surgery and help me estimate how soon you will be able to be discharged from treatment. I am going to use this instrument, called a goniometer, to measure your movement. I will need you to lie on this table on your back so that I can perform the measurement."

Positioning the Patient: Measuring Joint Range of Motion

Proper positioning of the patient during measurement is critical to accurate measurement. The choice of a preferred patient position for measurement of motion at each joint is based on several criteria. For a position to be considered optimal, all criteria should be met. Although this is not an exhaustive list, the major criteria in selecting a preferred patient position for measurement of range of motion are as follows:

1. **The joint should be placed in the zero starting position.** The zero starting position for almost all joints is with that joint in the anatomical position (described previously). The only joint that is not placed in the anatomical position to start is the forearm, which is placed midway between full pronation and full supination (the neutral position of the forearm). When a joint is positioned in the zero starting position, the joint is considered to be at 0 degrees range of motion.

2. **The joint should be positioned such that the proximal segment of the joint is most easily stabilized.** This positioning allows maximal isolation of the intended motion.

3. **The bony landmarks to be used to align the measurement tool should be palpable and in proper alignment.** In some cases, this necessitates placing more proximal joints out of anatomical position. For example, when measuring flexion of the wrist, the shoulder is abducted to 90 degrees, the elbow flexed to 90 degrees, and the forearm is pronated in order to place the bony landmarks for goniometric alignment in a linear relationship.

4. **The joint to be measured should be free to move through its complete available range of motion.** Motion should not be blocked by external objects, such as the examining table, or by internal forces, such as muscle tightness. An example of the latter is positioning the patient in the prone position to measure knee flexion. As tension in the rectus femoris muscle can limit knee flexion when the hip is extended (patient positioned prone), a better position for this measurement is with the

patient supine. Such a position allows free flexion of the hip during knee flexion, thus eliminating potential restriction of knee flexion by rectus femoris tightness.

5. **The patient must be able to assume the position.** In some cases, this criterion cannot be met, and an alternative position must be used. In any instance in which an alternative position is used, the examiner should design the position so that it adheres to the previous four criteria as closely as possible.

The amount of range of motion measured may vary significantly depending on the position in which the patient is placed during the measurement. Two studies have demonstrated a statistically significant difference in the amount of range of motion obtained from a joint when the position in which the joint was measured was altered. A significantly higher amount of shoulder abduction was obtained when active or passive shoulder abduction was measured with the patient in the supine, as compared with the sitting, position.[82] Similarly, when hip lateral rotation was measured with the patient in both the seated and the prone positions, significantly more motion was obtained in the prone position.[87] Preferred patient positions are provided for each joint measurement technique described in this text. Whenever a position other than the preferred position is used, careful documentation should be made of the exact position chosen. In this way, techniques used in range of motion measurements can be duplicated by others, and more accurate comparisons of measurements taken on separate occasions, or by different examiners, can be made.

Further Exploration: Preferred Patient Position

The following activities are designed to help the student evaluate and design preferred patient positions for measurement of range of motion.

1. Select a technique for the measurement of joint range of motion from the text (e.g., shoulder lateral rotation). Apply the criteria listed to the preferred patient position described. How well does the position meet the criteria listed? Repeat this exercise for the techniques of several other motions.
2. Analyze the following scenarios, devising a preferred patient position in each situation. Once your preferred position is complete, apply the criteria listed. How well does your devised position meet the criteria? Make modifications to your devised position as needed, so that it adheres more closely to the criteria.
   A. Mr. Barnes suffered a spinal cord injury 2 years previously, currently has a decubitus ulcer on his sacrum, and is unable to sit or lie supine. How would you alter the preferred patient position for Mr. Barnes to perform the following measurements? (Refer to the techniques in Chapters 3 to 5 and Chapter 11 for information on the standard method for performing each measurement.)
      i. Shoulder flexion
      ii. Wrist extension
      iii. Forearm pronation
      iv. Hip abduction
      v. Hip lateral rotation
   B. Mrs. Kelley is 8 months pregnant and unable to lie on her right side because of pressure placed by the baby on her inferior vena cava. She is also unable to lie prone. How would you alter the preferred patient position for Mrs. Kelley in order to perform the fol-

lowing measurements? (Refer to the techniques in Chapters 3 and 11 for information on the standard method for performing each measurement.)

 i. Hip extension (consider both right and left sides)
 ii. Shoulder extension (consider both right and left sides)

Positioning the Patient: Measuring Muscle Length

Please note that the preparation for measurement and instructions to the patient are similar whether one is measuring range of motion or examining muscle length. However, positioning of the patient differs for the two types of measurement. When examining muscle length, the following guidelines for patient positioning should be followed:

1. **The muscle to be measured should be placed in the fully elongated position.** In the measurement of muscle length, the examiner is most concerned about the final, elongated position of the muscle and not as concerned about the measurement from the zero starting position (as would be appropriate for measurement of joint range of motion). In some instances the movement is initiated from the zero position to demonstrate to the subject the motion desired, but in most cases the muscle is placed in the elongated position, and the measurement is taken.

2. **As much as possible, the muscle should be isolated across one, or possibly two, joints.** Composite tests measuring movement across three or more joints should not be used. (Refer to the earlier section of this chapter on the history of muscle length testing.)

3. **The bony landmarks to be used to align the measurement tool should be palpable and in proper alignment.** In some cases, this necessitates placing more proximal joints out of anatomical position. For example, when measuring muscle length of the extensor digitorum communis muscle, the shoulder is abducted to 70 to 90 degrees, the forearm pronated, and the fingers flexed to place the bony landmarks for goniometric alignment in a linear relationship.

4. **Motion should not be blocked by external objects such as the support surface or a pillow.**

5. **The patient must be able to assume the position.** In some cases, this criterion cannot be met, and an alternative position must be used. In any instance in which an alternative position is used, the examiner should design the position so that it adheres to the previous four criteria as closely as possible.

Stabilization

Accurate measurement of joint range of motion and muscle length requires stabilization of the proximal bony segment of the joint being measured. Failure to provide adequate stabilization will prevent isolation of the intended motion and may allow the patient to substitute motion at another joint for the motion requested. For example, a patient who lacks forearm pronation may abduct and medially rotate the shoulder in an attempt to substitute for the lack of forearm motion. If the examiner fails to stabilize the humerus in an adducted position during measurement of forearm pronation, the patient may perform the substitute motion, and the measurement of forearm pronation would then be falsely inflated.

Lack of sufficient stabilization also may affect the reliability of measurements of range of motion or muscle length testing. Ekstrand et al.[30] performed range of motion and muscle length testing of selected lower extremity joints in adult male subjects using a modified goniometer and a Leighton flexometer. Standardized testing procedures were employed, and the motions were repeated on two occasions, 2 months apart. On the first occasion, the subjects were positioned on a soft, padded surface, while on the second occasion, measurements were made with the subject positioned on a hard wooden board. Results demonstrated a significantly lower intratester variability for both range of motion and muscle length measurements when patients were measured while positioned on a hard surface compared with a soft surface.

The ease with which the proximal joint segment is stabilized varies from joint to joint. In some instances, the patient's weight assists in stabilizing the proximal joint segment, but the examiner should always stabilize the proximal segment manually as well. In general, smaller segments, such as the forearm, are easier to stabilize than are larger segments, such as the pelvis. Some motions (e.g., shoulder flexion, hip flexion) cannot be isolated completely,[9] and in those cases, the examiner must realize that the motion measured is, at a minimum, a combination of motion at the joint being measured and motion at the next most proximal articulation.

Directions and illustrations for stabilization are provided for each range of motion and muscle length testing technique found in this text. The examiner should be very careful to provide the stabilization indicated when performing each measurement technique. Failure to do so could result in inaccurate and unreliable results.

Estimating Range of Motion and Determining End-Feel

Once the patient is positioned and the proximal joint segment is stabilized, the examiner should move the joint passively through the available range of motion. This maneuver accomplishes a variety of objectives. First, by moving the patient through the range of motion to be measured, the patient is made aware of the exact movement to be performed and can cooperate more fully and accurately with the procedure. Second, a rough estimation of the patient's available range of motion can be made by the examiner. Estimating the patient's range of motion provides the examiner with a self-check against gross errors in reading the goniometer. For example, if the examiner estimates that the patient has 125 degrees of elbow flexion but reads 58 degrees on the goniometer, then an error obviously has been made in the measurement (in this case, the wrong scale on the goniometer has been read). Estimating the patient's range of motion prior to measurement is a particularly valuable technique for the novice examiner, as novices are prone to errors in reading the measurement device. Finally, moving the patient passively through the range of motion allows the examiner to note any limitations to full range of motion, such as those caused by pain, muscle tightness, or other reasons.

Clues to the cause of range of motion limitations may be obtained by examining the quality of the resistance at the end of range of motion. Each joint has a characteristic feel to the resistance encountered at the end of normal range of motion. Typical end-feels encountered at the end of normal range of motion are the bony, capsular, muscular, and soft-tissue end-feels.[25, 51] These end-feels are described in the activities that follow this section and are defined for each joint in the introductory material for Chapters 3 to 5,

8 and 9, and 11 to 13. Chapters 6 and 14 describe measurement of muscle length of the upper and lower extremities, respectively. Given that the muscles are placed in the fully elongated position for these measurements, the end-feel is muscular.

Other end-feels are encountered only in situations of joint pathology. These include the empty, muscle-spasm, and springy block end-feels. Although explanations of these end-feels are beyond the scope of this text, definitions can be found in any basic musculoskeletal examination text.[25] Deviation from the expected end-feel when performing passive range of motion at a joint should alert the examiner that further examination of the joint is warranted.

Further Exploration: Identifying End-Feels

BONY END-FEEL: ELBOW EXTENSION

The bony end-feel occurs when the approximation of two bones stops the range of motion at a joint. The quality of the resistance felt is very hard and abrupt, and further motion is impossible.

1. Position the subject in the supine or sitting position.
2. Grasp the posterior aspect of the subject's distal humerus in one hand and the anterior aspect of the distal forearm in the other hand.
3. Flex the subject's elbow slightly, then gently return it to the fully extended position, repeating this maneuver several times.
4. While performing the passive movement described in step 3, pay close attention to the feel of the resistance at the point of full elbow extension. The resistance should feel hard and abrupt—a bony end-feel.

CAPSULAR END-FEEL: HIP MEDIAL ROTATION

The capsular end-feel occurs when the joint capsule and the surrounding noncontractile tissues limit the range of motion at a joint. The quality of the resistance felt is firm but not hard. There is a very slight "give" to the movement, as would be felt when stretching a piece of leather.

1. Position the subject in the sitting position.
2. Place one hand on the subject's knee and the other hand over the subject's medial malleolus.
3. Passively rotate the subject's hip medially by moving the subject's leg laterally (keeping the knee stationary) until firm resistance is felt. From this point, oscillate the subject's leg medially and laterally very slightly without allowing the knee to move.
4. While performing the passive movement described in step 3, pay close attention to the feel of the resistance at the point of full medial rotation of the hip. The resistance should feel firm and leathery—a capsular end-feel.

MUSCULAR END-FEEL: KNEE EXTENSION WITH HIP FLEXION

The muscular end-feel occurs when muscular tension limits the range of motion at a joint. The quality of the resistance felt is firm, although not as firm as with the capsular end-feel, and somewhat springy.

1. Position the subject in the supine position.
2. Place one hand on the anterior aspect of the subject's knee and the

other hand on the posterior aspect of the subject's foot, cupping the subject's heel.

3. Flex the subject's hip completely. Then slowly extend the subject's knee until resistance is felt. From this point, gently oscillate the leg into full extension and then into slight flexion.

4. While performing the passive movement described in step 3, pay close attention to the feel of the resistance at the end point of knee extension. The resistance should feel firm and slightly springy—a muscular end-feel.

SOFT-TISSUE END-FEEL: KNEE FLEXION

1. Position the subject in the supine position.

2. Place one hand on the anterior aspect of the subject's knee, and grasp the subject's ankle with the other hand.

3. Flex the subject's knee completely (slight hip flexion is allowed during this procedure, but only enough to allow full flexion of the knee) until the subject's calf is stopped by his or her posterior thigh. From this point, oscillate the leg into, and slightly out of, full knee flexion and slight extension.

4. While performing the passive movement described in step 3, pay close attention to the feel of the resistance at the end point of knee extension. The resistance, caused by the compression of the soft tissue of the calf and posterior thigh, should feel mushy or soft—a soft-tissue end feel.

Palpating Bony Landmarks and Aligning the Measurement Device

Accurate palpation of landmarks and precise alignment of the measurement device with those landmarks are critical to the correct measurement of joint range of motion and muscle length. Bony landmarks are used for alignment of the measurement device whenever possible, since bony structures are more stable and are less subject to change in position because of factors such as edema or muscle atrophy.

Aligning the Goniometer

Three landmarks, as a minimum, are used to align the goniometer. Two landmarks are used to align the arms of the goniometer, one landmark for the stationary arm and one for the moving arm. The stationary arm is generally aligned with the midline of the stationary segment of the joint, while the moving arm is aligned with the midline of the moving segment of the joint. The bony landmarks provided for alignment of the goniometer arms are generally target points on the bones of the stationary and moving joint segments. While the arms of the goniometer may not actually cross these bony targets once the instrument is aligned, the examiner should sight the midline of each goniometer arm so that it points directly at the corresponding bony target.

The third bony landmark provides a point for alignment of the fulcrum of the goniometer. The fulcrum of the goniometer is placed over a point that is near the axis of rotation of the joint. However, since the axis of rotation for most joints is not stationary but moves during motion of the joint, the goniometer's fulcrum often will not remain aligned over its corresponding bony landmark throughout the range of motion. Because the joint axis is not stationary, **the landmark for alignment of the fulcrum of the goniometer is the least important of the three landmarks for goniometer alignment.** To assure accurate alignment, priority should be given to alignment of the stationary and moving arms of the goniometer. Once the examiner is satisfied that the goniometer is aligned correctly, a reading should be taken from the scale of the goniometer at the beginning of the range of motion (see "Determining and Recording the Range of Motion with the Goniometer," discussed subsequently).

Aligning the Inclinometer

Only one bony landmark per measurement is needed for alignment of the standard inclinometer, and, therefore, the measurement device is not subject to errors in estimating multiple anatomical landmarks for one measurement. An inclinometer with a two-point contact base is preferred because this type of base best maintains contact over convex surfaces of the body. Because of its ease of use, the inclinometer has gained favor for the measurement of the spine.

The inclinometer has not been used as frequently as the goniometer to measure the extremities because of difficulties in stabilizing the instrument along the different anatomical contours of the body, especially on smaller joints. Additionally, any attempt to strap the inclinometer to the extremity introduces problems of soft-tissue variability, edema, and slippage.

Aligning the Tape Measure

With the tape measure, specific landmarks also are established prior to measurement. These landmarks may be only anatomical, such as the distance between the tip of the chin and the sternal notch. Or the landmarks may combine an anatomical landmark with the support surface on which the subject is sitting or lying, such as the perpendicular distance between the tip of the olecranon fossa and the support surface in a subject lying supine with hands clasped behind the head.

Determining and Recording the Range of Motion with the Goniometer

Determination of the patient's range of motion is accomplished by comparing the reading taken from the goniometer with the patient in the starting position with a second reading that is taken once the patient has completed the AROM or PROM. Before this second reading is taken, the goniometer alignment must be rechecked. Bony landmarks must be palpated again at the end of the patient's range of motion, and the arms and the fulcrum of the goniometer readjusted as necessary, so that alignment is once again accurate. Failure to confirm accurate goniometer alignment prior to reading the instrument may result in gross errors in range of motion measurement.

When the scale of the goniometer is read, the reading is taken at the point where the midline of the end of the moving arm crosses the scale of the protractor portion of the instrument. Many goniometers are imprinted with more than one scale, and the scales may encircle the protractor portion of the instrument in opposing directions. The examiner must pay careful attention to make sure that the correct scale is being read (see points 4, 5, 6, and 7 under "Moving arm" in Box 1–1).

After readings have been taken from the goniometer at the beginning and the end of the patient's movement, the examiner is ready to document the range of motion. Several items must be noted in the record of the patient's range of motion. These items include:

- Patient's name and identifying information
- Date measurement was taken
- Identification of person taking measurement
- Type of motion measured (AROM or PROM)
- Any alteration in patient's position (from preferred patient position) during measurement
- Beginning and ending readings from the goniometer for each motion measured

This information provides sufficient details should any question arise regarding the patient's range of motion at a particular joint. Additionally, information regarding the type of motion measured and any alterations in normal procedure allow other examiners to reproduce the technique should someone other than the original examiner need to measure the patient's range of motion.

When readings taken from the goniometer are recorded, both the beginning and ending readings should be reported, even if the beginning reading is 0 degrees. The beginning reading tells anyone who needs information from the patient's record where the range of motion begins. Two patients may both have 110 degrees of elbow flexion, but the motion in Patient A may start at 0 degrees and progress to 110 degrees of flexion, whereas the motion in Patient B may start at 25 degrees of flexion and progress to 135 degrees. Recording either patient's motion as 110 degrees would not allow anyone examining either patient's record to know where the motion began and where it ended. To avoid confusion on the part of those reading the patient's record, the use of a single number to record the range of motion should be avoided (except in certain cases—see "Single Motion Recording Technique," discussed later).

Occasionally, the goniometer will not read 0 degrees at the beginning of the range of motion, even when the patient is at the 0-degree starting position for that motion. An example of this phenomenon occurs during the measurement of hip abduction and adduction. At the beginning of these two motions, the alignment of the goniometer is such that the stationary and moving arms of the instrument make a 90-degree angle with each other. Thus, at the 0-degree starting position for hip abduction and adduction, the scale of the goniometer reads 90 degrees. This reading is taken as equivalent to 0 degrees, and the reading from the goniometer at the end of the range of motion is added to, or subtracted from, 90 degrees to obtain the range of motion. For example, in a patient who had 20 degrees of hip adduction, the goniometer would read 90 degrees at the beginning of the range of motion and 110 degrees at the end of the range of motion. Subtract: $110 - 90 = 20$. Therefore, the patient's hip adduction range of motion is recorded as 0 to 20 degrees hip adduction.

Several methods of recording range of motion exist. Two methods are presented here, and the reader may choose which method to use. However, in a clinical situation where multiple individuals are measuring and recording ranges of motion, a standardized method of recording these measurements should be agreed on by all individuals involved. Otherwise, a great deal of confusion is likely to result among those using the patient's record as the basis for decision making.

Single Motion Recording Technique

One method of recording joint range of motion involves separately documenting the range of each motion at each joint. Thus, when range of motion at the shoulder is recorded, shoulder flexion is documented separately from shoulder extension, and shoulder lateral rotation is documented separately from shoulder medial rotation. Both the beginning and the ending readings from the goniometer are recorded for each motion measured. An example of single motion recording of range of motion is provided in Figure 1–18.

Mrs. Stephenson is able to actively move her right shoulder from the 0-degree starting position to 165 degrees in the direction of shoulder flexion, and to 35 degrees in the direction of shoulder extension. Her range of motion would be documented as in Figure 1–18.

For some motions, the patient may not be able to attain the 0-degree starting position for the movement. In such cases, the patient is limited in one motion and completely lacks the opposing motion. For example, suppose Mrs. Stephenson is unable to attain the 0-degree starting position for elbow extension, but instead lacks 15 degrees of full extension (in other words, her elbow is in 15-degree flexion as she begins the flexion movement). Suppose further that she is able to move from this starting position to 140 degrees of elbow flexion. Mrs. Stephenson's elbow flexion is documented as shown in the chart in Figure 1–19, since she began the motion at 15 degrees and ended it at 140 degrees. In the case of elbow *extension*, Mrs. Stephenson has no *range* of motion because she is unable to attain the 0-degree starting position for the movement. Therefore, elbow extension for Mrs. Stephenson is documented as −15 degrees, as shown in Figure 1–19, indicating that she lacks 15 degrees of attaining the 0-degree starting position for elbow

Fig. 1–18.

			JOINT RANGE OF MOTION	Patient: *Nicole Stephenson* Age: *68* Indicate: AROM *X* PROM ____		
LEFT						**RIGHT**
			Date/Examiner's Initials	*01/03/02 NBR*		
			Shoulder			
			Flexion	*0°–165°*		
			Extension	*0°–35°*		
			Abduction			
			Adduction			
			Medial Rotation			
			Lateral Rotation			

Fig. 1–19.

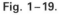

				LEFT			RIGHT		

JOINT RANGE OF MOTION

Patient: *Nicole Stephenson*
Age: *68*
Indicate:
    AROM *X*
    PROM _____

				RIGHT		
			Date/Examiner's Initials	*01/03/02 NBR*		
			Elbow/Forearm			
			Flexion	*15°–140°*		
			Extension	*–15°*		
			Pronation			
			Supination			

extension. Only in cases in which the patient has no motion in a given direction is a single number used to document range of motion.

Now suppose that Mrs. Stephenson's knee range of motion is measured, and the examiner discovers that Mrs. Stephenson is able to attain the 0-degree starting position for knee extension. She also can actively move her knee 10 degrees in the direction of extension and 145 degrees in the direction of flexion. In this case, Mrs. Stephenson's knee extension is recorded as 0 to 10 degrees knee *hyperextension*. When the normal amount of extension at a joint is 0 degrees, motion into extension beyond 0 degrees is documented as *hyperextension*. The use of the term *hyperextension* reflects that the motion is in excess of the normal amount of extension expected at that joint. In this case knee flexion is documented as 0 to 145 degrees flexion, since the starting position for flexion is 0 degrees. Even though Mrs. Stephenson is able to attain more than 0 degrees of extension, the extra motion is not included in the documentation for knee flexion, since the flexion movement begins at 0 (Fig. 1–20).

Fig. 1–20.

JOINT RANGE OF MOTION

Patient: *Nicole Stephenson*
Age: *68*
Indicate:
    AROM *X*
    PROM _____

				LEFT			RIGHT		

				RIGHT		
			Date/Examiner's Initials	*01/03/02 NBR*		
			Knee			
			Flexion	*0°–145°*		
			Extension	*0°–10°*		

Further Exploration: Documenting Range of Motion Using Single Motion Recording Technique

Using the charts that follow, practice documenting range of motion by recording the motion for each of the patients presented below.

1. Ms. Atchley is able to begin from the 0-degree starting position and actively move her knee 8 degrees in the direction of extension and 140 degrees in the direction of flexion. Record Ms. Atchley's knee flexion and extension range of motion (Fig. 1–21).
2. Mr. Taman is unable to attain the 0-degree starting position for hip flexion and extension. He begins the motion of hip flexion with his hip at 12 degrees of flexion and is able to actively move from there to 118 degrees of flexion. He is unable to move past 12 degrees of flexion toward the direction of extension. Record Mr. Taman's hip flexion and extension range of motion (Fig. 1–22).
3. Ms. Lusby is unable to abduct her shoulder to 90 degrees. Therefore, the examiner measures Ms. Lusby's shoulder rotation with her shoulder positioned in 45 degrees of abduction. From that position, she is able to attain the 0-degree starting position for shoulder rotation and to actively move her shoulder 60 degrees in the direction of medial rotation and 48 degrees in the direction of lateral rotation. Record Ms. Lusby's shoulder rotation range of motion. What notation should be made of Ms. Lusby's altered position for testing (Fig. 1–23)?

A wide variety of forms exist to use for recording range of motion. Appendix B provides a sampling of forms that can be used in the clinical setting.

Sagittal Frontal Transverse Rotational (SFTR) Recording Technique

A second method of recording joint range of motion records all motions that occur in a given plane together. For example, all motions occurring at the shoulder in the sagittal plane are recorded on the same line in the patient's record. Motions occurring in the frontal plane are then recorded, followed by motions occurring in the transverse plane, and so forth. When motion for

Fig. 1–21.

JOINT RANGE OF MOTION				Patient: _Elizabeth Atchley_
				Age: _20_
				Indicate: AROM _____ PROM _____

LEFT				RIGHT		
			Date/Examiner's Initials			
			Knee			
			Flexion			
			Extension			

Fig. 1–22.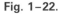

			JOINT RANGE OF MOTION		

Patient: _David Tamon_
Age: _46_
Indicate:
  AROM _____
  PROM _____

LEFT					**RIGHT**		
			Date/Examiner's Initials				
			Hip				
			Flexion				
			Extension				
			Abduction				
			Adduction				
			Medial Rotation				
			Lateral Rotation				

each plane of movement is recorded, a sequence of three numbers is used. The first number represents the extreme of motion in one direction, the second number represents the starting position, and the third number represents the extreme of motion in the opposite direction. For each plane of motion, movements are listed in the following order:

Fig. 1–23.

			JOINT RANGE OF MOTION		

Patient: _Danielle Lusby_
Age: _32_
Indicate:
  AROM _____
  PROM _____

LEFT					**RIGHT**		
			Date/Examiner's Initials				
			Shoulder				
			Flexion				
			Extension				
			Abduction				
			Adduction				
			Medial Rotation				
			Lateral Rotation				

Fig. 1–24.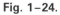

JOIN RANGE OF MOTION				Patient: _Nicole Stephenson_		
				Age: _68_		
				Indicate:		
				AROM _X_		
				PROM _____		

LEFT					**RIGHT**	
			Date/Examiner's Initials	01/03/02 NBR		
			Elbow/Forearm: S	0°–15°–140°		
			Elbow/Forearm: R			

Sagittal plane:	Extension/Starting position/Flexion
	Plantarflexion/Starting position/Dorsiflexion
Frontal plane:	Abduction/Starting position/Adduction
	Lateral flexion to left/Starting position/Lateral flexion to right
Transverse plane:	Horizontal abduction/Starting position/Horizontal adduction
Rotation:	Lateral rotation/Starting position/Medial rotation
	Supination/Starting position/Pronation
	Eversion/Starting position/Inversion
	Rotation to left/Starting position/Rotation to right

To use the example of Mrs. Stephenson that was provided previously, under the SFTR system, Mrs. Stephenson's range of motion would be documented thus:

- Shoulder S: 35°–0°–165°
- Elbow S: 0°–15°–140°
- Knee S: 10°–0°–145°

The notation for elbow motion indicates that Mrs. Stephenson is unable to move the elbow into extension and that she begins flexion at 15 degrees of flexion rather than at the 0-degree starting position. In other words, she has a 15-degree elbow flexion contracture. The chart in Figure 1–24 shows how

Fig. 1–25.

JOINT RANGE OF MOTION				Patient: _Elizabeth Atchley_		
				Age: _20_		
				Indicate:		
				AROM _____		
				PROM _____		

LEFT					**RIGHT**	
			Date/Examiner's Initials			
			Knee: S			

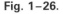

Fig. 1–26.

JOINT RANGE OF MOTION

Patient: _David Tamon_
Age: _46_
Indicate:
AROM _____
PROM _____

		LEFT		RIGHT		
			Date/Examiner's Initials			
			Hip:S			
			Hip:F			
			Hip:R			

Mrs. Stephenson's elbow range of motion is documented using the SFTR method.

On some occasions, motion at a joint is measured with the joint in some position other than the anatomical 0-degree starting position. In these cases, the SFTR system allows easy notation of the altered position. For example, if hip rotation is measured with the hip positioned in 90 degrees of flexion, a notation of the hip's position can made in the hip rotation record as follows: Hip R (S90): 32°–0°–28°. The designation (S90) indicates that the hip was positioned at 90 degrees in the sagittal plane when the hip rotation measurement was taken.

Further Exploration: Documenting Range of Motion Using SFTR Recording Technique

Using the information already provided for the sample patients Ms. Atchley, Mr. Taman, and Ms. Lusby, document the range of motion of each patient using the SFTR technique in the charts provided in Figures 1–25, 1–26, and 1–27.

Fig. 1–27.

JOINT RANGE OF MOTION

Patient: _Danielle Lusby_
Age: _32_
Indicate:
AROM _____
PROM _____

		LEFT		RIGHT		
			Date/Examiner's Initials			
			Shoulder:S			
			Shoulder:F			
			Shoulder:R			

Fig. 1–28.

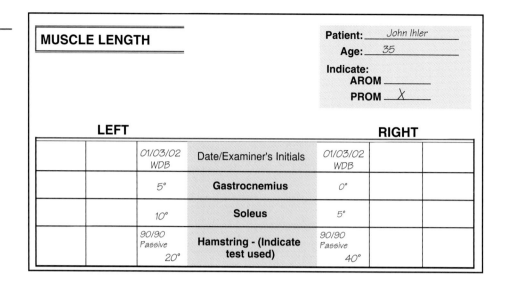

Determining and Recording Muscle Length

As indicated previously, in the measurement of muscle length, the examiner is most concerned about the final, elongated position of the muscle and not as concerned about the measurement from the zero starting position (as would be appropriate for measurement of joint range of motion). Therefore, for the measurement of muscle length, the muscle to be examined is placed in the elongated position and the measurement is taken using the suggested instrument (as is described in detail in Chapters 6 and 14). This actual measurement is the only information that is documented.

Assume that Mr. Ihler is a 35-year-old weekend tennis player with a diagnosis of patellar tendinitis in the right knee. Measurement of muscles on his right side indicates 0 degrees for the gastrocnemius, 5 degrees for the soleus, and 40 degrees from full knee extension for the hamstrings (using the passive 90/90 test described later in Chapter 14). Measurement of flexibility on his left side indicates 5 degrees for the gastrocnemius, 10 degrees for the soleus, and 20 degrees from full knee extension for the hamstrings. His muscle length data is documented as in Figure 1–28.

A wide variety of forms exist to use for recording muscle length data. Appendix B provides a sampling of forms that can be used in the clinical setting.

References

1. Allander E, Bjornsson OJ, Olafsson O, et al.: Normal range of joint movements in shoulder, hip, wrist and thumb with special reference to side: A comparison between two populations. Int J Epidemiol 1974;3:253–261.
2. American Academy of Orthopaedic Surgeons: Joint Motion: Method of Measuring and Recording. Chicago, American Academy of Orthopaedic Surgeons, 1965
3. American Medical Association: Guides to the Evaluation of Permanent Impairment, 4th ed. Chicago, 1993.
4. Armstrong AD, MacDermid JC, Chinchalkar S, et al.: Reliability of range-of-motion measurement in the elbow and forearm. J Shoulder Elbow Surg 1998;7:573–580.
5. Åstrom M, Arvidson T: Alignment and joint motion in the normal foot. J Orthop Sports Phys Ther 1995;22:216–222.
6. Bailey DS, Perillo JT, Forman M: Subtalar joint neutral. J Am Podiatr Med Assoc 1984;74:59–64.

7. Barrow HM, McGee R, Tritschler KA: Practical Measurement in Physical Education and Sports. Philadelphia, Lea & Febiger, 1989.
8. Bennett JG, Bergmanis LE, Carpenter JK, Skowlund HV. Range of motion of the neck. Phys Ther 1963;43:45–47.
9. Bohannon RW, Gajdosik RL, LeVeau BF: Relationship of pelvic and thigh motions during unilateral and bilateral hip flexion. Phys Ther 1985;65:1501–1504.
10. Bohannon RW, Tiberio D, Zito M: Selected measures of ankle dorsiflexion range of motion: Differences and intercorrelations. Foot Ankle Int 1989;10:99–103.
11. Brodie DA, Bird HA, Wright V: Joint laxity in selected athletic populations. Med Sci Sports Exerc 1982;14:190–193.
12. Brody DM: Running injuries. Clin Symp 1980;32:2–26.
13. Brosseau L, Tousignant M, Budd J, et al.: Intratester and intertester reliability and criterion validity of the parallelogram and universal goniometers for active knee flexion in healthy subjects. Physiother Res Int 1997;2:150–166.
14. Buell T, Green DR, Risser J: Measurement of the first metatarsophalangeal joint range of motion. J Am Podiatr Med Assoc 1988;78:439–448.
15. Cave EF, Roberts SM: A method for measuring and recording joint function. J Bone Joint Surg 1936;18:455–465.
16. Chiu H, Su FC, Wang S, et al.: The motion analysis system and goniometry of the finger joints. J Hand Surg 1998;23B:788–791.
17. Clapper MP, Wolf SL: Comparison of the reliability of the Orthoranger and the standard goniometer for assessing active lower extremity range of motion. Phys Ther 1988;68: 214–218.
18. Clark GR, Willis LA, Fish WW, Nichols PJ. Assessment of movement at the glenohumeral joint. Orthopaedics 1974;7:55–71.
19. Clark WA: A system of joint measurements. J Orthop Surg 1920;2:687–700.
20. Clark WA: A protractor for measuring rotation of joints. J Orthop Surg 1921;3:154–155.
21. Clarkson HM: Musculoskeletal Assessment: Joint Range of Motion and Manual Muscle Strength, 2nd ed. Baltimore, Williams & Wilkins, 2000.
22. Clemente CD (ed): Gray's Anatomy, 13th ed. Philadelphia, Lea & Febiger, 1985.
23. Cleveland DE: Diagrams for showing limitations of movements through joints. Can Med Assoc J 1918;8:70–72.
24. Cureton TK: Flexibility as an aspect of physical fitness. Res Q 1941;12:381–383.
25. Cyriax J: Textbook of Orthopaedic Medicine, 8th ed. London, Bailliere Tindall, 1982.
26. Darcus HD, Salter N: The amplitude of pronation and supination with the elbow flexed to a right angle. J Anat 1953;87:169–184.
27. Donatelli R: The Biomechanics of the Foot and Ankle. Philadelphia, F.A. Davis, 1990.
28. Donnery J, Spencer RB: The biplane goniometer: A new device for measurement of ankle dorsiflexion. J Am Podiatr Med Assoc 1988;78:348–351.
29. Dorinson SM, Wagner ML: An exact technic for clinically measuring and recording joint motion. Arch Phys Med 1948;29:468–475.
30. Ekstrand J, Wiktorsson M, Oberg B, Gillquist J. Lower extremity goniometer measurements: A study to determine their reliability. Arch Phys Med Rehabil 1982;63:171–175.
31. Ellis B, Bruton A, Goddard JR: Joint angle measurement: A comparative study of the reliability of goniometry and wire tracing for the hand. Clin Rehabil 1997;11:314–320.
32. Ellis MI, Stowe J: The hip. Clin Rheum Dis 1982;8:655–685.
33. Enwemeka C: Radiographic verification of knee goniometry. Scand J Rehabil Med 1986;18: 47–49.
34. Fairbank J, Pynsent PB, Phillips H: Quantitative measurements of joint mobility in adolescents. Ann Rheum Dis 1984;43:288–294.
35. Fish DR, Wingate L: Sources of goniometric error at the elbow. Phys Ther 1985;65: 1666–1670.
36. Fleischman EA: The Structure and Measurement of Physical Fitness. Englewood Cliffs, NJ: Prentice-Hall, 1964.
37. Fletcher J: Range of Motion, Chapter 2. In Bandy WD, Sanders B. Therapeutic Exercise: Techniques for Intervention. Baltimore: Lippincott, Williams, & Wilkins, 2001.
38. Fox RF: Demonstration of the mensuration apparatus in use at the Red Cross Clinic for the physical treatment of officers. Proc R Soc Med 1917;10:63.
39. Fox RF, van Breeman J. Chronic Rheumatism, Causation, and Treatment. London, Churchill Livingstone, 1934, p 327.
40. Gajdosik RL, Bohannon RW: Clinical measurement of range of motion: Review of goniometry emphasizing reliability and validity. Phys Ther 1987;67:1867–1872.
41. Gifford HC: Instruments for measuring joint movements and deformities in fracture treatment. Am J Surg 1914;28:237–238.
42. Glanville AD, Kreezer G. The maximum amplitude and velocity of joint movements in normal male human adults. Hum Biol 1937;9:197–201.
43. Goodwin J, Clark C, Deakes J, et al.: Clinical methods of goniometry: A comparative study. Disabil Rehabil 1992;14:10–15.

44. Greene WB, Heckman JD: The Clinical Measurement of Joint Motion. Rosemont, Ill, American Academy of Orthopaedic Surgeons, 1994.

45. Gunal I, Kose N, Erdogan O: Normal range of motion of the joints of the upper extremity in male subjects, with special reference to side. J Bone Joint Surg 1996;78:1404–1404.

46. Haley ET: Range of hip rotation and torque of hip rotator muscle groups. Am J Phys Med 1953;32:261–270.

47. Hamilton GF, Lachenbruch PA: Reliability of goniometers in assessing finger joint angle. Phys Ther 1969;49:465–469.

48. Hand JG. A compact pendulum arthrotomer. J Bone Joint Surg 1938;20:494–497.

49. Harris ML: A factor analytic study of flexibility. Res Q 1969;40:62–70.

50. Hewitt D: The range of active motion at the wrist of women. J Bone Joint Surg 1928;10:775–787.

51. Hertling D, Kessler RM: Management of Common Musculoskeletal Disorders. Philadelphia, JB Lippinocott, 1996.

52. Holmes C: Joint mobilization, Chapter 4. In Bandy WD, Sanders B. Therapeutic Exercise: Techniques for Intervention. Baltimore, Lippincott, Williams, & Wilkins, 2001.

53. Hubley-Kozey CL: Testing flexibility, Chapter 7. In MacDougall JD et al.: Physiological Testing of the High-Performance Athlete. Champaign, Ill: Human Kinetics Books, 1991.

54. Joseph, J: Range of movement of the great toe in men. J Bone Joint Surg 1954;36B:450–457.

55. Karpovich PV, Karpovich GP: Electrogoniometer: New device for study of joints in action. Fed Proc 1959;18:79.

56. Kebaetse M, McClure P, Pratt NA: Thoracic position effect on shoulder range of motion, strength, and three-dimensional scapular kinematics. Arch Phys Med Rehabil 1999;80;945–950.

57. Kendall FP, McCreary EK, Provance PG: Muscles: Testing and Function, 4th ed. Baltimore, Williams & Wilkins, 1993.

58. Kraus H: Backache, Stress, and Tension. New York: Simon and Schuster, 1965.

59. Lea RD, Gerhardt JJ: Current concepts review: Range of motion measurements. J Bone Joint Surg 1995;77A:784–798.

60. Leighton JR: An instrument and technic for the measurement of range of joint motion. Arch Phys Med 1955;36:571.

61. Loebl WY. Measurement of spinal posture and range of spinal movement. Ann Phys Med 1967;9:103–110.

62. Lundberg A, Kalin B, Selvik G: Kinematics of the ankle/foot complex: Plantarflexion and dorsiflexion. Foot Ankle Int 1989A;9:194–200.

63. Lundberg A, Svensson OK, Bylund D, et al.: Kinematics of the ankle/foot complex—Part 2: Pronation and supination. Foot Ankle Int 1989B;9:248–253.

64. Lundberg A, Svennson OK, Nèmeth G et al.: The axis of rotation of the ankle joint. J Bone Joint Surg Br 1989C;71-B:94–99.

65. Mann RA. Principles of examination of the foot and ankle. In Mann RA, Surgery of the Foot, 5th ed. St. Louis, Mosby, 1986.

66. Moore ML: The measurement of joint motion: Part IB—introductory review of the literature. Phys Ther Rev 1949;29:195–205.

67. Morrey BF, Askew LJ, Chao EYS: A biomechanical study of normal functional elbow motion. J Bone Joint Surg 1981;63:872–877.

68. Mundale MO, Hislop HJ, Babideau RJ et al.: Evaluation of extension of the hip. Arch Phys Med Rehabil 1956;37:75–80.

69. Muwanga CL, Dove AF: The measurement of ankle movements—a new method. Injury 1985;16:312–314.

70. Nicol AC: Measurement of joint motion. Clin Rehabil 1989;3:1–9.

71. Noer HR, Pratt DR: A goniometer designed for the hand. J Bone Joint Surg 1958;40-A:1154–1156.

72. Norkin CC, White DJ: Measurement of Joint Motion: A Guide to Goniometry, 2nd ed. Philadelphia, F.A. Davis, 1995.

73. Petherick M, Rheault W, Kimble, et al.: Concurrent validity and intertester reliability of universal and fluid based goniometer for active elbow range of motion. Phys Ther 1988;68:966–969.

74. Reese NR, Bandy WD: Unpublished data. 2000.

75. Resch S, Ryd L, Stenström A, et al.: Measuring hallux valgus: A comparison of conventional radiographic and clinical parameters with regard to measurements accuracy. Foot Ankle Int 1995;10:267–270.

76. Rheault W, Miller M, Nothnagel P, et al. Intertester reliability and concurrent validity of fluid-based and universal goniometer for active knee flexion. Phys Ther 1988;68:1676–1678.

77. Robinson WH: Joint range. J Orthop Surg 1921;3:41–51.

78. Rome, K: Ankle joint dorsiflexion measurement studies. A review of the literature. J Am Podiatr Med Assoc 1996;86:205–211

79. Root ML, Orien WP, Weed JH: Clinical biomechanics: Normal and abnormal function of the foot, vol. 2. Los Angeles, Clinical Biomechanics Corp., 1977.

80. Rosén NG: A simplified method of measuring amplitude of motion in joints. J Bone Joint Surg 1922;20:570–579.
81. Rowe CR: Joint measurement in disability evaluation. Clin Orthop 1964;32:43–53.
82. Sabari JS, Maltzer I, Lubarsky D, et al.: Goniometric assessment of shoulder range of motion: Comparison of testing in supine and sitting positions. Arch Phys Med Rehabil 1998;79:647–651.
83. Safaee-Rad R, Shwedyk E, Quanbury A, et al.: Normal functional range of motion of upper limb joints during performance of three feeding activities. Arch Phys Med Rehabil 1990;71:505–509.
84. Salter N: Methods of measurement of muscle and joint function. J Bone Joint Surg 1955;37B:474–491.
85. Schenker WW. Improved method of joint motion measurement. NY J Med 1956;56:539–542
86. Silver D: Measurement of the range of motion in joints. J Bone Joint Surg 1923;21:569–578.
87. Simoneau CC, Hoenig KJ, Lepley JE, Papanek PE: Influence of hip position and gender on active hip internal and external rotation. J Orthop Sports Phys Ther 1998;28:158–164.
88. Smith DS: Measurement of joint range—An overview. Clin Rheum Dis 1982;8):523–531.
89. Smith JR, Walker JM: Knee and elbow range of motion in healthy older individuals. Phys Occup Ther in Geriatr 1983;2:31–38.
90. Smith LK, Weiss EL, Lehmkuhl LD: Brunnstrom's Clinical Kinesiology, 5th ed. Philadelphia, F.A. Davis, 1996.
91. Soderberg GL: Kinesiology: Application to Pathological Motion, 2nd ed. Baltimore, Williams & Wilkins, 1997.
92. Stuberg W, Temme J, Kaplan P, et al.: Measurement of tibial torsion and thigh-foot angle using goniometry and computed tomography. Clin Orthop 1991;272:208–212.
93. Wakeley CPG: A new form of goniometer. The Lancet 1918;23:300.
94. Watkins MA, Riddle DL, Lamb RL, Personius WJ: Reliability of goniometric measurements and visual estimates of knee range of motion obtained in a clinical setting. Phys Ther 1991;71:90–96.
95. Weseley MS, Koval R, Kleiger B: Roentgen measurement of ankle flexion—extension motion. Clin Orthop 1969;65:167–174.
96. West CC: Measurement of joint motion. Arch Phys Med 1945;26:414–425.
97. West CC: Measurement of joint motion. Arch Phys Med Rehabil 1952;25:414.
98. Wiechec FJ, Krusen FH: A new method of joint measurement and a review of the literature. Am J Surg 1939;43:659–668.
99. Wilson GD, Stasch WH: Photographic record of joint motion. Arch Phys Med 1945;26:361–362.
100. Yang RS. A new goniometer. Orthop Rev 1992;21:877–882.
101. Youdas JW, Carey TR, Garrett TR: Reliability of measurement of cervical spine range of motion—Comparison of three methods. Phys Ther 1991;71:98–104.
102. Youdas JW, Bogard CL, Suman VJ: Reliability of goniometric measurements and visual estimates of ankle joint range of motion obtained in a clinical setting. Arch Phys Med Rehabil 1993;74:1113–1118.
103. Zachazewski JE: Flexibility for Sports, Chapter 13. In Sanders B. Sports Physical Therapy. Norwalk, Conn, Appleton & Lange, 1990.
104. Zankel HT: A new method of measurement of range of motion of joints. Arch Phys Med 1951;32:227–228.

MEASUREMENT of RANGE of MOTION and MUSCLE LENGTH: CLINICAL RELEVANCE

Chapter 1 introduced the background necessary to measure joint range of motion and muscle length using standardized procedures. The purpose of this chapter is to educate the individual collecting data on range of motion and muscle length regarding the meaning of that information. The clinician must be aware of the strengths and weaknesses of referring to data as "normative." The reader needs to understand both the changes that occur with age and the differences that exist between men and women, as well as among different cultures and occupations. Finally, if the measurements are not accurate, then the information gained from the data collected is literally worthless. The clinician must not only be aware of the need for accurate measurements, but also have an understanding of the reliability and validity of the procedures and instruments being used. After reading Chapter 2, readers should have a better understanding of the clinical relevance of the data collected in measuring range of motion and muscle length to better educate their patients and to guide their intervention.

NORMATIVE DATA FOR RANGE OF MOTION AND MUSCLE LENGTH

Numerous individuals and groups have provided "norms" for range of motion of the joints of the spine and extremities (see Appendix C). However, the validity of most of these "norms" is suspect for one reason or another. Many individuals and groups who have provided "norms" for range of motion have done so without substantiating the source of the "normative" data. For example, the long-used and accepted "norms" for range of motion provided by the American Academy of Orthopaedic Surgeons (AAOS)[3] were published without an explanation of how the data were obtained or any description of the population from which the data came. The newest edition of the AAOS joint motion manual repeats many of the 1965 "norms" and provides other normative data that are derived from studies with small or nonrandomized samples.[25] Likewise, the American Medical Association does not describe the source for its published "norms" for range of motion.[4] Instead of providing unsubstantiated normative data for the various movements, Appendix C attempts to provide "norms" for range of motion for movements of the extremities and the spine based on available published literature.

FACTORS AFFECTING RANGE OF MOTION

CHANGES IN RANGE OF MOTION WITH AGE

Lower Extremity

Normal range of motion in the joints is not static but changes across the life span, from birth until the later decades of life (Tables 2–1 and 2–2). Studies in the pediatric population have demonstrated increased hip flexion, abduction, and rotation range of motion in infants and young children compared with the adult population (Table 2–3).* Extension of the hip is decreased in neonates, resulting in a hip flexion contracture that appears to resolve by the age of 2 years.[9, 10, 15, 19, 26, 28, 44, 58, 59] A similar flexion contracture is seen at the knee of neonates,[10, 19, 58, 59] but this contracture appears to resolve fairly quickly, with knee extension approaching adult values by the time the infant reaches 3 to 6 months of age (see Table 2–2)[10, 31] and progressing to hyperextension in some children by 3 years of age. Studies of large groups of children in China, England, and Scotland revealed hyperextension of the knee in young children that disappeared sometime between the ages of 6 and 10 years.[12, 51, 60]

The range of ankle and foot motion in neonates also differs from adult values, with components of both pronation and supination showing increased motion compared with adults. Motion of the dorsiflexion and eversion components of pronation as well as of the inversion component of supination have been shown to be increased in neonates (see Table 2–2).[19, 58, 59] The amount of plantarflexion in neonates has been reported as decreased (compared with adult values) by some authors[31, 58, 59] and as equal to adult ranges by other investigators.[19]

Changes in range of motion also have been reported in the elderly population. A significant decrease in the amount of hip motion (abduction, adduction,

Table 2–1. CHANGES IN UPPER EXTREMITY RANGE OF MOTION: BIRTH TO 84 YEARS OF AGE				
SHOULDER	**Birth–2 yr***	**18 mo–19 yr†**	**20–54 yr†**	**60–84 yr‡**
Flexion	172°–180°	168° ± 4°	165° ± 5°	165° ± 10°
Extension	79°–89°	68° ± 8°	57° ± 8°	44° ± 12°
Abduction	177°–187°	185° ± 4°	183° ± 9°	165° ± 19°
Medial Rotation	72°–90°	71° ± 5°	67° ± 4°	63° ± 15°
Lateral Rotation	123°	108° ± 7°	100° ± 8°	81° ± 15°
ELBOW	**Birth–2 yr**	**18 mo–19 yr**	**20–54 yr**	**60–84 yr**
Flexion	148°–158°	145° ± 5°	141° ± 5°	144° ± 10°
Extension	−2°	1° ± 4°	0° ± 3°	−4° ± 4°
FOREARM	**Birth–2 yr**	**18 mo–19 yr**	**20–54 yr**	**60–84 yr**
Pronation	90°–96°	77° ± 5°	75° ± 5°	71° ± 11°
Supination	81°–93°	83° ± 3°	81° ± 4°	74° ± 11°
WRIST	**Birth–2 yr**	**18 mo–19 yr**	**20–54 yr**	**60–84 yr**
Flexion	88°–96°	78° ± 6°	75° ± 7°	64° ± 10°
Extension	82°–89°	76° ± 6°	74° ± 7°	63° ± 8°
Abduction (radial deviation)		22° ± 4°	21° ± 4°	19° ± 6°
Adduction (ulnar deviation)		37° ± 4°	35° ± 4°	26° ± 7°

* Watanabe et al.[58]
† Boone et al.[9]
‡ Walker et al.[57]

---

*See references 9, 10, 15, 19, 26, 28, 44, 54, 58, 59.

Table 2–2. CHANGES IN LOWER EXTREMITY RANGE OF MOTION: BIRTH TO 84 YEARS OF AGE

HIP	Birth–2 yr*	18 mo–19 yr[†]	25–39 yr[‡]	40–59 yr[‡]	60–84 yr[§]
Flexion	136°	123° ± 6°	122° ± 12°	120° ± 14°	111° ± 12°
Extension	−1°	7° ± 7°	22° ± 8°	18° ± 7°	−11° ± 4°
Abduction	57°	52° ± 9°	44° ± 11°	42° ± 11°	24° ± 8°
Adduction	17° ± 4°ʹ	28° ± 4°	26° ± 4°[†]	26° ± 4°[†]	15° ± 4°
Medial Rotation	38°	50° ± 6°	33° ± 7°	31° ± 8°	22° ± 6°
Lateral Rotation	70°	51° ± 6°	34° ± 8°	32° ± 8°	32° ± 6°
KNEE	**Birth–2 yr**	**18 mo–19 yr**	**25–39 yr**	**40–59 yr**	**60–84 yr**
Flexion	148°–159°	144° ± 5°	134° ± 9°	132° ± 11°	133° ± 6°
Extension	−4°	−2° ± 3°	−1° ± 2°[†]	−1° ± 2°[†]	−1° ± 2°
ANKLE/FOOT	**Birth–2 yr**	**18 mo–19 yr**	**25–39 yr**	**40–59 yr**	**60–84 yr**
Dorsiflexion**	48°	13° ± 5°	12° ± 4°[†]	12° ± 4°[†]	10° ± 5°
Plantarflexion[††]	56°	58° ± 6°	54° ± 6°[†]	54° ± 6°ʹ	29° ± 7°
Inversion**	99° ± 6°[¶]	38° ± 5°	36° ± 4°[†]	36° ± 4°[†]	30° ± 11°
Eversion[††]	82° ± 9°[¶]	22° ± 5°	19° ± 5°[†]	19° ± 5°[†]	13° ± 6°

* Watanabe et al.[58]
[†] Boone & Azen, 1979.[9]
[‡] Roach & Miles.[49]
[§] Walker et al.[57].
ʹ Forero et al.[26] (neonates).
[¶] Drews et al.[19] (neonates).
** Component of pronation.
[††] Component of supination.

medial rotation, and lateral rotation) was reported in male and female subjects aged 60 to 84 years as compared with mean values reported by the AAOS (see Table 2–2).[3, 54] However, these reported decreases in range of motion in the hip joints of older adults were not substantiated by Roach and Miles,[49] who reported on data from the first National Health and Nutrition Examination

Table 2–3. CHANGES IN HIP RANGE OF MOTION FROM BIRTH TO 2 YEARS: SELECTED SOURCES

AGE	FLEXION	EXTENSION	ABDUCTION	MEDIAL ROTATION	LATERAL ROTATION
Neonates					
Drews et al.[19]		−28° ± 6°*	56° ± 10°[†]	80° ± 9°[‡]	114° ± 10°[‡]
Forero et al.[26]	128° ± 5°	−30° ± 4°[§]	39° ± 5°[†]	76° ± 6°[‡]	92° ± 3°[‡]
Haas et al.[28]		−30° ± 8°[§]	76° ± 12°[‡]	62° ± 13°[‡]	89° ± 14°[‡]
Watanabe et al.[58]	120°	−25°	48°	21°	77°
1–3 Months					
Watanabe et al. (4 wk)[58]	138°	−12°	51°	24°	66°
Coon et al. (6 wk)[15]		−19° ± 6°[§]		24° ± 5°ʹ	48° ± 11°ʹ
Coon et al. (3 mo)[15]		−7° ± 4°[§]		26° ± 3°ʹ	45° ± 5°ʹ
4–8 Months					
Coon et al. (6 mo)[15]		−7° ± 4°[§]		21° ± 4°ʹ	46° ± 5°ʹ
Watanabe et al. (4–8 mo)[58]	136°	−4°	55°	39°	66°
9–12 Months					
Phelps et al. (9 mo)[44]		−10° ± 3°[¶]	59° ± 7°[†]	41° ± 8°ʹ	56° ± 7°ʹ
Watanabe et al. (8–12 mo)[58]	138°	3°	60°	38°	79°
1 Year					
Phelps et al.[44]		−9° ± 5°[¶]	54° ± 8°[†]	44° ± 9°ʹ	58° ± 9°ʹ
Watanabe et al.[58]	141°	15°	66°	49°	74°
2 Years					
Phelps et al.[44]		−3° ± 3°[¶]	60° ± 7°[†]	52° ± 10°ʹ	47° ± 9°ʹ
Watanabe et al.[58]	143°	21°	63°	59°	58°

* Measured with subject sidelying, contralateral hip flexed.
[†] Measured with subject supine, hip and knee extended.
[‡] Measured with subject supine, hips and knees flexed to 90°.
[§] Measured with subject supine, contralateral hip flexed.
ʹ Measured with subject prone, hip extended, knee flexed to 90°.
[¶] Measured with subject prone, both hips flexed over end of table.

Survey (NHANES I). In their analysis of 1313 of the original 1892 subjects (aged 25 to 74 years) on whom hip and knee range of motion measurements were taken as part of NHANES I, Roach and Miles[49] reported that, generally, differences in the mean range of motion between younger (aged 25 to 39) and older (aged 60 to 74) age groups were small, ranging from 3 to 5 degrees. The only motion of the hip that did appear to decrease in range with aging, according to Roach and Miles,[49] was hip extension, which showed a greater than 20% decline between the youngest (aged 25 to 39) and oldest (aged 60 to 74) age groups.

The apparent discrepancy in reported results between the Walker et al.[57] study and the Roach and Miles[49] study is probably due to differences in the age groups studied. The sample population in the Walker et al.[57] study included subjects with ages up to 84 years, whereas no subjects over the age of 74 were included in the data reported by Roach and Miles.[49] In a study that focused on subjects between the ages of 70 and 92 years, James and Parker[32] reported progressive decreases in all lower extremity joint motions with increasing age, with the most pronounced decreases in motion occurring after age 80. The largest changes in range of motion occurred with ankle dorsiflexion (knee extended) and hip abduction. Thus one could presume, by analyzing the three aforementioned studies, that lower extremity range of motion does show a decline with increasing age, but that decline is probably not significant until the ninth decade.

Some motions of the lower extremities have been reported to decline in range at earlier ages. Decreased range of motion of the first metatarsophalangeal joint after age 45 has been reported both for flexion and for extension of that joint.[11] Loss of extension range of motion appears to be both more marked and more significant in terms of potential loss of function.[11]

Upper Extremity

Range of motion of many upper extremity joints also appears to differ in infants and young children compared with adults (see Table 2–1). Measurements reported in a study of over 300 Japanese infants and children from birth to 2 years of age demonstrated an increased range of shoulder extension and lateral rotation, forearm pronation, and wrist flexion, along with a decreased range of elbow extension, in this age group compared with adults.[58] The amount of shoulder lateral rotation present in the neonate appears to decrease as the child ages, with the range of shoulder rotation approaching adult levels by the age of 2 years (Table 2–4). As a child ages, elbow extension range of motion also changes to approach adult levels, but more quickly than does the range of shoulder lateral rotation. The limitation in elbow extension seen in the neonate appears to

Table 2–4. UPPER EXTREMITY MOTIONS DEMONSTRATING SIGNIFICANT CHANGE IN AMPLITUDE DURING THE FIRST TWO YEARS*		
AGE	SHOULDER LATERAL ROTATION	ELBOW EXTENSION
Birth (*n* = 62)	134°	−14°
2–4 weeks (*n* = 57)	126°	−6°
4–8 months (*n* = 54)	120°	0°
8–12 months (*n* = 45)	124°	1°
1 year (*n* = 64)	116°	3°
2 years (*n* = 57)	118°	5°

* Source: Watanabe et al.[58]

resolve by the age of 3 to 8 months (see Table 2–4),[31, 58] progresses to hyperextension in many children by the age of 2 to 3 years,[13, 58, 60] and then gradually resolves to adult levels. A limitation in shoulder abduction also has been reported in neonates, but by only one investigator on a fairly small sample of subjects.[31] The limitation in shoulder abduction had disappeared in these infants by 3 months of age.

Decreases in upper extremity range of motion in older adults also have been reported (see Table 2–1). Walker et al.[57] reported a significant decrease in the amount of shoulder and wrist extension present in older males only, and a decrease in the amount of forearm supination present in older females, compared with mean values reported by the AAOS for all motions.[3] Statistically significant decreases with increasing age were reported for wrist flexion, wrist extension, and shoulder rotation range of motion in a group of 720 subjects, aged 33 to 70 years.[2] These subjects represented a subgroup of a population surveyed in Iceland and Sweden.

Decreases in other upper extremity motions (shoulder flexion, abduction, medial rotation, and lateral rotation) were reported by Downey et al.[18] in a group of 106 subjects aged 61 to 93 years. However, these decreases were based on comparison with means published by the AAOS in 1965, many of which have since changed. Comparison of values obtained by Downey et al.[18] with current AAOS means[27] reveals decreases only in shoulder abduction and lateral rotation in the group of older subjects.

Lumbar Spine

An investigation by van Adrichem and van der Korst[56] examined the changes that occur as children age from 6 to 18 years. Using a tape measure, the authors measured lumbar flexion in 248 children and reported that as the child became older and progressed to adulthood, flexion range of motion increased.

Four studies[21, 24, 36, 40] examined lumbar range of motion across the age span by categorizing subjects into 10-year increments and comparing the amount of lumbar motion in each age group. In one of the earliest studies, Loebl[36] used an inclinometer to measure lumbar flexion and extension in 176 individuals between the ages of 15 and 84 years and reported that a decrease in range of motion is "readily demonstrated." Similarly, Moll and Wright[40] used the tape measure technique to measure flexion, extension, and lateral flexion in 237 subjects (ages 18 to 71 years) and reported that an initial increase in lumbar motion occurred from the ages 15-to-24 decade to the ages 25-to-34 decade, followed by "a progressive decrease in advancing age." However, statistical support for the conclusions reported by both Loebl[36] and Moll and Wright[40] is unclear.

Examining flexion (using a tape measure), extension (using a goniometer), and lateral flexion (using a goniometer) in 172 primarily male subjects (only four subjects were female) between the ages of 20 and 82 years, Fitzgerald et al.[24] reported that lumbar motion decreased across the age span, with the difference being statistically significant at 20-year intervals. Reporting similar results after measuring flexion (with a tape measure), extension (with a goniometer), and lateral flexion (with a goniometer) in 109 females, Einkauf et al.[21] reported significant differences between the two youngest decades (ages 20 to 29 and ages 30 to 39) and the two oldest decades (ages 60 to 69 and ages 70 to 84). Additionally, Einkauf et al.[21] reported that extension showed the greatest decrease in motion with increasing age. Table 2–5 provides information on normative data related to lumbar range of motion with increased age derived from the research by Fitzgerald et al.[24] and Einkauf et al.[21]

Table 2–5. NORMATIVE RANGE OF MOTION OF THORACIC AND LUMBAR SPINE USING THE TAPE MEASURE (FLEXION ONLY) AND GONIOMETER (EXTENSION AND LATERAL FLEXION): AGE 40–80+ YEARS

AGE (YEARS)	SAMPLE SIZE		FLEXION (CM)		EXTENSION (DEGREES)		RIGHT LATERAL FLEXION (DEGREES)		LEFT LATERAL FLEXION (DEGREES)	
	A	B	A	B	A	B	A	B	A	B
40–49	16	17	3 (±.8)	6 (±1.0)	31 (±9)	21 (±8)	27 (±7)	29 (±5)	29 (±5)	28 (±7)
50–59	44	15	3 (±1.0)	6 (±1.0)	27 (±8)	22 (±7)	25 (±6)	31 (±6)	26 (±6)	28 (±5)
60–69	27	16	2 (±.7)	5 (±1.0)	17 (±8)	19 (±5)	20 (±5)	24 (±8)	20 (±5)	22 (±6)
70–84	9	15	2 (±.7)	5 (±1.0)	17 (±9)	18 (±4)	18 (±5)	24 (±4)	19 (±6)	20 (±4)

A = Measurement of flexion used Schober technique; all other measurements via goniometer (Fitzgerald et al.[24]).
B = Measurement of flexion used modified Schober; all other measurements via goniometer (Einkauf et al.[21]).

Cervical Spine

Although inconsistencies related to the effects of aging on joint range of motion in other joints may exist, agreement exists in the literature that range of motion of the cervical spine decreases in aging adults. Using an inclinometer attached by straps to the head and under the chin, Kuhlman[33] compared a group of 20- to 30-year-old subjects ($n = 31$) with a group of 70- to 90-year-old individuals ($n = 42$) for cervical flexion, extension, lateral flexion (right and left measured separately), and rotation (right and left measured separately). The authors reported that "the elderly group had significantly less motion than the younger group for all six motions measured." Furthermore, the authors reported that the loss of motion was greatest for cervical extension and least for cervical flexion.[33]

Review of the literature provides several studies that support the conclusions reported by Kuhlman.[33] Two studies used the cervical range of motion (CROM) device to examine changes in the cervical motion that occur with age. Examining combined flexion/extension, combined right/left lateral flexion, and combined right/left rotation in 90 subjects with an age range of 21 to 60 years, Nilsson et al.[42] reported that results indicated "significant differences between range of motion in different age groups for all directions of movement, in the sense that range of motion decreased with increasing age." Examining cervical flexion, extension, lateral flexion, and rotation in subjects categorized in 10-year increments across eight decades, Youdas et al.[61] examined 337 individuals ranging in age from 11 to 97 years. The authors concluded that males and females should expect a loss of 3 to 5 degrees for all cervical ranges of motion per 10-year increase in age. Table 2–6 provides the only published data on normative ranges of motion related to cervical motion with increased age.

Table 2–6. NORMATIVE RANGE OF MOTION OF CERVICAL SPINE USING CROM*: AGE 40–97†

AGE (YEARS)	FLEXION (DEGREES)	EXTENSION (DEGREES)	LEFT LATERAL FLEXION (DEGREES)	RIGHT LATERAL FLEXION (DEGREES)	LEFT ROTATION (DEGREES)	RIGHT ROTATION (DEGREES)
40–49	50 (±11)	70 (±13)	38 (±9)	40 (±10)	63 (±8)	67 (±8)
50–59	46 (±9)	63 (±13)	35 (±6)	36 (±6)	60 (±9)	61 (±8)
60–69	41 (±8)	61 (±12)	32 (±6)	31 (±8)	58 (±8)	59 (±9)
70–79	39 (±9)	54 (±12)	26 (±8)	27 (±7)	50 (±8)	52 (±10)
80–89	40 (±9)	50 (±13)	23 (±7)	25 (±6)	49 (±10)	50 (±9)
90–97	36 (±10)	53 (±18)	24 (±7)	22 (±8)	49 (±12)	48 (±12)

* Cervical Range of Motion Device.
† Data from Youdas et al.[61]

Two studies using similar three-dimensional devices to measure cervical range of motion also divided subjects into categories of 10-year intervals. Examining 150 subjects for combined flexion/extension, combined right/left lateral flexion, and combined right/left rotation from age 20 to "older than 60 years," Dvorak et al.[20] reported that range of motion decreased as age increased, "with the most dramatic decrease in range of motion occurring between the 30–39th and 40–49th decades." Similarly, Trott et al.[55] examined cervical flexion, extension, lateral flexion (right and left measured separately), and rotation (right and left measured separately) in 120 subjects aged 20 to 59 years and reported that "age had a significant effect on all the primary movements."

Grouping subjects ranging in age from 12 to 79 years into seven groups by age using 10-year increments ($n = 70$), Lind et al.[35] reported that radiographic examination indicated that "the motion in all three planes [flexion/extension, lateral flexion, and rotation] decreased with age." This decrease was significant and began in the third decade. Additionally, results reported by Lind et al.[35] are also consistent with a report by Kuhlman[33] that "in the sagittal plane, extension motion decreased more than motion in flexion."

An investigation by Mayer et al.[39] is the only study to report that no age-related differences occurred in the measurement of cervical flexion, extension, lateral flexion (right and left measured separately), and rotation (right and left measured separately) using a double inclinometer method. However a review of the study's procedures indicated that the authors compared the youngest 50% of the subjects with the oldest 50% of the subjects ($n = 58$). Although the age range of the subjects was reported as 17 to 62 years, no data were provided as to the mean age of each group. Therefore, the mean age of each group being compared in this study is unknown, and any conclusions of this study are unclear.[39]

DIFFERENCES IN RANGE OF MOTION BASED ON SEX

Lower Extremity

The amount of range of motion present in the joints of males and females appears to differ, but not with respect to all joints. However, in almost all cases cited, the greater amount of range of motion is found in the female population. In a study of 60 college-age subjects in which the influences of hip position and gender on hip rotation were investigated, females demonstrated a statistically greater range of active hip medial and lateral rotation compared with males.[52] Similar differences between the sexes regarding the range of hip rotation available were reported by James and Parker[32] in a sample of elderly (ages 70 to 92) males and females. Increased medial, but not lateral, hip rotation in females also has been reported by Walker et al.,[57] in a study of 60 male and female subjects aged 60 to 84 years, and in a study by Svenningsen et al.,[54] who studied 761 Norwegian subjects ranging in age from 4 years to adulthood (the 20s). Other motions of the hip that have been reported as being increased in females compared with males are hip flexion in adolescents, young adults,[54] and elderly females (ages 70 to 92),[32] and hip abduction in all age groups from age 4 to young adulthood.[54]

Two studies of older adults[32, 57] have reported a statistically increased range of knee flexion in female compared with male subjects. However, in one study, the difference did not exceed the inter-rater error for that measurement.[57] A greater amount of ankle plantarflexion also appears to be present in women compared with men across all adult age groups.[32, 41, 57] Conversely, there appears to be some indication that ankle dorsiflexion range of motion becomes significantly higher in males than in females for persons older than 70 years.[41]

Upper Extremity

Some motions of the upper extremity also appear to differ according to sex. In a study of 720 adult subjects from Sweden and Iceland,[2] significantly greater ranges of shoulder medial and lateral rotation were reported in females compared with males. These differences in shoulder lateral, but not medial, rotation were substantiated in a group of older male and female subjects.[57] Additionally, the older female subjects, who were between the ages of 60 and 84 years, demonstrated significantly more shoulder flexion, extension, and abduction than did their male counterparts.[57]

Differences in elbow range of motion between male and female subjects have been demonstrated in older adults in two studies. Both studies examined similar age groups (55 to 84 years compared with 60 to 84 years), and both demonstrated a significantly increased amount of elbow flexion in female compared with male subjects.[53, 57] One study also reported a significantly higher amount of elbow extension in female subjects.[57]

Wrist and hand motions also appear to differ in male compared with female subjects. Allander et al.[2] reported significantly higher ranges of wrist flexion and extension in females than in male adults. Increased wrist extension and adduction (ulnar deviation) in females, but not increased wrist flexion, were reported in a sample of older adults.[57] In a study of 120 young adults (ages 18 to 35 years), Mallon et al.[38] demonstrated increased active and passive extension at all joints of the fingers (metacarpophalangeal, proximal interphalangeal, and distal interphalangeal) in female subjects compared with males. Details of studies investigating differences in range of motion according to sex are found in Appendix C.

Lumbar Spine

Only two studies have investigated the differences between boys and girls in range of motion of the lumbar spine prior to adulthood. Using a tape measure to measure flexion and lateral flexion, Haley et al.[29] compared 142 females with 140 males between the ages of 5 and 9 years and reported that girls were significantly more flexible than boys. Conversely, van Adrichem and van der Korst[56] used a tape measure to measure lumbar flexion on children between the ages of 6 and 18 years and reported that no significant difference existed between boys ($n = 149$) and girls ($n = 149$).

Macrae and Wright[37] also used a tape measure to measure lumbar flexion, but on an older (age 18 to 71 years) sample of 195 females and 147 males. The authors reported that, regardless of age, males had significantly more lumbar flexion than females. More flexion in males than in females was supported in a later study by Moll and Wright,[40] who compared the difference in 119 males and 118 females, also using a tape measure. In addition, Moll and Wright[40] reported that males had more lumbar mobility than females for extension, but that females had more motion for lateral flexion than males.

In the only study to examine the difference in lumbar rotation related to sex, Boline et al.[8] examined lumbar rotation in 25 individuals with a mean age of 33 years. Using an inclinometer to compare the amount of rotation in

14 males with the amount of rotation in 11 females, the authors reported that no significant difference existed between males and females for right and left rotation.

Cervical Spine

Lind et al.[35] radiographically examined cervical range of motion in 35 male and in 35 female subjects. Using three measurement devices (CROM device, radiography, and a computerized tracking system), Ordway et al.[43] examined 20 subjects (11 female, 9 male) for cervical flexion and extension. The authors of both studies reported that no significant differences were found between males and females for any of the measurement devices.

Mayer et al.[39] used the double inclinometer method to compare the cervical range of motion of 28 males (age range 17 to 61 years) with the range of motion of 30 females (age range 19 to 62 years) and reported that, regardless of age, the only sex-specific difference in range of motion occurred in cervical extension; the authors reported that females possessed greater range of motion than males. No significant sex-related differences were found for cervical flexion, lateral flexion, and rotation.

Using an inclinometer attached to the top of the head with a head adapter and an adjustable headband and cloth chinstrap, Kuhlman[33] reported that "females had higher mean cervical range of motion than males for all cervical motion examined." In actuality, these differences between males and females were statistically significant only for cervical extension, lateral flexion (right and left), and rotation (right and left); no significant difference related to sex was found for cervical flexion.

Nilsson et al.[42] used the CROM device to compare 59 females with 31 males with an age range of 20 to 60 years. Although the authors concluded that differences were found between males and females, their results indicated that range of motion for lateral flexion (right and left total lateral flexion combined) was the only motion for which females had a statistically greater range than males. Results of statistical analyses comparing males and females for cervical flexion/extension (combined) and rotation (left and right total rotation combined) were not reported. Youdas et al.[61] also used the CROM device, comparing cervical range of motion between 171 females and 166 males ranging in age from 11 to 97 years. The authors concluded that across all ages, females had greater ranges of motion than males for all cervical motions.

Using a three-dimensional recording of cervical motion made with a computer-integrated electrogoniometric device, Trott et al.[55] examined differences in range of motion between 60 males and 60 females. Results of the study indicated "a gender difference in cervical range of motion that was reported at all decades, where women had a larger range of motion in all cardinal planes than men."

Using a measurement device similar to the one used by Trott et al.,[55] Dvorak et al.[20] measured three-dimensional motion of the cervical spine using computer-integrated potentiometers. Comparing cervical range of motion in 86 males and 64 females ranging in age from 20 to "older than 60" years they found that within each decade, females showed a significantly greater range than did males for all cervical motions.

Studies comparing the cervical range of motion of males with that of females are not as consistent as investigations related to changes that occur in cervical ranges of motion with advancing age. However, although reports are inconsistent as to whether a difference exists between the cervical range of motion of males compared with females, a review of the literature indicates that no study has reported that males have a greater cervical range of motion than females. In other words, the investigations reviewed related to cervical range of motion reported either that no difference in range of motion existed between sexes, or that females had a greater range of motion than males.

DIFFERENCES IN RANGE OF MOTION BASED ON CULTURE AND OCCUPATION

Differences in range of motion among individuals have been attributed both to culture and to occupation. Range of motion of lower extremity joints has been shown to be significantly increased in populations of Chinese and Saudi Arabian subjects compared with British and Scandinavian subjects, respectively.[1, 30] All lower extremity joint motions, with the exception of hip adduction, were reported to be significantly higher in a group of 50 Saudi Arabian males[1] when their mean ranges of motion were compared with those of a group of 105 males of the same age group from Sweden.[48] Higher ranges of hip flexion, abduction, medial rotation, and lateral rotation were reported in a group of 500 Chinese subjects over the age of 54 years, compared with values for hip range of motion in British adults.[30] In both instances in which cultural differences in range of motion were noted, the authors were unable to define the cause for the differences. Suppositions included biologic differences such as capsular laxity; differences in activities of daily living, as many individuals in China and Saudi Arabia squat and kneel routinely during daily activities; and differences in measurement techniques between the studies.[1, 30]

Occupation, whether vocational or recreational, also appears to be related to changes in range of motion at various joints. A study of 30 senior female classical ballet dancers along with age-matched controls revealed significantly higher ranges of hip flexion, extension, lateral rotation, and abduction, and significantly lower ranges of hip medial rotation and adduction in the dancers compared with the control subjects.[46] Shoulder motion, particularly rotation, but also abduction, has been reported as differing from normal values in certain athletes. Competitive tennis players and swimmers demonstrate increased shoulder lateral rotation and decreased shoulder medial rotation when their mean values are compared with published norms for those motions.[6, 7, 14, 23] Swimmers also have been reported to have increased shoulder abduction range of motion compared with published norms for shoulder abduction.[7]

RELIABILITY AND VALIDITY

RELIABILITY

The usefulness of a measurement device for the examination of a patient's range of motion and muscle length depends on the extent to which the device can be used by the clinician to accurately perform the activity, called reliability. Throughout this text, information is presented on the reliability of the various techniques described. Reliability concerns whether or not the same trait can be measured consistently on repeated measurements. In other words, reliability is "the extent to which measurements are repeatable."[17]

To establish reliability for a measurement device, a test-retest design is frequently used. Using a test-retest design, a sample of subjects is measured on two occasions, keeping all testing variables as constant as possible during each test session. For example, if the reliability of the goniometer to measure knee flexion is to be tested, knee flexion range of motion would be measured on two (or more) occasions. The goniometer would be considered reliable if the range of motion measurements of knee flexion taken on the two occasions were similar.

Frequently, a clinical measurement requires the observation of a human observer, or a *rater*. Two types of reliability are important when dealing with clinical measurement; intrarater reliability and inter-rater reliability. Intrarater reliability is "the consistency with which one rater assigns scores to a single set of responses on two [or more] separate occasions."[17] To return to the example of measuring knee flexion range of motion, a check of intrarater reliability would involve one tester, or rater, examining knee flexion range of motion of 30 individuals on two occasions and comparing the results. Information obtained from the study would indicate whether the rater is reliable within ("intra") himself or herself.

Inter-rater reliability is the "consistency of performances among different raters or judges in assigning scores to the same objects or responses . . . determined when two or more raters judge the performance of one group of subjects at the same point in time."[17] An example of inter-rater reliability is to have two testers, or raters, measure knee flexion range of motion on 30 individuals on one occasion and compare the results. Inter-rater reliability is especially important if more than one clinician is going to be measuring range of motion of a particular patient.

Quantification

In order to quantify reliability, both the relationship and the agreement between repeated measurements must be examined. Domholdt[17] referred to the assessment of the relationship between repeated measurements as assessing *relative reliability* and the examination of the magnitude of the difference between repeated measurements as assessing *absolute reliability*.

Relative Reliability

Relative reliability "is based on the idea that if a measurement is reliable, individual measurements within a group will maintain their position within the group on repeated measurements."[17] For example, an individual with a large amount of shoulder range of motion on an initial measurement compared with a sample would be expected to have a large amount of range of motion when compared with a sample on subsequent measurements.

The most commonly used statistic to analyze relative reliability of measurement is the correlation coefficient. The assumption is that relative reliability is established if the paired measurements correlate highly. A common method for interpreting the correlation coefficient and, therefore, the reliability of the measurement, is to examine the strength of the relationship. Correlation coefficients range from −1.0 to +1.0; a perfect positive relationship (+1.0) indicates that a higher value on one variable is associated with a higher value on the second variable.[17]

Reliability is rarely perfect; therefore, correlation coefficients of 1.0 are rare. A review of the literature related to the measurement of range of motion and muscle length reveals that several authors suggest that in order to achieve acceptable reliability, a correlation of at least .80 is necessary.[16, 22, 25, 34, 47]

The Pearson product moment correlation (referred to as Pearson's *r*) has traditionally been used to analyze the strength of the correlation and, hence, reliability. However, the Pearson correlation is limited because, although it is quite appropriate for measuring the association between two variables (relative reliability), it cannot measure agreement between the two variables (absolute reliability).

Absolute Reliability

The Pearson correlation coefficient only provides information regarding relative reliability of a measurement. Information about the variability of a score with repeated measurements that is caused by measurement error also is important in the assessment of reliability of range of motion and muscle length tests. Reliability should examine not only the consistency of the rank of the score, but also the degree of similarity between repeated scores. This consistency between scores (also referred to as *agreement*) is referred to as absolute reliability.[17]

One method used to accommodate the fact that the Pearson correlation does not measure absolute reliability is to supplement the information obtained with the Pearson correlation with follow-up testing. Several tests exist to determine absolute reliability, with two of the most common tests being the paired *t* test and the standard error of the measurement.

THE *t* TEST

One way to extend the reliability analysis beyond the Pearson correlation measuring relative reliability is to conduct a *t* test. The *t* test is the most basic standard procedure for comparing the difference between group means.[17, 45] For example, suppose the goal of a study is to determine whether the measurement of knee flexion range of motion using a goniometer is the same for Examiner #1 and Examiner #2 (intertester reliability). Each examiner measures 30 subjects. First, a Pearson correlation can be calculated to determine relative reliability for each tester. Second, each tester can obtain mean scores for each group and perform a *t* test to compare the two groups. If the *t* test that is performed to compare the means of the two samples indicates a significant difference, the researchers can conclude that the population means are different from one another. This significant difference between the two testers would call into question the intertester reliability. Conversely, if the results of the *t* test indicate that no significant difference exists, the researcher can assume that any difference between the two examiners occurred by chance, and conclude that agreement exists between the two examiners. For a more detailed discussion of the *t* test, the reader is referred to texts written by Domholdt[17] and by Portney and Watkins.[45]

STANDARD ERROR OF THE MEASUREMENT (SEMm)

A second way to examine for absolute reliability of a measurement is to calculate the standard error of the measurement (SEMm), defined as "the range in which a single subject's true score could be expected to lie when measurement error is considered."[5] In fact Rothstein and Echternach[50] suggested that the SEMm is the "ideal statistic for estimating the error associated with reliability."

The SEMm is an estimate of the amount of error that would occur if repeated measurements were taken on the same subjects. Given that it is not practical to take repeated measurements 25 to 30 times to establish the actual SEMm, the value is estimated from the following formula:

$$SEMm = SD \sqrt{1 - r}$$

where SD is the standard deviation and r is the correlation coefficient. The more reliable a measure, the smaller the errors would be, and the SEMm would be low. As indicated by the formula, the magnitude of the SEMm is directly related to the standard deviation (as the standard deviation decreases, the SEMm decreases) and indirectly related to the correlation coefficient (as the correlation approaches 1.0, the SEMm approaches 0).[17, 45]

The SEMm is based on the standard deviation and has properties similar to those of the standard deviation. Once the SEMm is calculated, it can be concluded that a repeated measurement would fall within 1 SEMm of the mean 68% of the time, and within 2 SEMm of the mean 95% of the time. For example, if the mean value of the range of shoulder flexion obtained by an examiner measuring 30 individuals were 160 degrees and the SEMm were 2 degrees, then a 95% chance exists that the true value of shoulder flexion would fall between 156 and 164 degrees (2 SEMm above and below the mean). In this example, absolute reliability would be considered very good. If, on the other hand, data collected indicated a mean value of shoulder flexion of 160 degrees and a SEMm of 10 degrees, then a 95% chance exists that the true value of shoulder flexion would fall between 140 and 180 degrees. In this second example, absolute reliability would be in question because the amount of measurement error was so large. Again, both Portney and Watkins[45] and Domholdt[17] are excellent sources for more detailed information on the SEMm, as well as on statistical analysis in general.

Intraclass Correlation (ICC)

Portney and Watkins[45] expressed concern over using both a Pearson correlation and a follow-up test because such analyses do not provide a single index to describe reliability. Using a Pearson correlation and a follow-up test, "the scores may be consistent but significantly different, or they may be poorly correlated but not significantly different. How should these results be interpreted?" A correlation analysis that accounts for both absolute and relative reliability is the intraclass correlation coefficient (ICC), considered by some as the preferred correlation coefficient to be used when examining reliability.[45] The ICC is calculated using variance estimates obtained from an analysis of variance, thereby reflecting both relative and absolute reliability in one index. Domholdt[17] described the ICC as a "family of coefficients" that allows analysis of reliability with at least six different ICC formulas classified using two numbers in parentheses. Portney and Watkins[45] described three models of the ICC, with each model being expressed in two possible forms (for a total of six), depending on whether the scores collected as part of a study are single ratings or mean ratings.

For a detailed discussion of the three models, the reader is referred to Portney and Watkins.[45] For the purpose of this textbook, if "it is important to demonstrate that a particular measurement tool can be used with confidence by all clinicians, then Model 2 should be used. This approach [Model 2] is appropriate for clinical studies and methodological research, to document that a measurement tool has broad application."[45]

The various types of ICCs are classified by using two numbers in parentheses. The first number designates the model (1, 2, 3) and the second number indicates the form. If the form is to use a single measurement, the number is 1; if the form is the mean of more than one measurement, a constant (k) is used. For example, ICC (2, 1) indicates model 2 is used using single measurement (not mean) scores.[45]

VALIDITY

A measurement instrument must not only be reliable; the device also must be valid. Domholdt[17] has defined validity as the "appropriateness, meaningfulness, and usefulness of the test scores." In other words, validity deals with whether an instrument is truly measuring what the device is intended to measure.

Several types of validity exist and are described in Table 2–7. For purposes of determining the validity of measurements obtained with the devices presented in this text, the most appropriate type of validity is concurrent validity (a subcategory of criterion-related validity). For example, the gold standard for measurement of flexion of the spine can be considered the radiologic examination. If measurement of flexion of the spine using an inclinometer is found to be consistent with the amount of flexion of the spine measured with an x-ray, validity is established, and the inclinometer can be said to measure what it was purported to measure (flexion of the spine). Of course, the validity of the measurement is dependent on the assumption that radiographic analysis of flexion of the spine is an accurate gold standard.

Quantification

Criterion-related validity can be quantified by using correlation coefficients and follow-up tests, as appropriate, similar to those described in the Reliability section of this chapter. The process for interpreting statistical analyses related to validity is the same as for interpreting the reliability coefficient.

RELIABILITY AND VALIDITY: CRITERION FOR INCLUSION

Subsequent chapters of this text describe techniques for the measurement of range of joint motion and length of muscles of the extremities, spine, and

---

Table 2–7. TYPES OF MEASUREMENT VALIDITY

Face validity: Indicates that an instrument appears to test what it is supposed to test. The weakest form of measurement validity.

Content validity: Indicates that the items that make up an instrument adequately sample the universe of content that defines the variable being measured. Most useful with questionnaires and inventories.

Criterion-related validity: Indicates that the outcomes of one instrument, the target test, can be used as a substitute measure for an established gold standard criterion test. Can be tested as concurrent or predictive validity.

  Concurrent validity: Establishes validity when two measures are taken at relatively the same time. Most often used when the target test is considered more efficient than the gold standard and, therefore, can be used instead of the gold standard.

  Predictive validity: Establishes that the outcome of the target test can be used to predict a future criterion score or outcome.

    Prescriptive validity: Establishes that the interpretation of a measurement is appropriate for determining effective intervention.

Construct validity: Establishes the ability of an instrument to measure an abstract construct and the degree to which the instrument reflects the theoretical components of the construct.

From Portney LG, Watkins MP: Foundations of Clinical Research: Applications to Practice, 2nd ed. Upper Saddle River, NJ, Prentice-Hall, 2000, with permission.

temporomandibular joint. Additionally, Chapters 7, 10, and 15 present available information regarding the reliability and validity of these measurement techniques. The criterion for inclusion of an article in these chapters was that the study examining reliability or validity provides an analysis of both *relative* and *absolute* reliability or validity. For example, if a Pearson correlation was performed (relative reliability) and no follow-up testing was performed for absolute reliability, the study was not included in the chapter, unless an exception for inclusion could be rationalized. Exceptions to this criterion include if an article is the *only* study investigating a specific technique, or if the study is the *original* study of a specific technique commonly used in the clinic.

On the other hand, if a Pearson correlation and follow-up analysis were used or an ICC was used, the study was included in these chapters. However, no interpretive comments are made on reliability or validity related to the information presented in these chapters. As an example, if in providing two indexes for reliability (i.e., a Pearson correlation and a *t* test), contradictory views are presented, no interpretations are presented to clarify the results. Although presenting both indexes may cause confusion in the interpretation of the results, "uncertainty based on complete information is preferable to a sense of certainty based on incomplete information."[17]

These chapters on reliability and validity of measurement techniques are presented as a reference in order for readers to possess the information needed to choose measurement devices and techniques best suited for their own clinical situations. Additionally, it is hoped that gaps in the literature on specific techniques or devices will stimulate much-needed additional research in the area of measurement of joint range of motion and muscle length.

References

1. Ahlberg A, Moussa M, Al-Nahdi M: On geographical variations in the normal range of joint motion. Clin Orthop 1988;234:229–231.
2. Allander E, Bjornsson OJ, Olafsson O, et al.: Normal range of joint movements in shoulder, hip, wrist and thumb with special reference to side: A comparison between two populations. Int J Epidemiol 1974;3:253–261.
3. American Academy of Orthopaedic Surgeons: Joint Motion: Method of Measuring and Recording. Chicago, American Academy of Orthopaedic Surgeons, 1965.
4. American Medical Association: Guides to the Evaluation of Permanent Impairment, 4th ed. Chicago, American Medical Association, 1993.
5. Anastasi A: Psychological Testing. New York, Macmillan, 1988.
6. Bak K, Magnusson SP: Shoulder strength and range of motion in symptomatic and pain-free elite swimmers. Am J Sports Med 1997;25:454–459.
7. Beach ML, Whitney SL, Dickoff-Hoffman SA: Relationship of shoulder flexibility, strength, and endurance to shoulder pain in competitive swimmers. J Orthop Sports Phys Ther 1992;16:262–268.
8. Boline PD, Keating JC, Haas M, Anderson AV: Interexaminer reliability and discriminant validity of inclinometric measurement of lumbar rotation in chronic low-back pain patients and subjects without low-back pain. Spine 1992;17:335–338.
9. Boone DC, Azen SP, Lin C, et al.: Reliability of goniometric measurements. Phys Ther 1978;58:1355–1390.
10. Broughton NS, Wright J, Menelaus MB: Range of knee motion in normal neonates. J Pediatr Orthop 1993;13:263–264.
11. Buell T, Green DR, Risser J: Measurement of the first metatarsophalangeal joint range of motion. J Am Podiatr Med Assoc 1988;78:439–448.
12. Cheng JCY, Chan PS, Chiang SC: Angular and rotational profile of the lower limb in 2,630 Chinese children. J Pediatr Orthop 1991;11:154–161.
13. Cheng JCY, Chan PS, Hui PW: Joint laxity in children. J Pediatr Orthop B 1991;11:752–755.
14. Chinn CJ, Priest JD, Kent BE: Upper extremity range of motion, grip strength, and girth in highly skilled tennis players. Phys Ther 1974;54:474–482.
15. Coon V, Donato G, Honser C, et al.: Normal ranges of hip motion in infants six weeks, three months and six months of age. Clin Orthop 1975;110:256–260.

16. Currier DP: Elements of Research in Physical Therapy, 2nd ed. Baltimore, Williams & Wilkins, 1984.
17. Domholdt E: Physical Therapy Research: Principles and Applications. Philadelphia, WB Saunders, 2000.
18. Downey PA, Fiebert I, Stackpole-Brown JB: Shoulder range of motion in persons aged sixty and older. Phys Ther 1991;71:S75.
19. Drews JE, Vraciu JK, Pellino G: Range of motion of the joints of the lower extremities of newborns. Phys Occup Ther Pediatr 1984;4:49–62.
20. Dvorak J, Antinnes JA, Panjabi M, et al.: Age and gender related normal motion of the cervical spine. Spine 1992;17:393–398.
21. Einkauf DK, Gohdes ML, Jensen GM, Jewell MJ: Changes in spinal mobility with increasing age in women. Phys Ther 1987;67:370–375.
22. Eleveru RA, Rothstein JM, Lamb RL: Goniometric reliability in a clinical setting: Subtalar and ankle measurements. Phys Ther 1988;68:672–677.
23. Ellenbecker TS, Roetert EP, Piorkowski PA, Schulz DA: Glenohumeral joint internal and external range of motion in elite tennis players. J Orthop Sports Phys Ther 1996;24:336–341.
24. Fitzgerald GK, Wynveen KJ, Rheault W, Rothschild B: Objective assessment with establishment of normal values for lumbar spinal range of motion. Phys Ther 1983;63:1776–1781.
25. Fleiss JJ, Cohen J: The equivalence of weighted Kappa and intraclass correlation coefficient as measures of reliability. Educ Psychol Meas 1973;33:613–619.
26. Forero N, Okamura LA, Larson MA: Normal ranges of hip motion in neonates. J Pediatr Orthop 1989;9:391–395.
27. Greene WB, Heckman JD: The Clinical Measurement of Joint Motion. Rosemont, Ill, American Academy of Orthopaedic Surgeons, 1994.
28. Haas SS, Epps CH, Adams JP: Normal ranges of hip motion in the newborn. Clin Orthop 1973;19:114–118.
29. Haley SM, Tada WL, Carmichael EM: Spinal mobility in young children—A normative study. Phys Ther 1986;66:1697–1703.
30. Hoaglund FT, Yau A, Wong WL: Osteoarthritis of the hip and other joints in southern Chinese in Hong Kong. J Bone Joint Surg Am 1973;55A:545–557.
31. Hoffer MM: Joint motion limitations in newborns. Clin Orthop 1980;148:94–96.
32. James B, Parker AW: Active and passive mobility of lower limb joints in elderly men and women. Am J Phys Med Rehabil 1989;68:162–167.
33. Kuhlman KA: Cervical range of motion in the elderly. Arch Phys Med Rehabil 1993;74:1071–1079.
34. Landis JR, Koch GG: The measurement of observer agreement for categorical data. Biometrics 1977;33:159–174.
35. Lind B, Sihlbom H, Nordwall A, Malchau H: Normal range of motion of the cervical spine. Arch Phys Med Rehabil 1989;70:692–695.
36. Loebl WY: Measurement of spinal posture and range of spinal movement. Ann Phys Med 1967;9:103–110.
37. Macrae IF, Wright V: Measurement of back movement. Ann Rheum Dis 1969;28:584–589.
38. Mallon WJ, Brown HR, Nunley JA: Digital ranges of motion: Normal values in young adults. J Hand Surg [Am] 1991;16:882–887.
39. Mayer T, Brady S, Bovasso E, et al.: Noninvasive measurement of cervical tri-planar motion in normal subjects. Spine 1993;18:2191–2195.
40. Moll JMV, Wright V: Normal range of motion: An objective clinical study. Ann Rheum Dis 1971;30:381–386.
41. Nigg BM, Fisher V, Allinger TL, et al.: Range of motion of the foot as a function of age. Foot Ankle 1992;13:336–343.
42. Nilsson N: Measuring passive cervical motion: A study of reliability. J Manipulative Physiol Ther 1995;18:293–297.
43. Ordway NR, Seymour R, Donelson RG, et al.: Cervical sagittal range-of-motion analysis using three methods. Spine 1997;22:501–508.
44. Phelps E, Smith LJ, Hallum A: Normal ranges of hip motion of infants between nine and 24 months of age. Dev Med Child Neurol 1985;27:785–792.
45. Portney LG, Watkins MP: Foundations of Clinical Research: Applications to Practice, 2nd ed. Upper Saddle River, NJ, Prentice-Hall, 2000.
46. Reid DC, Burnham RS, Saboe LA, Kushner SF: Lower extremity flexibility patterns in classical ballet dancers and their correlation to lateral hip and knee injuries. Am J Sports Med 1987:15:347–352.
47. Richman T, Madridis L, Prince B: Research methodology and applied statistics, part 3: Measurement procedures in research. Physiother Canada 1980;32:253–257.
48. Roaas A, Anderson G: Normal range of motion of the hip, knee and ankle joints in male subjects 30–40 years of age. Acta Orthop Scand 1982;53:205–208.
49. Roach KE, Miles TP: Normal hip and knee active range of motion: The relationship to age. Phys Ther 1991;71:656–665.

50. Rothstein JM, Echternach JL: Primer on Measurement: An Introductory Guide to Measurement Issues. Alexandria, Va, American Physical Therapy Association, 1993.

51. Silverman S, Constine L, Harvey W, Grahame R: Survey of joint mobility and in vivo skin elasticity in London schoolchildren. Ann Rheum Dis 1975;34:177–180.

52. Simoneau CC, Hoenig KJ, Lepley JE, Papanek PE: Influence of hip position and gender on active hip internal and external rotation. J Orthop Sports Phys Ther 1998;28:158–164.

53. Smith JR, Walker JM: Knee and elbow range of motion in healthy older individuals. Phys Occup Ther Geriatr 1983;2:31–38.

54. Svenningsen S, Terjesen T, Auflem M, et al.: Hip motion related to age and sex. Acta Orthop Scand 1989;60:97–100.

55. Trott PH, Pearcy MJ, Ruston SA, et al.: Three-dimensional analysis of active cervical motion: The effect of age and gender. Clin Biomech (Bristol, Avon) 1996:11:201–206.

56. van Adrichem JAM, van der Korst JK: Assessment of the flexibility of the lumbar spine. Scand J Rheumatol 1973;2:87–91.

57. Walker JM, Sue D, Miles-Elkousy N, et al.: Active mobility of the extremities in older subjects. Phys Ther 1984;64:919–923.

58. Watanabe H, Ogata K, Amano T, Okabe TL: The range of joint motions of the extremities in healthy Japanese people: The difference according to age. Cited in Walker, JM: Musculoskeletal development: A review. Phys Ther 1991:71:878.

59. Waugh KG, Minkel JL, Parker R, Coon VA: Measurement of selected hip, knee, and ankle joint motions in newborns. Phys Ther 1983;63:1616–1621.

60. Wynne-Davis R: Acetabular dysplasia and familiar joint laxity: Two etiological factors in congenital dislocation of the hip. J Bone Joint Surg (Br) 1970;52:704–716.

61. Youdas JW, Garrett TR, Suman VJ, et al.: Normal range of motion of the cervical spine: An initial goniometric study. Phys Ther 1992;72:770–780.

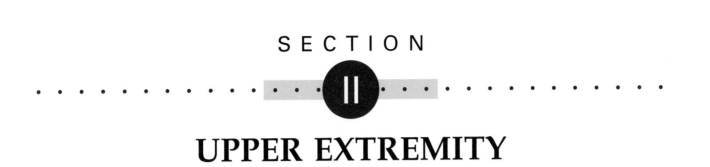

SECTION

II

UPPER EXTREMITY

3

MEASUREMENT of RANGE of MOTION of the SHOULDER

ANATOMY AND OSTEOKINEMATICS

The shoulder joint complex is composed of three synovial joints (glenohumeral, acromioclavicular, and sternoclavicular), along with the articulation between the ventral surface of the scapula and the dorsal thorax (herein referred to as the scapulothoracic articulation). Although other structures, such as the "subacromial joint,"[16] are occasionally included as part of the shoulder joint complex, a more conservative, four-articulation description of the complex is used in this text.[10]

Of the three synovial joints that are part of the shoulder joint complex, two, the acromioclavicular and the sternoclavicular, are classified as plane joints, and the glenohumeral joint is classified as a ball-and-socket joint.[3] Motion at each of the four articulations making up the shoulder complex occurs in all three of the cardinal planes. At the glenohumeral joint, motion is produced by gliding, rolling, and spinning of the convex head of the humerus against the shallow, concave surface of the glenoid fossa of the scapula.

Motions of the shoulder joint complex include flexion, extension, abduction, adduction, medial rotation, and lateral rotation. Many motions of the shoulder joint contain component motions occurring at all four articulations composing the shoulder complex. For example, elevation of the arm in the frontal plane (shoulder abduction) or sagittal plane (shoulder flexion) is accomplished by motions occurring at the glenohumeral joint (glenohumeral flexion or abduction), at the sternoclavicular joint (clavicular elevation), at the acromioclavicular joint (clavicular rotation), and at the scapulothoracic articulation (scapular abduction, elevation, and upward rotation). Shoulder elevation is produced by a combination of humeral and scapular motion, which has been described as occurring in varying ratios of glenohumeral to scapulothoracic motion. Although it is widely accepted that the relative contributions of glenohumeral and scapulothoracic movements vary throughout the range of shoulder elevation, the overall ratios of glenohumeral to scapulothoracic motion have been reported from as high as 2:1[9] to as low as 1.25:1,[1] with other ratios reported between those margins.[4, 7] The motion of the scapula is a result of motion occurring at the acromioclavicular and sternoclavicular joints, whereas humeral motion is produced at the glenohumeral joint. Since isolated glenohumeral motion does not occur during normal elevation of the shoulder past the first 30 or so degrees,[9, 15] no attempt is made to measure isolated glenohumeral flexion or abduction. Rather, flexion and abduction are measured as shoulder complex motions, allowing full excursion at all joints involved.

LIMITATIONS OF MOTION: SHOULDER JOINT

Since motions involving elevation of the shoulder are combined motions involving movement at acromioclavicular, glenohumeral, and sternoclavicular joints as well as at the scapulothoracic articulation, shoulder flexion and abduction are limited by anatomical structures located at multiple joints. For example, clavicular elevation, necessary for complete elevation of the shoulder, is limited by tension in the costoclavicular ligament.[3] At the glenohumeral joint, motion is limited primarily by muscular and capsuloligamentous structures. Elevation (flexion or abduction) is limited by tension in the inferior glenohumeral ligament and inferior joint capsule.[12] Extension is limited by the superior and middle glenohumeral ligaments.[16] Glenohumeral rotation is limited by ligamentous structures and by tension in muscles of the rotator cuff, with lateral rotation being limited by tension in the subscapularis muscle; in the anteroinferior joint capsule; and in the coracohumeral, superior and middle glenohumeral, and anterior band of the inferior glenohumeral ligaments.[5, 6, 13, 14] Medial rotation at the glenohumeral joint is limited by tension in the infraspinatus and teres minor muscles, in the posterior joint capsule, and in the posterior band of the inferior glenohumeral ligament.[13, 14] Thus, the normal end-feel for all motions of the shoulder joint complex is firm, as all motions are restricted by capsuloligamentous or musculotendinous structures. Information regarding normal ranges of motion for all motions of the shoulder is found in Appendix C.

TECHNIQUES OF MEASUREMENT: SHOULDER FLEXION/EXTENSION

Shoulder flexion is a composite of motions occurring at multiple joints making up the shoulder complex. Although some texts attempt to isolate the flexion that occurs at the glenohumeral joint and measure that motion alone, because such isolated movement does not occur past the first 30 or so degrees of shoulder flexion in normal motion, no such attempt to isolate glenohumeral motion is presented in this text.

The preferred patient positions for measuring shoulder flexion and extension are supine and prone, respectively, because of the greater stabilization of the spine that occurs in those positions compared with the other positions in which shoulder flexion and extension can be measured. Measurement of shoulder flexion and extension also can be performed with the patient in the standing, sitting, or sidelying positions. The American Academy of Orthopaedic Surgeons (AAOS) advocates measuring shoulder flexion and extension with the patient standing, but states, "If spine and pelvic motion cannot be controlled, external rotation and elevation should be assessed with the patient supine."[8] When shoulder flexion and extension are measured, regardless of the position used, care should be taken to prevent extension of the spine, in the case of shoulder flexion, or flexion of the spine, in the case of shoulder extension, which artificially inflate the resulting measurement and increase measurement error.

TECHNIQUES OF MEASUREMENT: SHOULDER ABDUCTION

As is the case for shoulder flexion, shoulder abduction is a composite movement, and no attempt is made in this text to isolate and measure the glenohumeral component of shoulder abduction. Again because of issues of stabilization in the spine, shoulder abduction is best measured with the patient in a supine position. Other positions for measuring abduction include standing, sitting, and prone, with standing being the position advocated by the AAOS.[8] During any measurement of shoulder abduction, regardless of the position used, care should be taken to prevent lateral flexion of the spine by the patient, as this motion artificially inflates the range of shoulder abduction obtained.

TECHNIQUES OF MEASUREMENT: SHOULDER MEDIAL/LATERAL ROTATION

The AAOS recommends measuring lateral rotation of the shoulder with the patient's shoulder placed in either 0 degrees or 90 degrees of abduction; medial rotation is measured with the shoulder in 90 degrees abduction.[8] Other authors have advocated a slightly abducted position of the shoulder during the measurement of medial/lateral rotation.[11] Since the amount of shoulder abduction used seems to affect the range of shoulder rotation obtained during measurement,[2, 11] a standardized technique for patient positioning should be followed for this, as for all other, goniometric procedures. In this text, shoulder medial and lateral rotation is measured with the patient positioned in 90 degrees of shoulder abduction. However, some patients with shoulder pathology are unable to attain 90 degrees of shoulder abduction, and in such cases alternative positioning may be required. When used, such alternative positioning should be clearly documented.

Shoulder Flexion

Fig. 3–1. Starting position for measurement of shoulder flexion. Bony landmarks for goniometer alignment (lateral aspect of acromion process, lateral midline of thorax, lateral humeral epicondyle) indicated by orange line and dots.

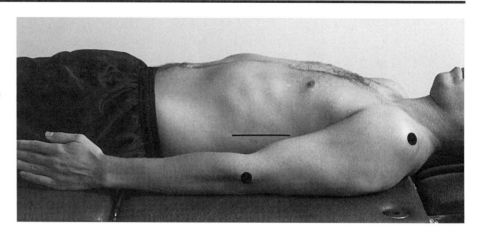

Patient position:	Supine with shoulder in 0 degrees flexion, elbow fully extended, forearm in neutral rotation with palm facing trunk (Fig. 3–1).
Stabilization:	Over anterosuperior aspect of ipsilateral shoulder, proximal to humeral head (Fig. 3–2).
Examiner action:	After instructing patient in motion desired, flex patient's shoulder through available range of motion (ROM) avoiding extension of spine. Return limb to starting position. Performing passive movement provides an estimate of ROM and demonstrates to patient exact motion desired (see Fig. 3–2).
Goniometer alignment:	Palpate the following bony landmarks (shown in Fig. 3–1) and align goniometer accordingly (Fig. 3–3).
Stationary arm:	Lateral midline of thorax.
Axis:	Midpoint of lateral aspect of acromion process.
Moving arm:	Lateral midline of humerus toward lateral humeral epicondyle.
	Read scale of goniometer.

Fig. 3–2. End of shoulder flexion ROM, showing proper hand placement for stabilizing thorax and flexing shoulder. Bony landmarks for goniometer alignment (lateral midline of thorax, lateral humeral epicondyle) indicated by orange line and dot.

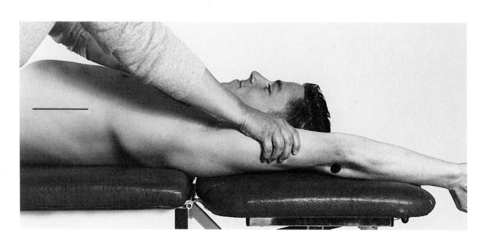

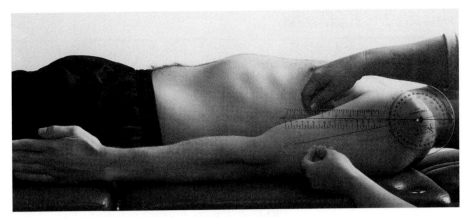

Fig. 3–3. Starting position for measurement of shoulder flexion, demonstrating proper initial alignment of goniometer.

Patient/Examiner action:	Perform passive, or have patient perform active, shoulder flexion (Fig. 3–4).
Confirmation of alignment:	Repalpate landmarks and confirm proper goniometric alignment at end of ROM, correcting alignment as necessary (see Note). Read scale of goniometer (Fig. 3–4).
Documentation:	Record patient's ROM.
Note:	No extension of spine should be allowed during measurement of shoulder flexion, to prevent artificial inflation of ROM measurements.
Alternative patient position:	Seated or sidelying; goniometer alignment remains same. Owing to decreased ability to stabilize trunk in these positions, great care must be taken to assure that stationary arm of goniometer remains aligned with lateral midline of thorax and that extension of spine does not occur. Failure to exercise such care will result in errors of measurement.

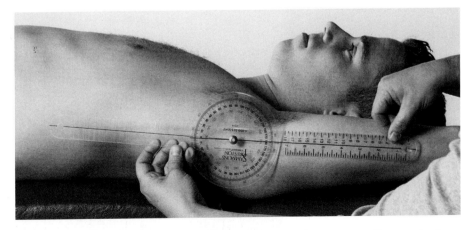

Fig. 3–4. End of shoulder flexion ROM, demonstrating proper alignment of goniometer at end of range.

Shoulder Extension

Fig. 3–5. Starting position for measurement of shoulder extension. Bony landmarks for goniometer alignment (lateral aspect of acromion process, lateral midline of thorax, lateral humeral epicondyle) indicated by orange line and dots.

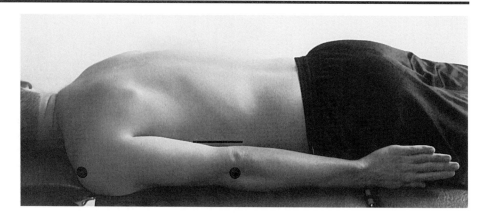

Patient position:	Prone with shoulder in 0 degrees flexion, elbow fully extended, forearm in neutral rotation with palm facing trunk (Fig. 3–5).
Stabilization:	Over posterosuperior aspect of ipsilateral shoulder, proximal to humeral head (Fig. 3–6).
Examiner action:	After instructing patient in motion desired, extend patient's shoulder through available ROM, avoiding rotation of trunk. Return limb to starting position. Performing passive movement provides an estimate of ROM and demonstrates to patient exact motion desired (see Fig. 3–6).
Goniometer alignment:	Palpate the following bony landmarks (shown in Fig. 3–5) and align goniometer accordingly (Fig. 3–7).
Stationary arm:	Lateral midline of thorax.
Axis:	Midpoint of lateral aspect of acromion process.
Moving arm:	Lateral midline of humerus toward lateral humeral epicondyle.

Read scale of goniometer.

Fig. 3–6. End of shoulder extension ROM, showing proper hand placement for stabilizing thorax and extending shoulder. Bony landmarks for goniometer alignment (lateral aspect of acromion process, lateral midline of thorax, lateral humeral epicondyle) indicated by orange line and dots.

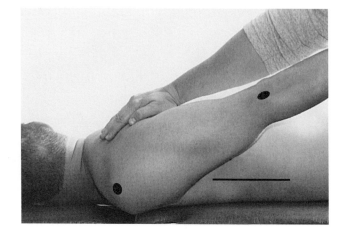

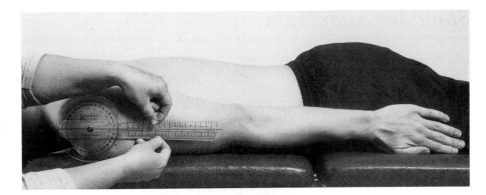

Fig. 3–7. Starting position for measurement of shoulder extension, demonstrating proper initial alignment of goniometer.

Patient/Examiner action: Perform passive, or have patient perform active, shoulder extension (Fig. 3–8).

Confirmation of alignment: Repalpate landmarks and confirm proper goniometric alignment at end of ROM, correcting alignment as necessary (see Note). Read scale of goniometer (Fig. 3–8).

Documentation: Record patient's ROM.

Note: No rotation of spine should be allowed during measurement of shoulder extension, to prevent artificial inflation of ROM measurements.

Alternative patient position: Seated or sidelying; goniometer alignment remains same. Owing to decreased ability to stabilize trunk in these positions, great care must be taken to assure that stationary arm of goniometer remains aligned with lateral midline of thorax and that flexion of spine does not occur. Failure to exercise such care will result in errors of measurement.

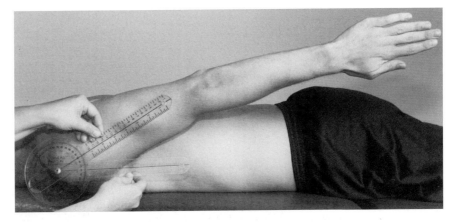

Fig. 3–8. End of shoulder extension ROM, demonstrating proper alignment of goniometer at end of range.

Shoulder Abduction

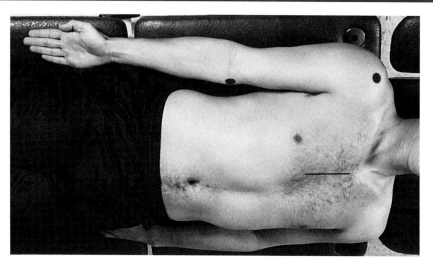

Fig. 3–9. Starting position for measurement of shoulder abduction with patient in the supine position. Bony landmarks for goniometer alignment (anterior aspect of acromion process, midline of sternum, medial humeral epicondyle) indicated by orange line and dots.

Patient position: Supine with arm at side, upper extremity in anatomical position (Fig. 3–9).

Stabilization: Over superior aspect of ipsilateral shoulder, proximal to humeral head (Fig. 3–10).

Examiner action: After instructing patient in motion desired, abduct patient's shoulder through available ROM, avoiding lateral trunk flexion. Return limb to starting position. Performing passive movement provides an estimate of the ROM and demonstrates to patient exact motion desired (see Fig. 3–10).

Fig. 3–10. End of shoulder abduction ROM, showing proper hand placement for stabilizing thorax and abducting shoulder. Bony landmarks for goniometer alignment (midline of sternum, medial humeral epicondyle) indicated by orange line and dot.

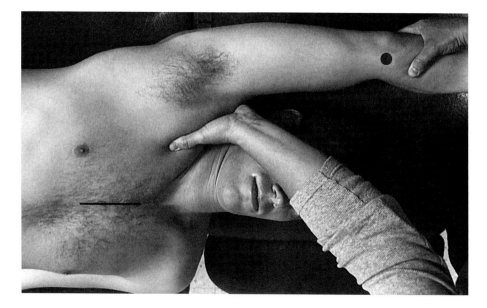

Fig. 3–11. Starting position for measurement of shoulder abduction, demonstrating proper initial alignment of goniometer.

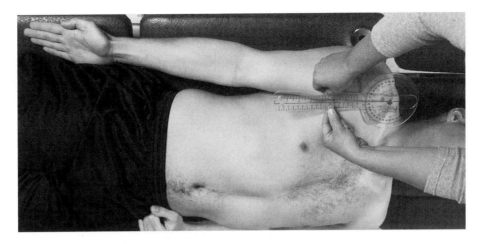

Goniometer alignment:	Palpate the following bony landmarks (shown in Fig. 3–9) and align goniometer accordingly (Fig. 3–11).
Stationary arm:	Parallel to sternum.
Axis:	Anterior aspect of acromion process.
Moving arm:	Anterior midline of humerus toward medial humeral epicondyle.

Read scale of goniometer.

Patient/Examiner action:	Perform passive, or have patient perform active, shoulder abduction (Fig. 3–12).
Confirmation of alignment:	Repalpate landmarks and confirm proper goniometric alignment at end of ROM, correcting alignment as necessary (see Note). Read scale of goniometer (Fig. 3–12).
Documentation:	Record patient's ROM.
Note:	No lateral flexion of spine should be allowed during measurement of shoulder abduction to prevent artificial inflation of ROM measurements.
Alternative patient position:	Seated; goniometer is aligned as follows: Stationary arm parallel to spinous process of vertebral column, axis with posterior aspect of acromion, and moving arm along posterior midline of humerus toward lateral humeral epicondyle.

Fig. 3–12. End of shoulder abduction ROM, demonstrating proper alignment of goniometer at end of range.

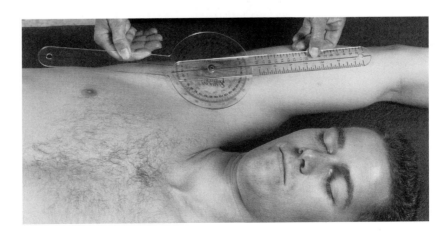

Shoulder Adduction

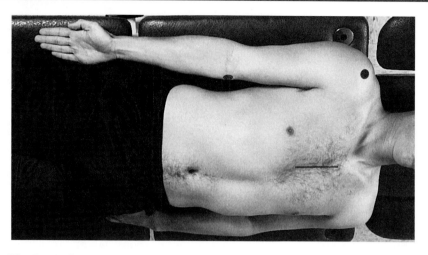

Fig. 3–13. Starting position for measurement of shoulder adduction with patient in the supine position. Bony landmarks for goniometer alignment (anterior aspect of acromion process, midline of sternum, medial humeral epicondyle) indicated by orange line and dots.

Patient position:	Supine with arm at side, upper extremity in anatomical position (Fig. 3–13).
Stabilization:	Over superior aspect of ipsilateral shoulder, proximal to humeral head (Fig. 3–14).
Examiner action:	After instructing patient in motion desired, adduct patient's shoulder through available ROM, avoiding lateral trunk flexion. Return limb to starting position. Performing passive movement provides an estimate of ROM and demonstrates to patient exact motion desired (see Fig. 3–14).

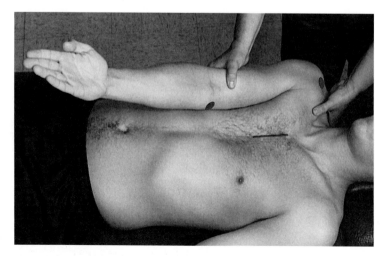

Fig. 3–14. End of shoulder adduction ROM, showing proper hand placement for stabilizing thorax and adducting shoulder. Bony landmarks for goniometer alignment (anterior aspect of acromion process, midline of sternum, medial humeral epicondyle) indicated by orange line and dots.

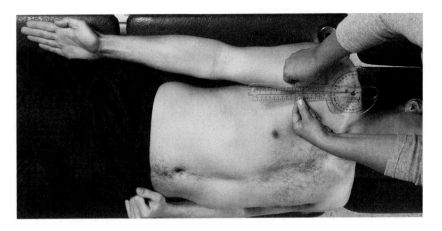

Fig. 3–15. Starting position for measurement of shoulder adduction, demonstrating proper initial alignment of goniometer.

Goniometer alignment:	Palpate the following bony landmarks (shown in Fig. 3–13) and align goniometer accordingly (Fig. 3–15).
Stationary arm:	Parallel to sternum.
Axis:	Anterior aspect of acromion process.
Moving arm:	Anterior midline of humerus in line with medial humeral epicondyle.
	Read scale of goniometer.
Patient/Examiner action:	Perform passive, or have patient perform active, shoulder adduction (Fig. 3–16).
Confirmation of alignment:	Repalpate landmarks and confirm proper goniometric alignment at end of ROM, correcting alignment as necessary (see Note). Read scale of goniometer (Fig. 3–16).
Documentation:	Record patient's ROM.
Note:	No lateral flexion of spine should be allowed during measurement of shoulder adduction to prevent artificial inflation of ROM measurements.
Alternative patient position:	Seated; goniometer alignment remains the same.

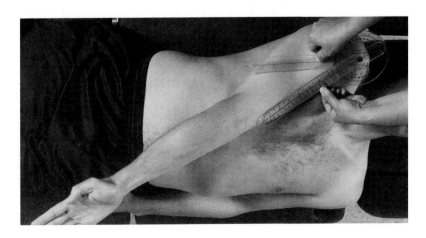

Fig. 3–16. End of shoulder adduction ROM, demonstrating proper alignment of goniometer at end of range.

Shoulder Lateral Rotation

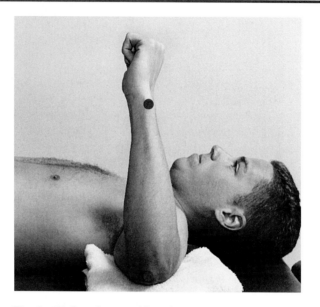

Fig. 3–17. Starting position for measurement of shoulder lateral rotation. Landmarks for goniometer alignment (olecranon and styloid processes of ulna) indicated by orange dots.

Patient position:	Supine with shoulder abducted to 90 degrees, elbow flexed to 90 degrees, forearm pronated, folded towel under humerus (Fig. 3–17).
Stabilization:	Place heel of hand over superior aspect of ipsilateral shoulder, proximal to humeral head; fingers over ipsilateral scapula (Fig. 3–18).
Examiner action:	After instructing patient in motion desired, laterally rotate patient's shoulder through available ROM, making sure the scapula does not lift off the table. Return limb to starting position. Performing passive movement provides an estimate of ROM and demonstrates to patient exact motion desired (see Fig. 3–18).

Fig. 3–18. End of shoulder lateral rotation ROM, showing proper hand placement for stabilizing thorax and laterally rotating shoulder. Landmarks for goniometer alignment (olecranon and styloid processes of ulna) indicated by orange dots.

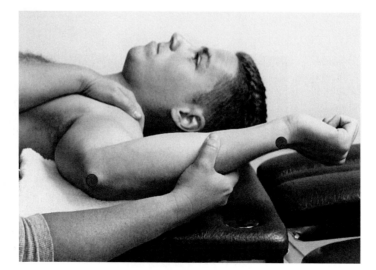

Fig. 3–19. Starting position for measurement of shoulder lateral rotation, demonstrating proper initial alignment of goniometer.

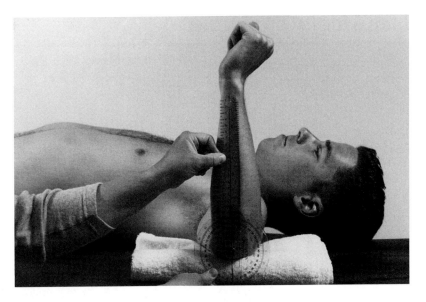

Goniometer alignment:	Palpate the following bony landmarks (shown in Fig. 3–17) and align goniometer accordingly (Fig. 3–19).
Stationary arm:	Perpendicular to floor.
Axis:	Olecranon process of ulna.
Moving arm:	Ulnar border of forearm toward ulnar styloid process.
	Read scale of goniometer.
Patient/Examiner action:	Perform passive, or have patient perform active, lateral rotation of the shoulder, stopping at the point of elevation of the scapula off the table (Fig. 3–20).
Confirmation of alignment:	Repalpate landmarks and confirm proper goniometer alignment at end of ROM, correcting alignment as necessary. Read scale of goniometer (Fig. 3–20).
Documentation:	Record patient's ROM.
Alternative patient position:	Prone; goniometer alignment remains same. Measurement also may be taken with shoulder positioned in less abduction. If such positioning is used, amount of abduction of shoulder must be documented.

Fig. 3–20. End of shoulder lateral rotation ROM, demonstrating proper alignment of goniometer at end of range.

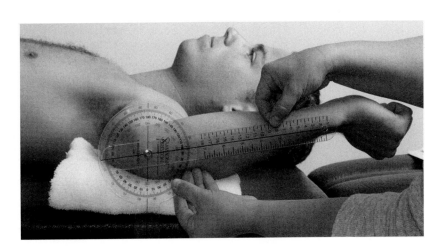

Shoulder Medial Rotation

Fig. 3–21. Starting position for measurement of shoulder medial rotation. Landmarks for goniometer alignment (olecranon and styloid processes of ulna) indicated by orange dots.

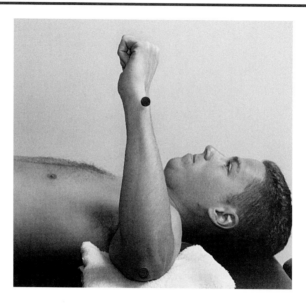

Patient position:	Supine with shoulder abducted to 90 degrees, elbow flexed to 90 degrees, forearm pronated, folded towel under humerus (Fig. 3–21).
Stabilization:	Place heel of hand over superior aspect of ipsilateral shoulder, proximal to humeral head, and fingers over ipsilateral scapula (Fig. 3–22).
Examiner action:	After instructing patient in motion desired, medially rotate patient's shoulder through available ROM, making sure the scapula does not lift off the table. Return limb to starting position. Performing passive movement provides an estimate of ROM and demonstrates to patient exact motion desired (see Fig 3–22).

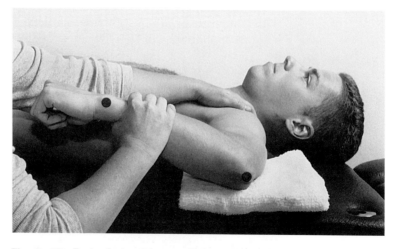

Fig. 3–22. End of shoulder medial rotation ROM, showing proper hand placement for stabilizing thorax and medially rotating shoulder. Landmarks for goniometer alignment (olecranon and styloid processes of ulna) indicated by orange dots.

Fig. 3–23. Starting position for measurement of shoulder medial rotation, demonstrating proper initial alignment of goniometer.

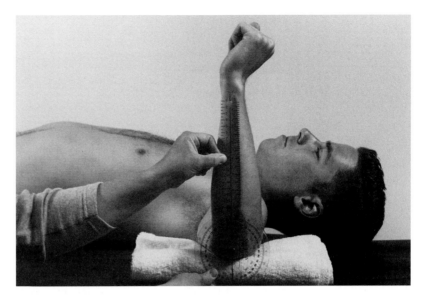

Goniometer alignment:	Palpate the following bony landmarks (shown in Fig. 3–21) and align goniometer accordingly (Fig. 3–23).
Stationary arm:	Perpendicular to floor.
Axis:	Olecranon process of ulna.
Moving arm:	Ulnar border of forearm toward ulnar styloid process.
	Read scale of goniometer.
Patient/Examiner action:	Perform passive, or have patient perform active, medial rotation of the shoulder, stopping at the point of elevation of the scapula off the table (Fig. 3–24).
Confirmation of alignment:	Repalpate landmarks and confirm proper goniometer alignment at end of ROM, correcting alignment as necessary. Read scale of goniometer (Fig. 3–24).
Documentation:	Record patient's ROM.
Alternative patient position:	Prone; goniometer alignment remains same. Measurement also may be taken with shoulder positioned in less abduction. If such positioning is used, amount of abduction of shoulder must be documented.

Fig. 3–24. End of shoulder medial rotation ROM, demonstrating proper alignment of goniometer at end of range.

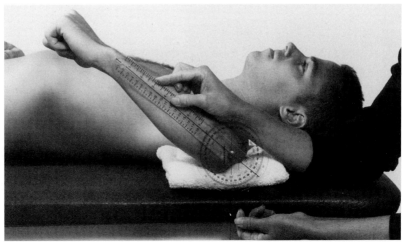

References

1. Bagg SD, Forrest WJ: A biomechanical analysis of scapular rotation during arm abduction in the scapular plane. Am J Phys Med Rehabil 1988;67:238–245.
2. Boone DC, Azen SP: Normal range of motion of joints in male subjects. J Bone Joint Surg 1979;61:756–759.
3. Clemente CD: Gray's Anatomy of the Human Body, 13th ed. Philadelphia, Lea & Febiger, 1985.
4. Doody SG, Freedman L, Waterland JC: Shoulder movements during abduction in the scapular plane. Arch Phys Med Rehabil 1970;51:595–604.
5. Edelson JG, Taitz C, Grishkan A: The coracohumeral ligament: Anatomy of a substantial but neglected structure. J Bone Joint Surg [Br] 1991;73-B:150–153.
6. Ferrari DA: Capsular ligaments of the shoulder: Anatomical and functional study of the anterior superior capsule. Am J Sports Med 1990;18:20–24.
7. Freedman L, Murro RR: Abduction of the arm in the scapular plane: Scapular and glenohumeral movements. J Bone Joint Surg 1966;48A:1503–1510.
8. Greene WB, Heckman JD: The Clinical Measurement of Joint Motion. Rosemont, Ill, American Academy of Orthopaedic Surgeons, 1994.
9. Inman VT, Saunders JB, Abbott LC: Observations of the function of the shoulder joint. J Bone Joint Surg 1944;26:1–30.
10. Kent BE: Functional anatomy of the shoulder complex: A review. J Am Phys Ther Assoc 1971:51;867–887.
11. MacDermid JC, Chesworth BM, Patterson S, Roth JH: Intratester and intertester reliability of goniometric measurement of passive lateral shoulder rotation. J Hand Ther 1999;12:187–192.
12. Morrey BF, An K: Biomechanics of the shoulder. In Rockwood CA, Matsen FA (eds): The Shoulder, vol 1. Philadelphia, WB Saunders, 1990.
13. O'Brien SJ, Neves MC, Arnoczky SP, et al.: The anatomy and histology of the inferior glenohumeral ligament complex of the shoulder. Am J Sports Med 1990; 18:449–456.
14. Ovesen J, Nielsen S: Stability of the shoulder joint: Cadaver study of stabilizing structures. Acta Orthop Scand 1985:56;149–151.
15. Poppen NK, Walker PS: Normal and abnormal motion of the shoulder. J Bone Joint Surg 1976;58-A:195–201.
16. Smith LK, Weiss EL, Lehmkuhl LD: Brunnstrom's Clinical Kinesiology, 5th ed. Philadelphia, F.A. Davis, 1996.

4

MEASUREMENT of RANGE of MOTION of the ELBOW and FOREARM

ELBOW JOINT

ANATOMY AND OSTEOKINEMATICS

Within the elbow joint capsule are three articulations, two that make up the elbow joint complex and one that is part of the forearm complex. The humeroradial and humeroulnar joints make up the joint complex known as the elbow. The humeroradial joint consists of the articulation between the convex capitulum of the distal humerus and the slightly concave proximal surface of the radial head. The articulation between the trochlea of the humerus and the trochlear notch of the ulna forms the humeroulnar joint. Both joints are located within a single joint capsule that is also shared by the proximal radioulnar joint.[2]

Although the elbow joint traditionally has been classified as a hinge joint, the hinge component occurs at the humeroulnar articulation, while the humeroradial joint is classified as a plane joint.[2] Motions available at the elbow are flexion and extension, which occur in a plane oriented slightly oblique to the sagittal plane, owing to the angulation of the trochlea of the humerus.[5] The axis of rotation for flexion and extension of the elbow is centered on the trochlea except at the extremes of flexion and extension, when the axis moves anteriorly and posteriorly, respectively.[7]

LIMITATIONS OF MOTION: ELBOW JOINT

Elbow flexion range of motion (ROM) is limited by soft tissue approximation between the structures of the anterior arm and the forearm, particularly during active flexion of the joint, or in the presence of sufficient arm and forearm muscle mass during passive flexion. Such soft tissue approximation produces a soft end-feel at the limits of elbow flexion range of motion. In cases where little muscle is present, elbow flexion may be limited by bony contact between the coronoid process of the ulna and the coronoid fossa of the humerus. In this case, the end-feel for elbow flexion would be bony. Elbow extension range of motion is limited by contact of the olecranon process of the ulna with the olecranon fossa of the humerus, which produces a hard end-feel at the limits of elbow extension.[5, 8] Information regarding normal range of motion for the elbow is located in Appendix C.

TECHNIQUES OF MEASUREMENT: ELBOW FLEXION/EXTENSION

Elbow flexion and extension may be measured with the patient in the upright (standing or sitting), supine, or sidelying positions. Because of the greater stability provided to the humerus, the supine position is preferred for measurement of range of motion. The American Academy of Orthopaedic Surgeons[4] recommends that the patient be in the upright position with the shoulder flexed to 90 degrees when measurements of elbow flexion and extension are taken. In patients with tightness of the long head of the triceps, such positioning may limit flexion of the elbow. Therefore, motions of the elbow joint should be measured with the shoulder maintained in the anatomical position.

FOREARM JOINTS

ANATOMY AND OSTEOKINEMATICS

Gray's Anatomy[2] describes three joints interconnecting the bones of the forearm: the proximal and distal radioulnar joints and the middle radioulnar union. The proximal radioulnar joint is located anatomically within the capsule of the elbow joint and consists of the articulation between the rim of the radial head and the fibro-osseous ring formed by the annular ligament and the radial notch of the ulna. The distal radioulnar joint is located anatomically at the wrist, although inside a separate joint capsule. This joint is formed by the articulation between the concave ulnar notch of the radius and the convex head of the ulna. Since the middle radioulnar union is classified as a syndesmosis, which, by definition, allows only limited motion at best, no further discussion of this component of the forearm is presented. Both the proximal and the distal radioulnar joints are classified as pivot joints, allowing rotation of the radius around the ulna in a transverse plane, thus producing the motions of pronation and supination of the forearm.

LIMITATIONS OF MOTION: FOREARM JOINTS

Supination of the forearm is limited by tension in ligamentous structures (anterior radioulnar ligament and oblique cord),[6] resulting in a firm end-feel for forearm supination. Limitation of forearm pronation is secondary to contact between the bones of the forearm (radius crossing over ulna) and to tension in the medial collateral ligament of the elbow.[3] Thus, the end-feel for forearm pronation is typically hard. Information regarding normal ranges of motion for forearm supination and pronation is located in Appendix C.

TECHNIQUES OF MEASUREMENT: FOREARM PRONATION/SUPINATION

Forearm pronation and supination typically are measured with the elbow positioned in 90 degrees of flexion and the shoulder fully adducted. In this position, the patient is prevented from substituting rotation of the shoulder for rotation of the forearm, and pronation and supination of the forearm can be easily visualized. Some authors recommend measuring forearm rotation with a rod or rod-like object held in the hand,[4] but errors of measurement have been shown to result from the use of such methods.[1] Therefore, goniometric techniques involving measurement of forearm rotation in this text will use the distal forearm rather than a hand-held object as the reference for the moving arm of the goniometer.

Elbow Flexion

Fig. 4–1. Starting position for measurement of elbow flexion. Bony landmarks for goniometer alignment (lateral aspect of acromion process, lateral humeral epicondyle, radial styloid process) indicated by orange dots.

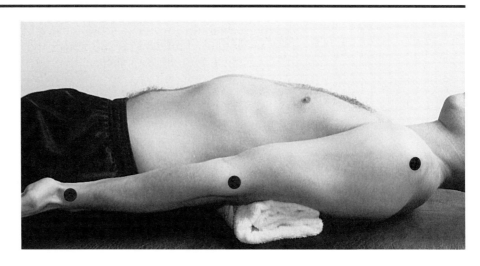

Patient position: Supine with upper extremity in anatomical position (see Note), folded towel under humerus, proximal to humeral condyles (Fig. 4–1).

Stabilization: Over posterior aspect of proximal humerus (Fig. 4–2).

Examiner action: After instructing patient in motion desired, flex patient's elbow through available ROM. Return limb to starting position. Performing passive movement provides an estimate of ROM and demonstrates to patient exact motion desired (see Fig. 4–2).

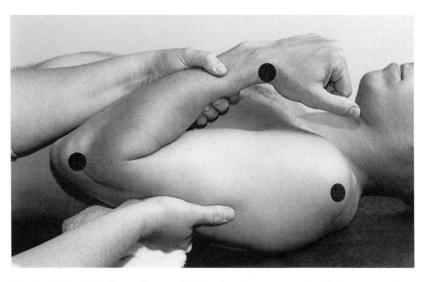

Fig. 4–2. End of elbow flexion ROM, showing proper hand placement for stabilizing humerus and flexing elbow. Bony landmarks for goniometer alignment (lateral aspect of acromion process, lateral humeral epicondyle, radial styloid process) indicated by orange dots.

Fig. 4–3. Starting position for measurement of elbow flexion, demonstrating proper initial alignment of goniometer.

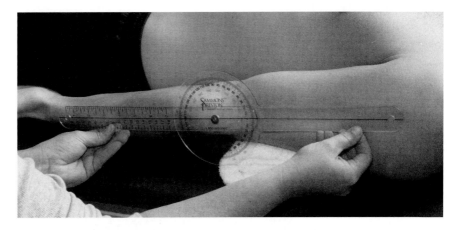

Goniometer alignment:	Palpate the following bony landmarks (shown in Fig. 4–1) and align goniometer accordingly (Fig. 4–3).
Stationary arm:	Lateral midline of humerus toward acromion process.
Axis:	Lateral epicondyle of humerus.
Moving arm:	Lateral midline of radius toward radial styloid process (see Note).
	Read scale of goniometer.
Patient/Examiner action:	Perform passive, or have patient perform active, elbow flexion (Fig. 4–4).
Confirmation of alignment:	Repalpate landmarks and confirm proper goniometric alignment at end of ROM, correcting alignment as necessary. Read scale of goniometer (Fig. 4–4).
Documentation:	Record patient's ROM.
Note:	Patient's forearm should be completely supinated at beginning of ROM, or beginning reading of goniometer will be inaccurate and make patient appear to lack full elbow extension.
Alternative patient position:	Seated or sidelying; towel not needed; goniometer alignment remains same. Stability of humerus decreased in these positions; thus, extra care must be taken to manually stabilize humerus.

Fig. 4–4. End of elbow flexion ROM, demonstrating proper alignment of goniometer at end of range.

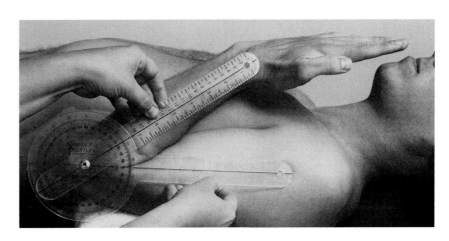

Elbow Extension

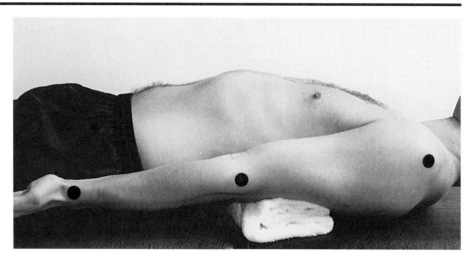

Fig. 4–5. Starting position for measurement of elbow extension. Bony landmarks for goniometer alignment (lateral aspect of acromion process, lateral humeral epicondyle, radial styloid process) indicated by orange dots.

Patient position: Supine with upper extremity in anatomical position (see Note), elbow extended as far as possible, folded towel under distal humerus, proximal to humeral condyles (Fig. 4–5).

Stabilization: None needed.

Examiner action: Determine if elbow is extended as far as possible by either: a) asking patient to straighten elbow as far as possible (if measuring active ROM); or, b) providing pressure across the elbow in the direction of extension (if measuring passive ROM) (Fig. 4–6).

Fig. 4–6. End of elbow extension ROM, showing proper hand placement for stabilizing humerus and extending elbow. Bony landmarks for goniometer alignment (lateral aspect of acromion process, lateral humeral epicondyle, radial styloid process) indicated by orange dots.

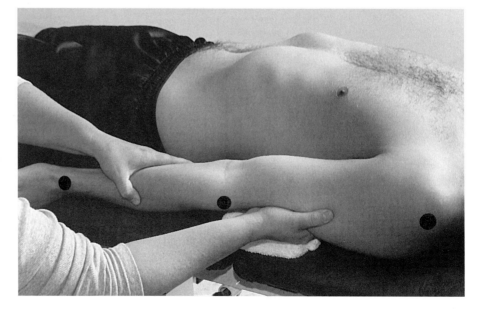

Fig. 4–7. Goniometer alignment for measurement of elbow extension.

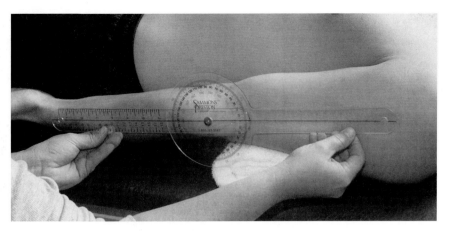

Goniometer alignment:	Palpate the following bony landmarks (shown in Fig. 4–5) and align goniometer accordingly (Fig. 4–7).
Stationary arm:	Lateral midline of humerus toward acromion process.
Axis:	Lateral epicondyle of humerus.
Moving arm:	Lateral midline of radius toward radial styloid process (see Note).
	Read scale of goniometer (Fig. 4–7).
Documentation:	Record patient's amount of elbow extension.
Note:	Patient's forearm should be completely supinated at beginning of ROM, or beginning reading of goniometer will be inaccurate and make patient appear to lack full elbow extension.
Alternative patient position:	Seated or sidelying; towel not needed; goniometer alignment remains same.

Forearm Supination

Fig. 4–8. Starting position for measurement of forearm supination. Bony landmarks for goniometer alignment (anterior midline of humerus and ulnar styloid process) indicated by orange line and dot.

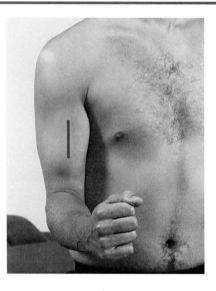

Patient position:	Seated or standing with shoulder completely adducted, elbow flexed to 90 degrees, forearm in neutral rotation (Fig. 4–8).
Stabilization:	Over lateral aspect of distal humerus, maintaining 0 degrees shoulder adduction (Fig. 4–9).
Examiner action:	After instructing patient in motion desired, supinate patient's forearm through available ROM, avoiding lateral rotation of shoulder or shoulder adduction past 0 degrees (see Note). Return limb to starting position. Performing passive movement provides an estimate of ROM and demonstrates to patient exact motion desired (see Fig. 4–9).
Goniometer alignment:	Palpate the following bony landmarks (shown in Fig. 4–8) and align goniometer accordingly (Fig. 4–10).
Stationary arm:	Parallel with anterior midline of humerus.
Axis:	On volar surface of wrist, in line with styloid process of ulna.*
Moving arm:	Volar surface of wrist, at level of ulnar styloid process.

Read scale of goniometer.

Fig. 4–9. End of forearm supination ROM, showing proper hand placement for stabilizing humerus against thorax and supinating forearm. Bony landmark for goniometer alignment (anterior midline of humerus) indicated by orange line.

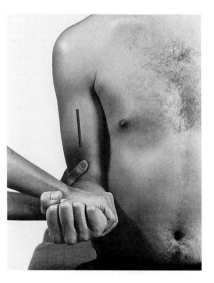

Fig. 4–10. Starting position for measurement of forearm supination, demonstrating proper initial alignment of goniometer.

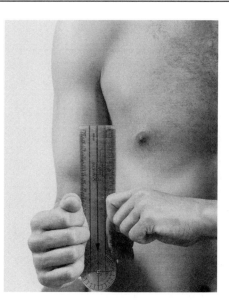

Patient/Examiner action:	Perform passive supination, or have patient perform active forearm supination (Fig. 4–11).
Confirmation of alignment:	Repalpate landmarks and confirm proper goniometric alignment at end of ROM, correcting alignment as necessary (see Note). Read scale of goniometer (Fig. 4–11).
Documentation:	Record patient's ROM.
Note:	No adduction or lateral rotation of shoulder should be allowed during measurement of forearm supination, to prevent artificial inflation of ROM measurements.

---

* Alignment of goniometer's axis opposite ulnar styloid process is possible at start of measurement of forearm supination (see Fig. 4–10). By end of supination ROM, axis of goniometer will have moved to a position superior and medial to ulnar styloid (see Fig. 4–11). Alignment of arms, and not axis, of goniometer is most critical element in this measurement.

Fig. 4–11. End of forearm supination ROM, demonstrating proper alignment of goniometer at end of range.

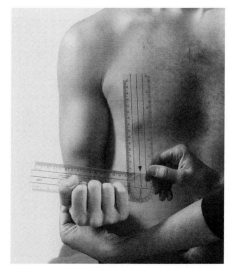

Forearm Pronation

Fig. 4–12. Starting position for measurement of forearm pronation. Bony landmarks for goniometer alignment (anterior midline of humerus and ulnar styloid process) indicated by orange line and dot.

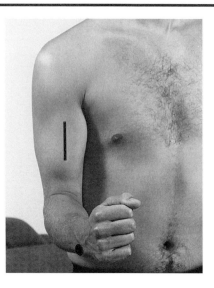

Patient position:	Seated or standing with shoulder completely adducted, elbow flexed to 90 degrees, forearm in neutral rotation (Fig. 4–12).
Stabilization:	Over lateral aspect of distal humerus, maintaining shoulder adduction (Fig. 4–13).
Examiner action:	After instructing patient in motion desired, pronate patient's forearm through available ROM, avoiding shoulder abduction and medial rotation (see Note). Return limb to starting position. Performing passive movement provides an estimate of ROM and demonstrates to patient exact motion desired (see Fig. 4–13).
Goniometer alignment:	Palpate the following bony landmarks (shown in Fig. 4–12) and align goniometer accordingly (Fig. 4–14).
Stationary arm:	Parallel with anterior midline of humerus.
Axis:	In line with, and just proximal to, styloid process of ulna.*
Moving arm:	Dorsum of forearm, just proximal to ulnar styloid process.

Read scale of goniometer.

Fig. 4–13. End of forearm pronation ROM, showing proper hand placement for stabilizing humerus against thorax and pronating forearm. Bony landmark for goniometer alignment (anterior midline of humerus) indicated by orange line.

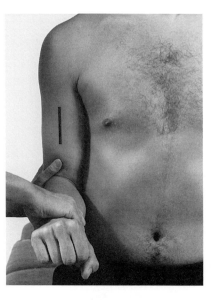

Fig. 4–14. Starting position for measurement of forearm pronation, demonstrating proper initial alignment of goniometer.

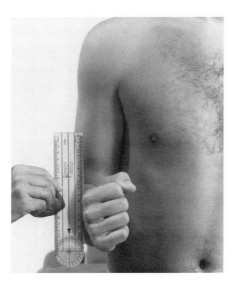

Patient/Examiner action:	Perform passive forearm pronation, or have patient perform active forearm pronation (Fig. 4–15).
Confirmation of alignment:	Repalpate landmarks and confirm proper goniometric alignment at end of ROM, correcting alignment as necessary (see Note). Read scale of goniometer (Fig. 4–15).
Documentation:	Record patient's ROM.
Note:	No abduction or medial rotation of shoulder should be allowed during measurement of forearm pronation, to prevent artificial inflation of ROM measurements.

---

* Alignmen of goniometer's axis with ulnar styloid process is possible at start of measurement of forearm pronation (see Fig. 4–14). By end of pronation ROM, axis of goniometer will have moved to a position superior and lateral to ulnar styloid (see Fig. 4–15). Alignment of arms, and not axis, of goniometer is most critical element in this measurement.

Fig. 4–15. End of forearm pronation ROM, demonstrating proper alignment of goniometer at end of range.

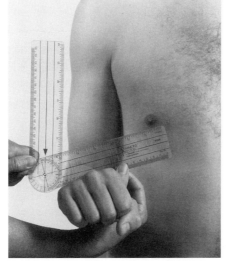

References

1. Amis AA, Miller JH: The elbow. Clin Rheum Dis 1982;8:571–594.
2. Clemente CD (ed): Gray's Anatomy of the Human Body. Philadelphia, Lea & Febiger, 1985.
3. Hotchkiss RN, Weiland AJ: Valgus stability of the elbow. J Orthop Res 1987;5:372–377.
4. Greene WB, Heckman JD: The Clinical Measurement of Joint Motion. Rosemont, Ill, American Academy of Orthopaedic Surgeons, 1994.
5. Kapandji IA: The Physiology of the Joints, vol. 1, Upper Limb, 5th ed. New York, Churchill Livingstone, 1982.
6. Levangie PK, Norkin CC: Joint Structure and Function: A Comprehensive Analysis, 3rd ed. Philadelphia, F.A. Davis, 2001.
7. London JT: Kinematics of the elbow. J Bone Joint Surg 1981;63A:529–535.
8. Smith LK, Weiss EL, Lehmkuhl LD: Brunnstrom's Clinical Kinesiology, 5th ed. Philadelphia, F.A. Davis, 1996.

MEASUREMENT of RANGE of MOTION of the WRIST and HAND

WRIST JOINT

ANATOMY AND OSTEOKINEMATICS

Although *Gray's Anatomy* designates the radiocarpal joint as "the wrist joint proper,"[4] other authors describe a wrist joint complex that includes the more distal midcarpal joint as well as the radiocarpal joint.[8] The radiocarpal joint consists of the articulation between the distal end of the radius and the radioulnar disk proximally, and the proximal row of carpal bones distally. The articulation between the proximal and distal rows of carpal bones makes up the midcarpal joint. Movement at both joints is necessary to achieve the full range of motion (ROM) of the wrist, which has been classified as a condyloid joint.[2] Motions present at the wrist include flexion, extension, abduction (radial deviation), and adduction (ulnar deviation).

LIMITATIONS OF MOTION: WRIST JOINT

With the fingers free to move, limitation of wrist flexion and extension range of motion is produced by passive tension in ligaments crossing the dorsal and volar surfaces of the wrist, respectively. Thus, the end-feel for passive flexion and extension of the wrist is firm. However, if the fingers are not free to move and are flexed, the position of the fingers will limit wrist flexion secondary to passive tension in the extrinsic finger extensors. Conversely, extension of the fingers will limit wrist extension owing to passive tension in the extrinsic finger flexors. Wrist adduction is limited by ligamentous structures (radial collateral ligament) and is associated with a capsular end-feel, whereas wrist abduction is limited by bony contact between the radial styloid process and and the trapezium, producing a bony end-feel at the limit of wrist abduction.[4, 6, 12] Information regarding normal ranges of motion for all movements of the wrist is found in Appendix C.

TECHNIQUES OF MEASUREMENT: WRIST JOINT

Recommended techniques for measuring flexion and extension of the wrist include positioning the goniometer along the radial, ulnar, and dorsal/volar surfaces of the wrist.[1, 5, 10, 11] In a multicenter study of wrist flexion and extension goniometry, LaStayo and Wheeler[7] compared the reliability of all three positioning techniques and found that the dorsal/volar technique was consistently more reliable than the other two (see Chapter 7 for a full description of this study). Therefore, in this text, the dorsal/volar positioning technique is presented as the technique of choice, with radial positioning used as an alternative technique for measuring wrist flexion and extension. Wrist abduction and adduction are measured using the standard technique of positioning the goniometer over the dorsal surface of the joint.[3, 5, 11]

FIRST CARPOMETACARPAL JOINT

ANATOMY AND OSTEOKINEMATICS

Unlike the carpometacarpal (CMC) joints of the fingers, the CMC joint of the thumb (1st CMC joint) has a high degree of mobility. This joint is classified as a saddle joint and is formed by the articulation between the trapezium and the base of the first metacarpal bone. Motions occurring at the 1st CMC joint include flexion, extension, abduction, adduction, rotation, and opposition. From the anatomical position, CMC flexion and extension occur in a plane parallel to the palm of the hand (frontal plane), whereas abduction and adduction occur in a plane positioned perpendicular to the palm (sagittal plane).[4] Rotation occurs as a result of rotation of the metacarpal around its longitudinal axis during flexion and extension of the 1st CMC joint and is normally not measured clinically. Opposition is a combination of flexion, medial rotation, and abduction of the 1st CMC joint.[4]

LIMITATIONS OF MOTION: FIRST CARPOMETACARPAL JOINT

Motions of the 1st CMC joint are limited by a variety of structures, including soft tissues, ligaments, muscles, and joint capsule. Carpometacarpal joint flexion may be limited by contact between the thenar muscle mass and the soft tissue of the palm, thereby producing a soft end-feel to the motion. When muscle mass of the thenar eminence is not well developed, limitation of CMC joint flexion is caused by tension in the extensor pollicis brevis and abductor pollicis brevis muscles as well as by tension in the dorsal aspect of the CMC joint capsule, causing the end-feel to be firm. Extension of the 1st CMC joint is limited primarily by tension in muscles (adductor pollicis, flexor pollicis brevis, 1st dorsal interosseous, opponens pollicis) as well as by tension in the anterior aspect of the CMC joint capsule, thus producing a firm end-feel to the motion. A firm end-feel also is present at the limits of CMC abduction owing to tension in the adductor pollicis and 1st dorsal interosseous muscles and secondary to stretch of the skin and connective tissue of the web space. Both opposition and adduction of the 1st CMC joint are limited by soft-tissue approximation, the former between the pad of the thumb and the base of the fifth digit, and the latter between the side of the thumb and the tissue overlying the second metacarpal.[3, 6, 11] Information regarding normal ranges of motion for all movements of the 1st CMC joint is found in Appendix C.

TECHNIQUES OF MEASUREMENT: FIRST CARPOMETACARPAL JOINT

A variety of methods to measure motion of the 1st CMC joint have been presented in the literature.[1, 3, 5] Reported norms for range of motion of this joint vary widely (see Appendix C), presumably because of differences in measurement techniques. Much of the variation in technique appears to be due, at least in part, to inconsistent terminology regarding motion of this joint. The majority of techniques used in this text are based on motions of the CMC joint as defined in *Gray's Anatomy*[4] and are similar to those techniques demonstrated in other goniometry texts.[3, 11]

Measurement of 1st CMC joint opposition, as described in other goniometry texts, involves the measurement of motions occurring at the 1st and 5th CMC joints, as well as motion occurring in at least one other joint of the 1st or 5th digits.[3, 11] To avoid measuring motion in any joint other than the 1st CMC joint, the technique described in this text for measuring 1st CMC opposition is one that was modified from two different techniques recommended by the American Academy of Orthopaedic Surgeons (AAOS)[5] and the American Medical Association (AMA).[1] The AAOS technique examines opposition by measuring the linear distance from the tip of the thumb to the base of the 5th metacarpal, stating that "opposition is usually considered complete when the tip of the thumb touches the base of the fifth finger."[5] Although the base (palmar digital crease) of the fifth digit provides a reproducible landmark against which 1st CMC joint opposition can be measured, included in this motion is measurement of metacarpophalangeal (MCP) and interphalangeal (IP) flexion of the thumb, which the AAOS considers part of opposition. The technique for examining opposition recommended by the AMA involves measuring the linear distance from the flexor crease of the thumb IP joint to the distal palmar crease over the 3rd metacarpal, without allowing flexion at the MCP or IP joints of the thumb.[1] While the flexor crease of the thumb IP joint provides a more reproducible landmark than the tip of the thumb, the distal palmar crease runs obliquely across the 3rd metacarpal, allowing a variety of points along which the distal end of the ruler may be placed during measurement (Fig. 5–1). Such a variety of possible placements could lend inconsistency to the results obtained when measuring opposition according to the AMA technique.

In an effort to use a technique that: 1) measures only opposition occurring at the 1st CMC joint; and 2) uses reproducible landmarks for both the proximal and the distal ends of the ruler, a technique that combines the best of the AAOS[5] and AMA[1] techniques is described in this text. The technique described herein examines 1st CMC joint opposition by measuring the linear distance between the flexor crease of the IP joint of the 1st digit (thumb) and

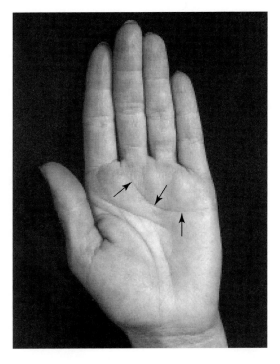

Fig. 5–1. Volar (palmar) surface of hand, demonstrating distal palmar crease (tip of arrows). Note oblique angle at which distal palmar crease crosses 3rd metacarpal.

the palmar digital crease of the 5th digit. Motion of the MCP and IP joints of the 1st and 5th digits is prevented during the measurement. Unfortunately, no standards for normal ROM are as yet available for this technique of measuring opposition.

METACARPOPHALANGEAL AND INTERPHALANGEAL JOINTS

ANATOMY AND OSTEOKINEMATICS

The metacarpophalangeal (MCP) joints of digits 1 through 5 are classified as condyloid joints and are formed by the articulation of the convex head of the metacarpal with the convex base of the proximal phalanx of the corresponding digit. Motions available at these joints are flexion, extension, abduction, and adduction. Some variation exists between the MCP joints of digits 2 through 5 and the 1st MCP joint (in the thumb), causing the range of abduction and adduction of the 1st MCP joint to be severely restricted.[4, 6]

Nine interphalangeal (IP) joints are present in the digits of the hand. Each finger possesses two IP joints: a proximal interphalangeal joint (PIP), which consists of the articulation of the convex head of the proximal phalanx with the concave base of the middle phalanx, and a distal interphalangeal joint (DIP), which consists of the articulation of the convex head of the middle phalanx with the concave base of the distal phalanx. The thumb possesses only a single IP joint, formed by the articulation of the convex head of the proximal phalanx with the concave base of the distal phalanx. Each of the IP joints of the hand is classified as a hinge joint and is thus able to perform the motions of flexion and extension.[4, 6]

LIMITATIONS OF MOTION: METACARPOPHALANGEAL AND INTERPHALANGEAL JOINTS

Flexion of the MCP joints increases in range as one moves from the 1st digit (the thumb) toward the 5th digit, and is restricted by a variety of structures, including tension in the collateral ligaments and posterior joint capsule and bony contact between the anterior aspects of the metacarpal head and the base of the proximal phalanx. Thus, depending on the particular individual, the end-feel for MCP joint flexion can be capsular or bony. Limitation of MCP joint extension is produced by tension in the anterior joint capsule and volar plate, producing a capsular end-feel to the motion. The range of MCP joint abduction is most pronounced in the 2nd and 5th digits, with less motion available in the 3rd and 4th digits and even less motion available in the 1st MCP joint (in the thumb). Owing to tightness of the collateral ligaments when the MCP joints are flexed, MCP abduction is least restricted when the MCP joints are extended and is severely limited-to-absent when the joints are flexed. The end-feel for MCP joint abduction is capsular, owing to tension produced by the collateral ligaments and the skin of the interdigital web spaces. Since MCP joint adduction is restricted primarily by soft-tissue contact with the adjacent digit, the end-feel for this motion is soft.[3, 6, 8]

Limitation of IP joint flexion depends on the joint being moved. Flexion at the PIP joint usually is limited by contact of the soft tissue covering the anterior aspects of the proximal and middle phalanges of digits 2 through 5, thus producing a soft end-feel to the motion. Flexion at the IP (thumb) and DIP (fingers) joints (and occasionally flexion at the PIP joints of the fingers) is limited by tension in the posterior joint capsule and collateral ligaments, resulting in a capsular end-feel for IP (thumb) and DIP (fingers) flexion. Extension of all IP joints is limited by tension in the anterior joint capsule and volar plate of the joint being moved; thus, a capsular end-feel results.[3, 6, 8] Information regarding normal ranges of motion for all movements of the MCP and IP joints of the hand is found in Appendix C.

TECHNIQUES OF MEASUREMENT: METACARPOPHALANGEAL AND INTERPHALANGEAL JOINTS

During goniometric measurement of MCP and IP joint motion, one must remain mindful of the fact that position of the proximal joints can greatly affect the range of motion of the more distal joints of the hand.[9] Tension in the extrinsic finger extensors, when more proximal joints such as the wrist are flexed, can restrict the amount of flexion available in distal joints, such as the MCP joints. Conversely, extension of the more proximal joints causes tension on the extrinsic finger flexors, which in turn restricts the amount of extension that can be obtained at more distal joints. Therefore, care should be taken to maintain the proximal joints of the wrist and hand in a neutral position during measurement of flexion and extension of the MCP and IP joints.

The standard technique for measuring MCP and IP joint flexion is with the goniometer positioned over the dorsal surface of the joint being examined.[1, 3, 5, 11] Extension of the MCP and IP joints may be measured with the goniometer positioned over either the dorsal[11] or the volar[3] surface of the joint. However, the soft tissue over the volar surface of the MCP joints may interfere with alignment of the goniometer during measurement of MCP extension using the volar positioning technique.

Wrist Flexion: Dorsal Alignment

Fig. 5–2. Starting position for measurement of wrist flexion using dorsal alignment technique. Bony landmarks for goniometer alignment (lateral epicondyle of humerus, lunate, dorsal midline of 3rd metacarpal) indicated by orange line and dots.

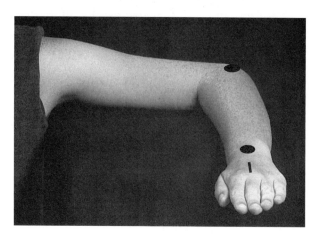

Patient position:	Seated, with shoulder abducted 90 degrees; elbow flexed 90 degrees; forearm pronated; arm and forearm supported on table; hand off table with wrist in neutral position (Fig. 5–2).
Stabilization:	Over dorsal surface of forearm (Fig. 5–3).
Examiner action:	After instructing patient in motion desired, flex patient's wrist through available ROM (see Note). Return wrist to neutral position. Performing passive movement provides an estimate of ROM and demonstrates to patient exact motion desired (see Fig. 5–3).
Goniometer alignment:	Palpate the following bony landmarks (shown in Fig. 5–2) and align goniometer accordingly (Fig. 5–4).
Stationary arm:	Dorsal midline of forearm toward lateral epicondyle of humerus.
Axis:	Lunate.
Moving arm:	Dorsal midline of 3rd metacarpal.

Read scale of goniometer.

Fig. 5–3. End of wrist flexion ROM, showing proper hand placement for stabilizing forearm and flexing wrist. Bony landmarks for goniometer alignment (lateral epicondyle of humerus, lunate, dorsal midline of 3rd metacarpal) indicated by orange line and dots.

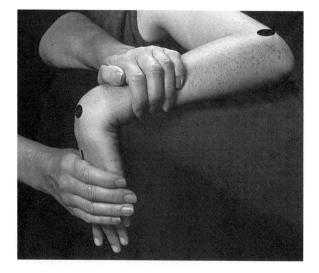

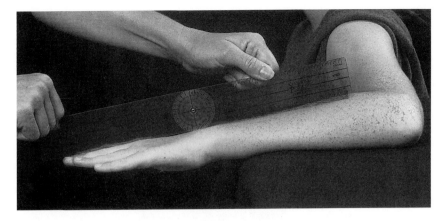

Fig. 5–4. Starting position for measurement of wrist flexion, demonstrating proper initial alignment of goniometer.

Patient/Examiner action:	Perform passive, or have patient perform active, wrist flexion (Fig. 5–5).
Confirmation of alignment:	Repalpate landmarks and confirm proper goniometric alignment at end of ROM, correcting alignment as necessary. Read scale of goniometer (Fig. 5–5).
Documentation:	Record patient's ROM.
Note:	Flexion of fingers should be avoided during measurement of wrist flexion to prevent limitation of motion by tension in extrinsic finger extensors.
Alternative patient position:	Patients unable to achieve 90 degrees of shoulder abduction may be positioned with shoulder adducted for this measurement. In such a case, stationary arm of goniometer should be aligned with dorsal midline of forearm toward bicipital tendon at elbow.
	Measurement may also be made with forearm in neutral rotation.

Fig. 5–5. End of wrist flexion ROM, demonstrating proper alignment of goniometer at end of range.

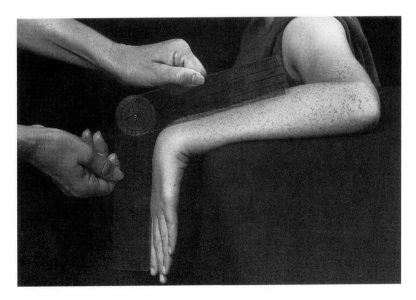

Wrist Flexion: Lateral Alignment

Fig. 5–6. Starting position for measurement of wrist flexion using lateral alignment technique. Bony landmarks for goniometer alignment (olecranon process of ulna, triquetrum, lateral midline of 5th metacarpal) indicated by orange line and dots.

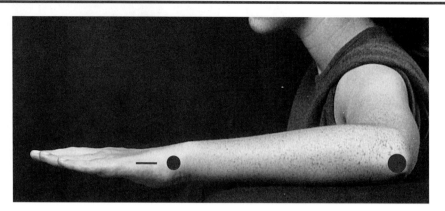

Patient position:	Seated, with shoulder abducted 90 degrees; elbow flexed 90 degrees; forearm pronated; arm and forearm supported on table; hand off table with wrist in neutral position (Fig. 5–6).
Stabilization:	Over dorsal surface of forearm (Fig. 5–7).
Examiner action:	After instructing patient in motion desired, flex patient's wrist through available ROM (see Note). Return wrist to neutral position. Performing passive movement provides an estimate of ROM and demonstrates to patient exact motion desired (see Fig. 5–7).
Goniometer alignment:	Palpate the following bony landmarks (shown in Fig. 5–6) and align goniometer accordingly (Fig. 5–8).
Stationary arm:	Lateral midline of ulna toward olecranon process.
Axis:	Triquetrum.
Moving arm:	Lateral midline of 5th metacarpal.
	Read scale of goniometer.

Fig. 5–7. End of wrist flexion ROM, showing proper hand placement for stabilizing forearm and flexing wrist. Bony landmarks for goniometer alignment (olecranon process of ulna, triquetrum, lateral midline of 5th metacarpal) indicated by orange line and dots.

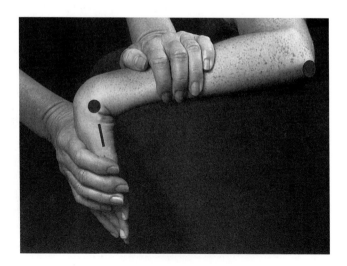

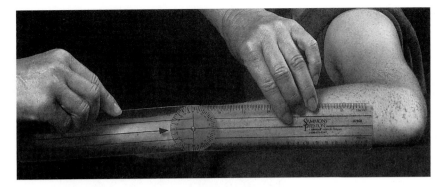

Fig. 5–8. Starting position for measurement of wrist flexion, demonstrating proper initial alignment of goniometer.

Patient/Examiner action:	Perform passive, or have patient perform active, wrist flexion (Fig. 5–9).
Confirmation of alignment:	Repalpate landmarks and confirm proper goniometric alignment at end of ROM, correcting alignment as necessary. Read scale of goniometer (Fig. 5–9).
Documentation:	Record patient's ROM.
Note:	Flexion of fingers should be avoided during measurement of wrist flexion to prevent limitation of motion by tension in extrinsic finger extensors.
Alternative patient position:	Patients unable to achieve 90 degrees of shoulder abduction may be positioned with shoulder adducted. In such a case, a dorsal alignment technique should be used, and the measurement also may be made with forearm in neutral rotation. Stationary arm of the goniometer should be aligned with the dorsal midline of the forearm toward the bicipital tendon at the elbow.

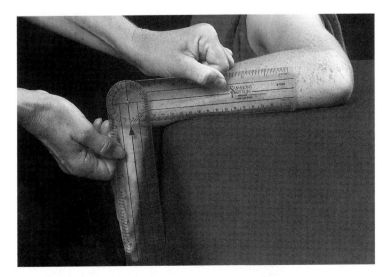

Fig. 5–9. End of wrist flexion ROM, demonstrating proper alignment of goniometer at end of range.

Wrist Extension: Volar Alignment

Fig. 5–10. Starting position for measurement of wrist extension using volar alignment technique. Bony landmarks for goniometer alignment (bicepital tendon at elbow, lunate, volar midline of 3rd metacarpal) indicated by orange line and dots.

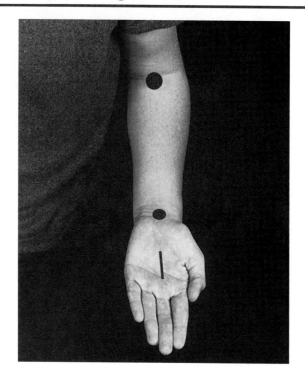

Patient position:	Seated, with shoulder adducted; elbow flexed 90 degrees; forearm supinated and supported on table; wrist and hand off table with wrist in neutral position (Fig. 5–10).
Stabilization:	Over ventral surface of forearm (Fig. 5–11).
Examiner action:	After instructing patient in motion desired, extend patient's wrist through available ROM (see Note). Return wrist to neutral position. Performing passive movement provides an estimate of ROM and demonstrates to patient exact motion desired (see Fig. 5–11).

Fig. 5–11. End of wrist extension ROM, showing proper hand placement for stabilizing forearm and extending wrist. Bony landmarks for goniometer alignment (bicepital tendon at elbow, lunate, volar midline of 3rd metacarpal) indicated by orange line and dots.

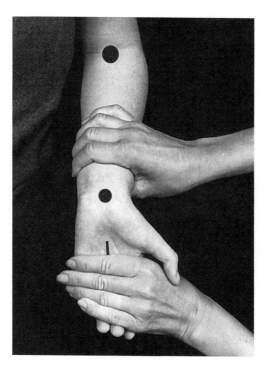

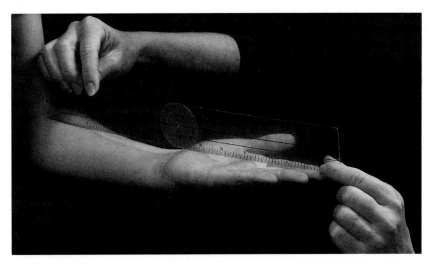

Fig. 5–12. Starting position for measurement of wrist extension, demonstrating proper initial alignment of goniometer.

Goniometer alignment:	Palpate the following landmarks (shown in Fig. 5–10) and align goniometer accordingly (Fig. 5–12).
Stationary arm:	Volar midline of forearm toward bicipital tendon at elbow.
Axis:	Lunate.
Moving arm:	Volar midline of 3rd metacarpal.
	Read scale of goniometer.
Patient/Examiner action:	Perform passive, or have patient perform active, wrist extension (Fig. 5–13).
Confirmation of alignment:	Repalpate landmarks and confirm proper goniometric alignment at end of ROM, correcting alignment as necessary. Read scale of goniometer (Fig. 5–13).
Documentation:	Record patient's ROM.
Note:	Extension of fingers should be avoided during measurement of wrist extension to prevent limitation of motion by tension in extrinsic finger flexors.
Alternative patient position:	Measurement also may be made with forearm in neutral rotation.

Fig. 5–13. End of wrist extension ROM, demonstrating proper alignment of goniometer at end of range.

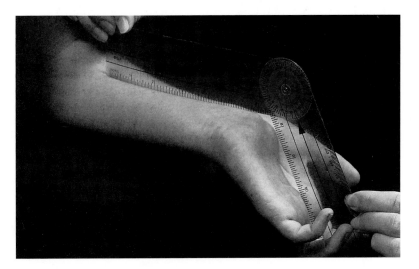

Wrist Extension: Lateral Alignment

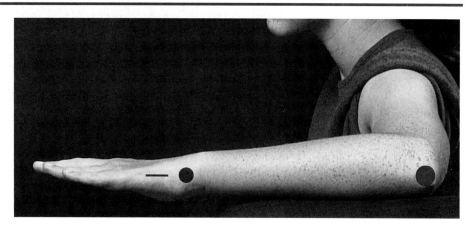

Fig. 5–14. Starting position for measurement of wrist extension using lateral alignment technique. Bony landmarks for goniometer alignment (olecranon process of ulna, triquetrum, lateral midline of 5th metacarpal) indicated by orange line and dots.

Patient position:	Seated, with shoulder abducted 90 degrees; elbow flexed 90 degrees; forearm pronated; arm and forearm supported on table; hand off table with wrist in neutral position (Fig. 5–14).
Stabilization:	Over dorsal surface of forearm (Fig. 5–15).
Examiner action:	After instructing patient in motion desired, extend patient's wrist through available ROM (see Note). Return wrist to neutral position. Performing passive movement provides an estimate of ROM and demonstrates to patient exact motion desired (see Fig. 5–15).
Goniometer alignment:	Palpate the following bony landmarks (shown in Fig. 5–14) and align goniometer accordingly (Fig. 5–16).
Stationary arm:	Lateral midline of ulna toward olecranon process.
Axis:	Triquetrum.
Moving arm:	Lateral midline of 5th metacarpal.
	Read scale of goniometer.

Fig. 5–15. End of wrist extension ROM, showing proper hand placement for stabilizing forearm and extending wrist. Bony landmarks for goniometer alignment (olecranon process of ulna, triquetrum, lateral midline of 5th metacarpal) indicated by orange line and dots.

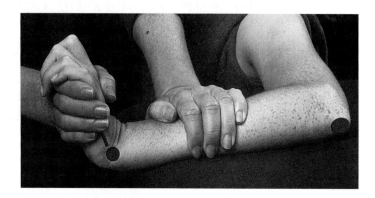

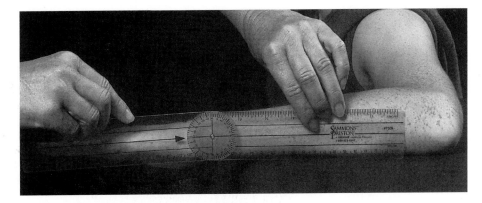

Fig. 5–16. Starting position for measurement of wrist extension, demonstrating proper initial alignment of goniometer.

Patient/Examiner action: Perform passive, or have patient perform active, wrist extension (Fig. 5–17).

Confirmation of alignment: Repalpate landmarks and confirm proper goniometric alignment at end of ROM, correcting alignment as necessary. Read scale of goniometer (Fig. 5–17).

Documentation: Record patient's ROM.

Note: Extension of fingers should be avoided during measurement of wrist extension to prevent limitation of motion by tension in extrinsic finger flexors.

Alternative patient position: Measurement also may be made with forearm in neutral rotation. In such a case, goniometer should be placed over volar surface of wrist with stationary arm aligned with midline of forearm toward bicipital tendon, axis over lunate, and moving arm aligned with volar midline of 3rd metacarpal.

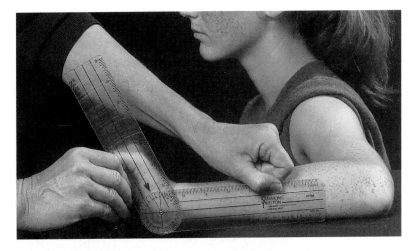

Fig. 5–17. End of wrist extension ROM, demonstrating proper alignment of goniometer at end of range.

Wrist Adduction: Ulnar Deviation

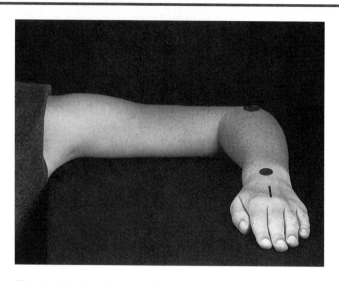

Fig. 5–18. Starting position for measurement of wrist adduction. Bony landmarks for goniometer alignment (lateral epicondyle of humerus, capitate, dorsal midline of 3rd metacarpal) indicated by orange line and dots.

Patient position:	Seated, with shoulder abducted 90 degrees; elbow flexed 90 degrees; forearm pronated; upper extremity (UE) supported on table; wrist and hand in neutral position (Fig. 5–18).
Stabilization:	Over dorsal surface of distal forearm (Fig. 5–19).
Examiner action:	After instructing patient in motion desired, adduct patient's wrist through available ROM. Return wrist to neutral position. Performing passive movement provides an estimate of ROM and demonstrates to patient exact motion desired (see Fig. 5–19).

Fig. 5–19. End of wrist adduction ROM, showing proper hand placement for stabilizing forearm and adducting wrist. Bony landmarks for goniometer alignment (lateral epicondyle of humerus, capitate, dorsal midline of 3rd metacarpal) indicated by orange line and dots.

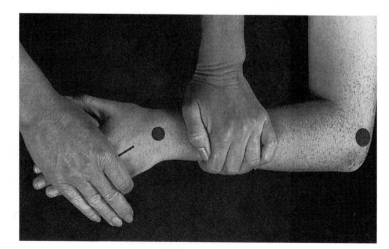

Fig. 5–20. Starting position for measurement of wrist adduction, demonstrating proper initial alignment of goniometer.

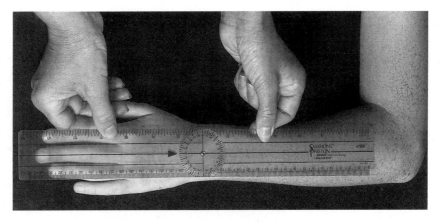

Goniometer alignment:	Palpate the following bony landmarks (shown in Fig. 5–18) and align goniometer accordingly (Fig. 5–20).
Stationary arm:	Dorsal midline of forearm toward lateral epicondyle of humerus.
Axis:	Capitate.
Moving arm:	Dorsal midline of 3rd metacarpal.
	Read scale of goniometer.
Patient/Examiner action:	Perform passive, or have patient perform active, wrist adduction (Fig. 5–21).
Confirmation of alignment:	Repalpate landmarks and confirm proper goniometric alignment at end of ROM, correcting alignment as necessary. Read scale of goniometer (Fig. 5–21).
Documentation:	Record patient's ROM.
Alternative patient position:	Patients unable to achieve 90 degrees of shoulder adduction may be positioned with shoulder adducted for this measurement. In such a case, stationary arm of goniometer should be aligned with dorsal midline of forearm toward bicipital tendon at elbow.

Fig. 5–21. End of wrist adduction ROM, demonstrating proper alignment of goniometer at end of range.

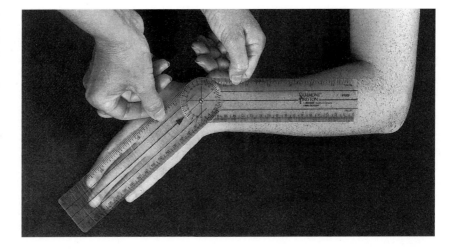

Wrist Abduction: Radial Deviation

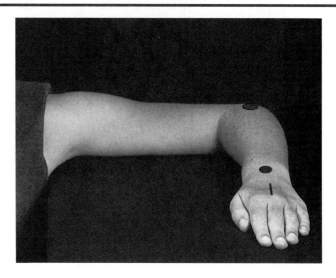

Fig. 5–22. Starting position for measurement of wrist abduction. Landmarks for goniometer alignment (lateral epicondyle of humerus, capitate, dorsal midline of 3rd metacarpal) indicated by orange line and dots.

Patient position: Seated, with shoulder abducted 90 degrees; elbow flexed 90 degrees; forearm pronated; UE supported on table; wrist and hand in neutral position (Fig. 5–22).

Stabilization: Over dorsal surface of distal forearm (Fig. 5–23).

Examiner action: After instructing patient in motion desired, abduct patient's wrist through available ROM. Return wrist to neutral position. Performing passive movement provides an estimate of the ROM and demonstrates to patient exact motion desired (Fig. 5–23).

Fig. 5–23. End of wrist abduction ROM, showing proper hand placement for stabilizing forearm and adducting wrist. Landmarks for goniometer alignment (lateral epicondyle of humerus, capitate, dorsal midline of 3rd metacarpal) indicated by orange line and dots.

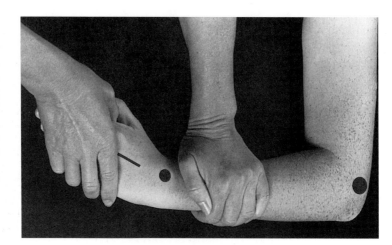

Fig. 5–24. Starting position for measurement of wrist abduction, demonstrating proper initial alignment of goniometer.

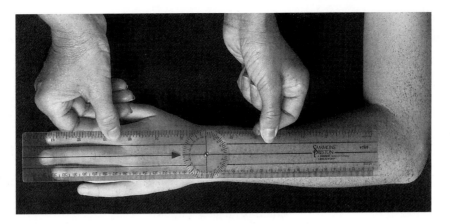

Goniometer alignment:	Palpate the following bony landmarks (shown in Fig. 5–22) and align goniometer accordingly (Fig. 5–24).
Stationary arm:	Dorsal midline of forearm toward lateral epicondyle of humerus.
Axis:	Capitate.
Moving arm:	Dorsal midline of 3rd metacarpal.

Read scale of goniometer.

Patient/Examiner action:	Perform passive, or have patient perform active, wrist abduction (Fig. 5–25).
Confirmation of alignment:	Repalpate landmarks and confirm proper goniometric alignment at end of ROM, correcting alignment as necessary. Read scale of goniometer (Fig. 5–25).
Documentation:	Record patient's ROM.
Alternative patient position:	Patients unable to achieve 90 degrees of shoulder abduction may be positioned with shoulder adducted for this measurement. In such a case, stationary arm of goniometer should be aligned with dorsal midline of forearm toward bicipital tendon at elbow.

Fig. 5–25. End of wrist abduction ROM, demonstrating proper alignment of goniometer at end of range.

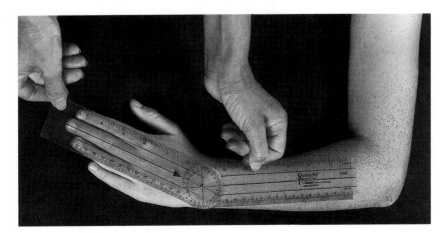

Metacarpophalangeal (MCP) Abduction

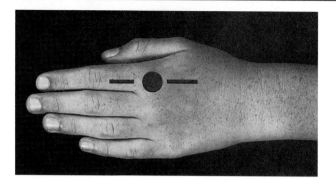

Fig. 5-26. Starting position for measurement of MCP abduction. Landmarks for goniometer alignment (dorsal midline of metacarpal, dorsum of MCP joint, dorsal midline of proximal phalanx) indicated by orange lines and dot.

Patient position: Seated, with forearm pronated; UE supported on table; wrist and hand in neutral position (Fig. 5-26).

Stabilization: Over metacarpals (Fig. 5-27).

Examiner action: After instructing patient in motion desired, abduct MCP joint to be examined through available ROM. Return finger to neutral position. Performing passive movement provides an estimate of ROM and demonstrates to patient exact motion desired (see Fig. 5-27).

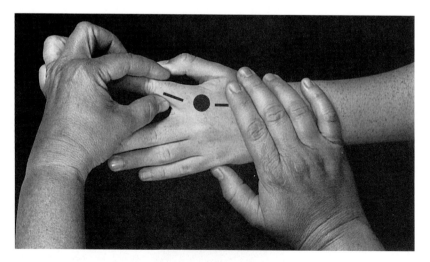

Fig. 5-27. End of MCP abduction ROM, showing proper hand placement for stabilizing metacarpals and abducting MCP joint. Landmarks for goniometer alignment (dorsal midline of metacarpal, dorsum of MCP joint, dorsal midline of proximal phalanx) indicated by orange lines and dot.

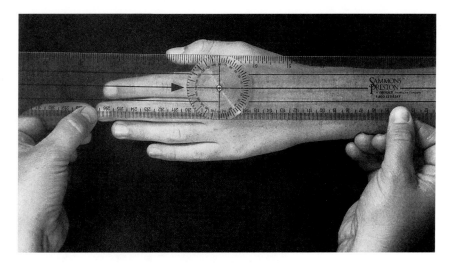

Fig. 5–28. Starting position for measurement of MCP abduction, demonstrating proper initial alignment of goniometer.

Goniometer alignment:	Palpate the following bony landmarks (shown in Fig. 5–26) and align goniometer accordingly (Fig. 5–28).
Stationary arm:	Dorsal midline of metacarpal.
Axis:	Dorsum of MCP joint.
Moving arm:	Dorsal midline of proximal phalanx.
	Read scale of goniometer.
Patient/Examiner action:	Perform passive, or have patient perform active, MCP abduction. (Fig. 5–29).
Confirmation of alignment:	Repalpate landmarks and confirm proper goniometric alignment at end of ROM, correcting alignment as necessary. Read scale of goniometer (Fig. 5–29).
Documentation:	Record patient's ROM.

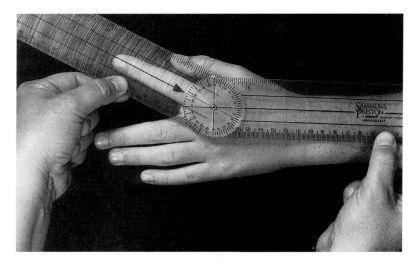

Fig. 5–29. End of MCP abduction ROM, demonstrating proper alignment of goniometer at end of range.

Metacarpophalangeal (MCP) or Interphalangeal (PIP or DIP) Flexion

Fig. 5–30. Starting position for measurement of MCP flexion. Landmarks for goniometer alignment (dorsal midline of metacarpal, dorsum of MCP joint, dorsal midline of proximal phalanx) indicated by orange lines and dot.

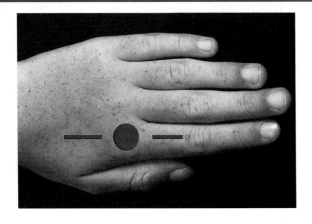

(Measurement of 2nd MCP joint shown.)

Patient position:	Seated, with UE supported on table; wrist and hand in neutral position* (Fig. 5–30).
Stabilization:	Over more proximal bone of joint (in this case, stabilization of a metacarpals is shown) (Fig. 5–31).
Examiner action:	After instructing patient in motion desired, flex joint to be examined through available ROM. Return finger to neutral position. Performing passive movement provides an estimate of ROM and demonstrates to patient exact motion desired (see Fig. 5–31).

---

* Proximal joints should remain in neutral position during measurement to prevent obstruction of full ROM by tension in extrinsic and intrinsic finger extensor muscles.

Fig. 5–31. End of MCP flexion ROM, showing proper hand placement for stabilizing metacarpals and flexing MCP joint. Landmarks for goniometer alignment (dorsal midline of metacarpal, dorsum of MCP joint, dorsal midline of proximal phalanx) indicated by orange lines and dot.

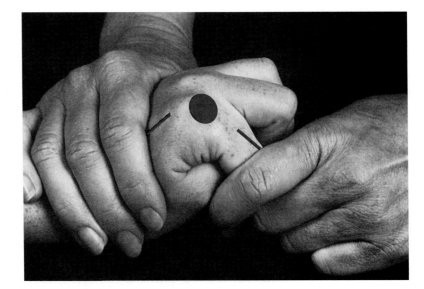

Fig. 5–32. Starting position for measurement of MCP flexion, demonstrating proper initial alignment of goniometer.

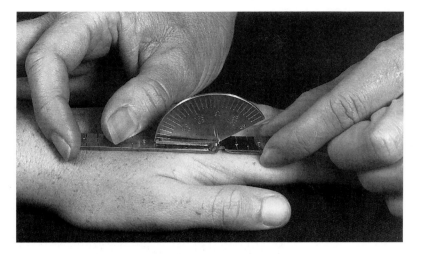

Goniometer alignment:	Palpate the following bony landmarks (shown in Fig. 5–30) and align goniometer accordingly (Fig. 5–32).
Stationary arm:	Dorsal midline of more proximal bone of joint (in this case, a metacarpal).
Axis:	Dorsum of joint being examined (in this case, MCP joint).
Moving arm:	Dorsal midline of more distal bone joint (in this case, a proximal phalanx).

Read scale of goniometer.

Patient/Examiner action:	Perform passive, or have patient perform active, flexion of the joint (Fig. 5–33).
Confirmation of alignment:	Repalpate landmarks and confirm proper goniometric alignment at end of ROM, correcting alignment as necessary. Read scale of goniometer (Fig. 5–33).
Documentation:	Record patient's ROM.
Note:	This technique may be used to measure flexion of the MCP, PIP, or DIP joints of the fingers. The figures shown here depict the measurement of MCP flexion of the 2nd digit (index finger).

Fig. 5–33. End of MCP flexion ROM, demonstrating proper alignment of goniometer at end of range.

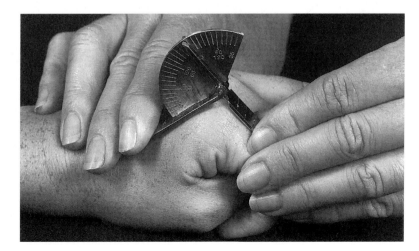

Metacarpophalangeal (MCP) or Interphalangeal (PIP or DIP) Extension

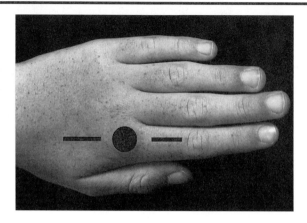

Fig. 5–34. Starting position for measurement of MCP extension. Landmarks for goniometer alignment (dorsal midline of metacarpal, dorsum of MCP joint, dorsal midline of proximal phalanx) indicated by orange lines and dot.

(Measurement of 2nd MCP joint shown.)

Patient position:	Seated, with UE supported on table; wrist and hand in neutral position* (Fig. 5–34).
Stabilization:	Over more proximal bone of joint being examined (in this case, stabilization of metacarpals is shown) (Fig. 5–35).
Examiner action:	After instructing patient in motion desired, extend MCP joint to be examined through available ROM. Return finger to neutral position. Performing passive movement provides an estimate of ROM and demonstrates to patient exact motion desired (see Fig. 5–35).

* Proximal joints should remain in neutral position during measurement to prevent obstruction of full ROM by tension in extrinsic or intrinsic finger flexor muscles.

Fig. 5–35. End of MCP extension ROM, showing proper hand placement for stabilizing metacarpals and extending MCP joint. Landmarks for goniometer alignment (dorsal midline of metacarpal, dorsum of MCP joint, dorsal midline of proximal phalanx) indicated by orange lines and dot.

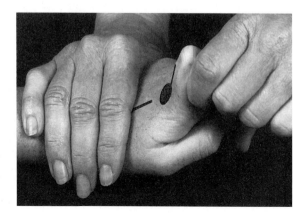

Fig. 5–36. Starting position for measurement of MCP extension, demonstrating proper initial alignment of goniometer.

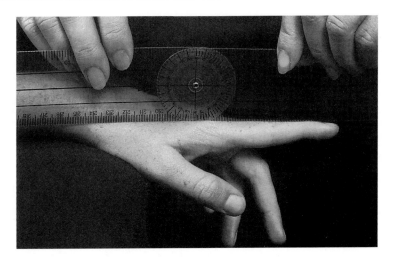

Goniometer alignment:	Palpate the following bony landmarks (shown in Fig. 5–34) and align goniometer accordingly (Fig. 5–36).
Stationary arm:	Dorsal midline of more proximal bone of joint (in this case, a metacarpal).
Axis:	Dorsum of joint being examined (in this case, MCP joint).
Moving arm:	Dorsal midline of more distal bone of joint (in this case, a proximal phalanx).

Read scale of goniometer.

Patient/Examiner action: Perform passive, or have patient perform active, extension of the joint (Fig. 5–37).

Confirmation of alignment: Repalpate landmarks and confirm proper goniometric alignment at end of ROM, correcting alignment as necessary. Read scale of goniometer (Fig. 5–37).

Documentation: Record patient's ROM.

Note: This technique may be used to measure extension of the MCP, PIP, or DIP joints of the fingers. The figures shown here depict the measurement of MCP extension of the 2nd digit (index finger).

FIG. 5–37. End of MCP extension ROM, demonstrating proper alignment of goniometer at end of range.

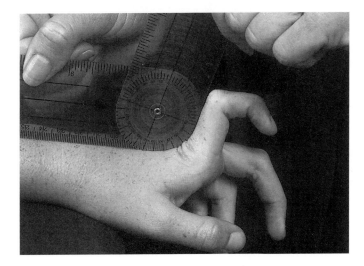

Carpometacarpal (First CMC) Abduction

Fig. 5–38. Starting position for measurement of 1st CMC abduction. Note that thumb is positioned alongside volar surface of 2nd metacarpal. Landmarks for goniometer alignment (lateral midline of 2nd metacarpal, radial styloid process, dorsal midline of 1st metacarpal) indicated by orange lines and dot.

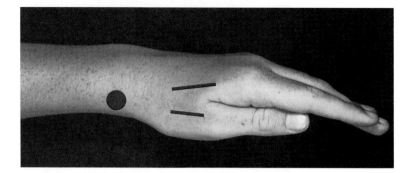

Patient position:	Seated, with forearm neutral; UE supported on table; wrist and hand in neutral position; thumb positioned along volar surface of 2nd metacarpal (Fig. 5–38).
Stabilization:	Over 2nd metacarpal (Fig. 5–39).
Examiner action:	After instructing patient in motion desired, abduct 1st CMC joint by grasping 1st metacarpal and moving thumb perpendicularly away from palm. Return thumb to starting position. Performing passive movement provides an estimate of ROM and demonstrates to patient exact motion desired (see Fig. 5–39).
Goniometer alignment:	Palpate the following bony landmarks (shown in Fig. 5–38) and align goniometer accordingly (Fig. 5–40).
Stationary arm:	Lateral midline of 2nd metacarpal.
Axis:	Radial styloid process.
Moving arm:	Dorsal midline of 1st metacarpal.
	Read scale of goniometer (see Note).

Fig. 5–39. End of 1st CMC abduction ROM, showing proper hand placement for stabilizing 2nd metacarpal and abducting 1st CMC joint. Landmarks for goniometer alignment (lateral midline of 2nd metacarpal, radial styloid process, dorsal midline of 1st metacarpal) indicated by orange lines and dot.

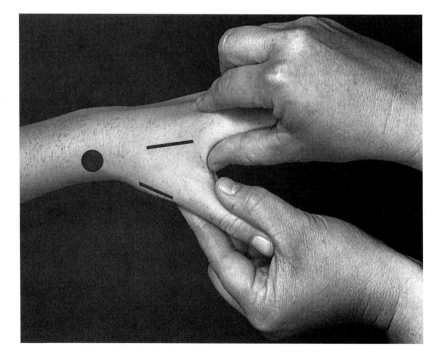

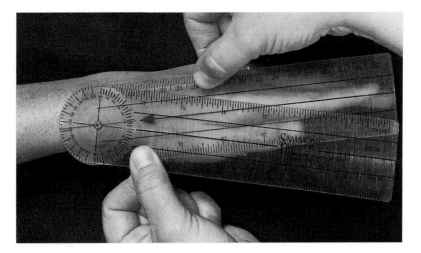

Fig. 5–40. Starting position for measurement of 1st CMC abduction, demonstrating proper initial alignment of goniometer.

Patient/Examiner action:	Perform passive, or have patient perform active, abduction of 1st CMC joint (Fig. 5–41).
Confirmation of alignment:	Repalpate landmarks and confirm proper goniometric alignment at end of ROM, correcting alignment as necessary (Fig. 5–41). Read scale of goniometer (see Note).
Documentation:	Calculate and record patient's ROM (see Note).
Note:	Goniometer will not read 0 degrees at beginning of 1st CMC abduction. However, this initial reading should be translated as 0 degrees starting position. Number of degrees of abduction through which joint moves is calculated by subtracting *initial* goniometer reading from *final* reading. Motion is then recorded as 0 degrees to X degrees 1st CMC abduction. For example, if goniometer reads 25 degrees at beginning of 1st CMC abduction, and 52 degrees at end of ROM, then 1st CMC abduction = 52° − 25°, or 0 degrees to 27 degrees 1st CMC abduction.

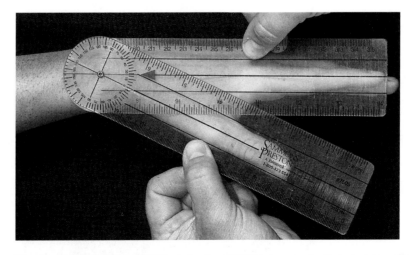

Fig. 5–41. End of 1st CMC abduction ROM, demonstrating proper alignment of goniometer at end of range.

Carpometacarpal (First CMC) Flexion

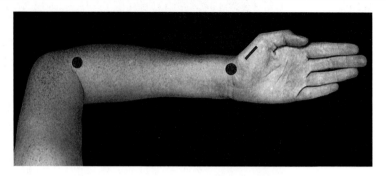

Fig. 5–42. Starting position for measurement of 1st CMC flexion. Note that thumb is positioned alongside lateral surface of 2nd metacarpal. Landmarks for goniometer alignment (radial head, ventral surface of 1st CMC joint, ventral midline of 1st metacarpal) indicated by orange line and dots.

Patient position:	Seated, with forearm supinated; UE supported on table; wrist and hand in neutral position; thumb positioned along lateral side of 2nd metacarpal (Fig. 5–42).
Stabilization:	Over ventral surface of wrist (Fig. 5–43).
Examiner action:	After instructing patient in motion desired, flex 1st CMC joint by grasping 1st metacarpal and moving thumb across palm. Return thumb to starting position. Performing passive movement provides an estimate of ROM and demonstrates to patient exact motion desired (see Fig. 5–43).
Goniometer alignment:	Palpate the following bony landmarks (shown in Fig. 5–56) and align goniometer accordingly (Fig. 5–44).
Stationary arm:	Ventral midline of radius toward radial head.
Axis:	Ventral surface of 1st CMC joint.
Moving arm:	Ventral midline of 1st metacarpal.
	Read scale of goniometer (See Note).

Fig. 5–43. End of 1st CMC flexion ROM, showing proper hand placement for stabilizing 2nd metacarpal and flexing 1st CMC joint. Landmarks for goniometer alignment (radial head, ventral surface of 1st CMC joint, ventral midline of 1st metacarpal) indicated by orange line and dots.

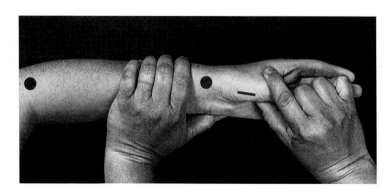

Fig. 5–44. Starting position for measurement of 1st CMC flexion, demonstrating proper initial alignment of goniometer.

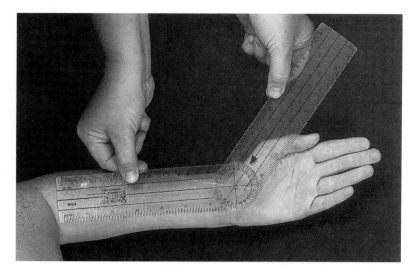

Patient/Examiner action: Perform passive, or have patient perform active, flexion of 1st CMC joint (Fig. 5–45).

Confirmation of alignment: Repalpate landmarks and confirm proper goniometric alignment at end of ROM, correcting alignment as necessary (Fig. 5–45). Read scale of goniometer (see Note).

Documentation: Calculate and record patient's ROM (see Note).

Note: Goniometer will not read 0 degrees at beginning of 1st CMC flexion. However, this initial reading should be translated as 0 degrees starting position. Number of degrees of flexion through which joint moves is calculated by subtracting *final* goniometer reading from *initial* reading. Motion is then recorded as 0 degrees to X degrees 1st CMC flexion. For example, if goniometer reads 36 degrees at beginning of 1st CMC flexion, and 4 degrees at end of ROM, then 1st CMC flexion = 36° − 4°, or 0 degrees to 32 degrees 1st CMC flexion.

Fig. 5–45. End of 1st CMC flexion ROM, demonstrating proper alignment of goniometer at end of range.

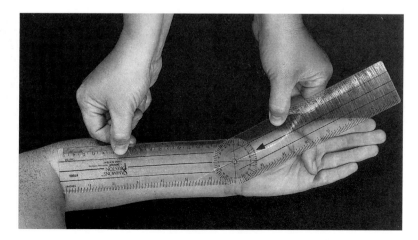

Carpometacarpal (First CMC) Extension

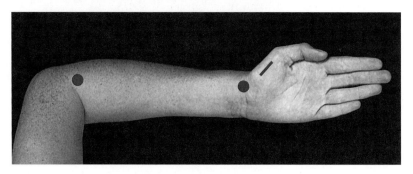

Fig. 5–46. Starting position for measurement of 1st CMC extension. Note that thumb is positioned alongside lateral surface of 2nd metacarpal. Landmarks for goniometer alignment (radial head, ventral surface of 1st CMC joint, ventral midline of 1st metacarpal) indicated by orange line and dots.

Patient position:	Seated, with forearm supinated; UE supported on table; wrist and hand in neutral position, thumb positioned along lateral side of 2nd metacarpal (Fig. 5–46).
Stabilization:	Over ventral surface of wrist (Fig. 5–47).
Examiner action:	After instructing patient in motion desired, extend 1st CMC joint by grasping 1st metacarpal and moving thumb away from, but parallel to, palm. Return thumb to starting position. Performing passive movement provides an estimate of ROM and demonstrates to patient exact motion desired (see Fig. 5–47).
Goniometer alignment:	Palpate the following bony landmarks (shown in Fig. 5–46) and align goniometer accordingly (Fig. 5–48).
Stationary arm:	Ventral midline of radius toward radial head.
Axis:	Ventral surface of 1st CMC joint.
Moving arm:	Ventral midline of 1st metacarpal.
	Read scale of goniometer (see Note).

Fig. 5–47. End of 1st CMC extension ROM, showing proper hand placement for stabilizing 2nd metacarpal and extending 1st CMC joint. Landmarks for goniometer alignment (radial head, ventral surface of 1st CMC joint, ventral midline of 1st metacarpal) indicated by orange line and dots.

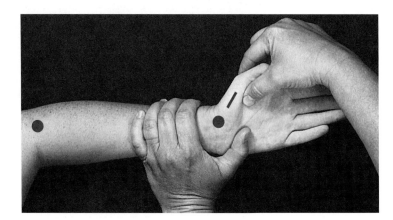

Fig. 5–48. Starting position for measurement of 1st CMC extension, demonstrating proper initial alignment of goniometer.

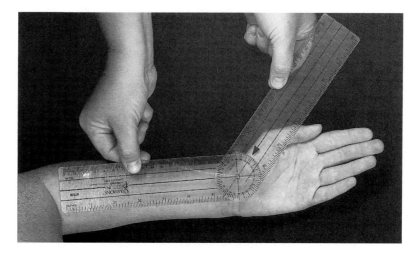

Patient/Examiner action:	Perform passive, or have patient perform active, extension of 1st CMC joint (Fig. 5–49).
Confirmation of alignment:	Repalpate landmarks and confirm proper goniometric alignment at end of ROM, correcting alignment as necessary (Fig. 5–49). Read scale of goniometer (see Note).
Documentation:	Calculate and record patient's ROM (see Note).
Note:	Goniometer will not read 0 degrees at beginning of 1st CMC extension. However, this initial reading should be translated as 0 degrees starting position. Number of degrees of extension through which joint moves is calculated by subtracting *initial* goniometer reading from *final* reading. Motion is then recorded as 0 degrees to X degrees 1st CMC extension. For example, if goniometer reads 36 degrees at beginning of 1st CMC extension, and 65 degrees at end of ROM, then 1st CMC extension = 65° − 36°, or 0 degrees to 29 degrees 1st CMC extension.

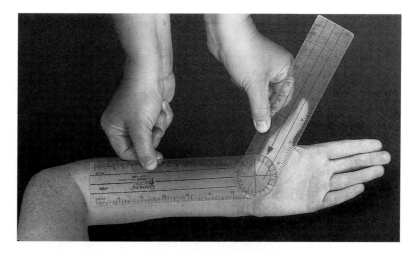

Fig. 5–49. End of 1st CMC extension ROM, demonstrating proper alignment of goniometer at end of range.

Carpometacarpal (First CMC) Opposition

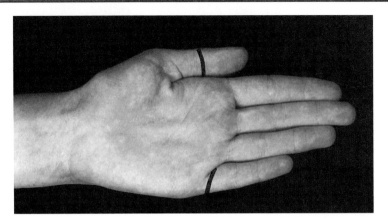

Fig. 5–50. Starting position for measurement of 1st CMC opposition. Note that thumb is positioned alongside lateral surface of 2nd metacarpal. Measurement is made with a ruler, rather than with a goniometer. Landmarks for alignment of ruler (palmar digital crease of 5th digit, flexor crease of IP joint of thumb) indicated by orange lines.

Patient position:	Seated, with forearm supinated; UE supported on table, wrist and hand in neutral position, thumb positioned along lateral side of 2nd metacarpal (Fig. 5–50).
Stabilization:	Over ventral surface of 5th metacarpal with one hand, and over MCP and IP joints of thumb with other hand, preventing flexion of MCP and IP joints of thumb (Fig. 5–51).
Examiner action:	After instructing patient in motion desired, move 1st CMC joint into opposition by bringing flexor crease of IP joint of patient's thumb toward palmar digital crease of 5th digit. No flexion of MCP or IP joints of thumb should be allowed. Return thumb to starting position. Performing passive movement provides an estimate of ROM and demonstrates to patient exact motion desired (see Fig. 5–51).

Fig. 5–51. End of 1st CMC opposition ROM, showing proper hand placement for stabilizing digits 2 through 5 and moving thumb into opposition toward 5th digit. Landmarks for goniometer alignment (palmar digital crease of 5th digit, flexor crease of IP joint of thumb) indicated by orange lines.

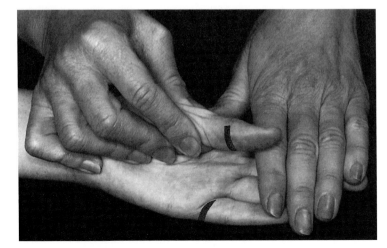

Fig. 5–52. End of 1st CMC opposition ROM, demonstrating proper alignment of ruler. Measurement is made of distance between flexor crease of IP joint of thumb and palmar digital crease of 5th digit.

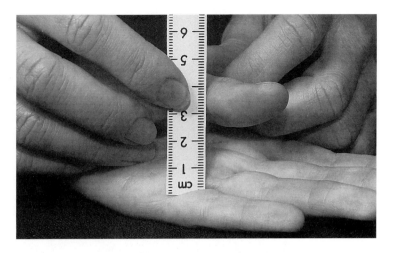

Instrument alignment:	Place end of ruler at palmar digital crease of 5th digit (Fig. 5–52).
Patient/Examiner action:	Perform passive, or have patient perform active, opposition of 1st CMC joint without flexing MCP or IP joints of thumb (see Fig. 5–52).
Measurement of motion:	Measure distance between flexor crease of IP joint of patient's thumb and palmar digital crease of 5th digit, keeping end of ruler in contact with palmar digital crease (see Fig. 5–52).
Documentation:	Record distance as measured.

Metacarpophalangeal (MCP) or Interphalangeal (IP) Flexion of Thumb

Fig. 5–53. Starting position for measurement of 1st MCP flexion (thumb). Note that CMC joint of thumb is positioned in slight abduction. Landmarks for goniometer alignment (dorsal midline of 1st metacarpal, dorsum of 1st MCP joint, dorsal midline of proximal phalanx) indicated by orange lines and dot.

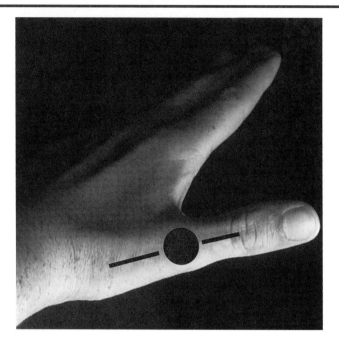

(Measurement of 1st MCP joint shown.)

Patient position:	Seated, with forearm neutral; UE supported on table; wrist in neutral position*; 1st CMC joint in slight abduction (Fig. 5–53).
Stabilization:	1st metacarpal (MCP) or proximal phalanx of thumb (IP). In this case, stabilization of 1st MCP is shown (Fig. 5–54).

---

* Proximal joints should remain in neutral position (not flexed or extended) during testing to prevent obstruction of full ROM by tension in thumb extensor muscles.

Fig. 5–54. End of 1st MCP flexion ROM, showing proper hand placement for stabilizing metacarpal and flexing 1st MCP joint. Landmarks for goniometer alignment (dorsal midline of 1st metacarpal, dorsum of 1st MCP joint, dorsal midline of proximal phalanx) indicated by orange lines and dot.

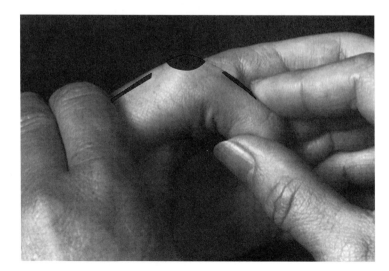

Fig. 5–55. Starting position for measurement of 1st MCP flexion, demonstrating proper initial alignment of goniometer.

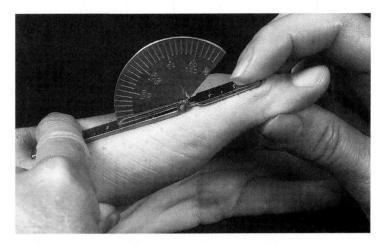

Examiner action:	After instructing patient in motion desired, flex joint through available ROM. Return thumb to neutral position. Performing passive movement provides an estimate of ROM and demonstrates to patient exact motion desired (see Fig. 5–54).
Goniometer alignment:	Palpate the following bony landmarks (shown in Fig. 5–53) and align goniometer accordingly (Fig. 5–55).
Stationary arm:	Dorsal midline of 1st metacarpal (MCP) or of proximal phalanx of thumb (IP).
Axis:	Dorsum of 1st MCP or IP joint.
Moving arm:	Dorsal midline of proximal phalanx of thumb (MCP) or distal phalanx of thumb (IP).
	Read scale of goniometer.
Patient/Examiner action:	Perform passive, or have patient perform active, flexion of joint to be measured (Fig. 5–56).
Confirmation of alignment:	Repalpate landmarks and confirm proper goniometric alignment at end of ROM, correcting alignment as necessary. Read scale of goniometer (Fig. 5–56).
Documentation:	Record patient's ROM.
Note:	This technique may be used to measure flexion of the MCP or IP joints of the thumb. The figures shown here depict the measurement of MCP flexion of the thumb.

Fig. 5–56. End of 1st MCP flexion ROM, demonstrating proper alignment of goniometer at end of range.

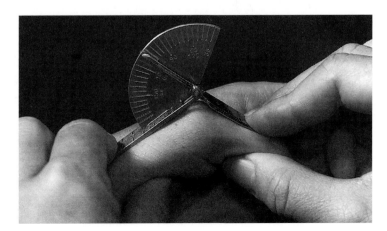

Metacarpophalangeal (MCP) or Interphalangeal (IP) Extension of Thumb

Fig. 5–57. Starting position for measurement of IP extension (thumb). Note that CMC joint of thumb is positioned in slight abduction. Landmarks for goniometer alignment (dorsal midline of proximal phalanx, dorsum of IP joint, dorsal midline of distal phalanx) indicated by orange lines and dot.

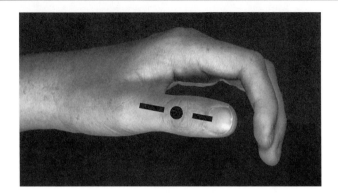

(Measurement of IP joint shown.)

Patient position:	Seated, with forearm neutral; UE supported on table; wrist in neutral position*; 1st CMC joint in slight abduction (Fig. 5–57).
Stabilization:	Over 1st metacarpal (MCP) or proximal phalanx of thumb (IP). In this case, stabilization of proximal phalanx is shown (Fig. 5–58).
Examiner action:	After instructing patient in motion desired, extend joint through available ROM. Return finger to neutral position. Performing passive movement provides an estimate of ROM and demonstrates to patient exact motion desired (see Fig. 5–58).

---

*Proximal joints should remain in neutral position during testing to prevent obstruction of full ROM by tension in flexor pollicis longus muscle.

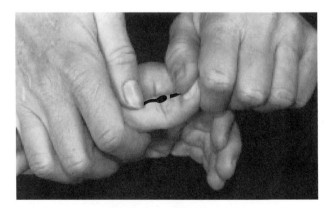

Fig. 5–58. End of IP extension ROM, showing proper hand placement for stabilizing proximal phalanx and extending IP joint. Landmarks for goniometer alignment (dorsal midline of proximal phalanx, dorsum of IP joint, dorsal midline of distal phalanx) indicated by orange lines and dot.

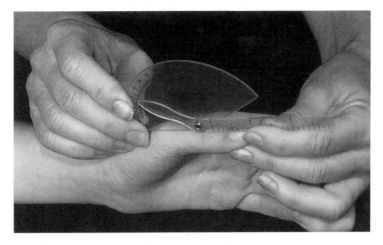

Fig. 5–59. Starting position for measurement of IP extension, demonstrating proper initial alignment of goniometer.

Goniometer alignment: Palpate the following bony landmarks (shown in Fig. 5–57) and align goniometer accordingly (Fig. 5–59).

  Stationary arm: Dorsal midline of 1st metacarpal (MCP) or of proximal phalanx of thumb (IP).

  Axis: Dorsum of 1st MCP or IP joint.

  Moving arm: Dorsal midline of proximal phalanx of thumb (MCP) or distal phalanx of thumb (IP).

Read scale of goniometer.

Patient/Examiner action: Perform passive, or have patient perform active, extension of joint to be measured (Fig. 5–60).

Confirmation of alignment: Repalpate landmarks and confirm proper goniometric alignment at end of ROM, correcting alignment as necessary. Read scale of goniometer (Fig. 5–60).

Documentation: Record patient's ROM.

Note: This technique may be used to measure extension of the MCP or IP joints of the thumb. The figures shown here depict the measurement of IP flexion of the thumb.

Fig. 5–60. End of IP extension ROM, demonstrating proper alignment of goniometer at end of range.

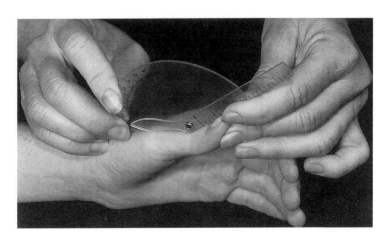

References

1. American Medical Association: Guides to the Evaluation of Permanent Impairment, 4th ed. American Medical Association, 1993.
2. Bird HA, Stowe J: The wrist. Clin Rheum Dis 1982;8:559–569.
3. Clarkson HM: Musculoskeletal Assessment: Joint Range of Motion and Manual Muscle Strength, 2nd ed. Baltimore, Williams & Wilkins, 2000.
4. Clemente CD (ed): Gray's Anatomy of the Human Body, 13th ed. Philadelphia, Lea & Febiger, 1985.
5. Greene WB, Heckman JD: The Clinical Measurement of Joint Motion. Rosemont, Ill, American Academy of Orthopaedic Surgeons, 1994.
6. Kapandji IA: The Physiology of the Joints, vol 1, Upper Limb, 5th ed. New York, Churchill Livingston, 1982.
7. LaStayo PC, Wheeler DL: Reliability of passive wrist flexion and extension goniometric measurements: A multicenter study. Phys Ther 1994;74:162–176.
8. Levangie PK, Norkin CC: Joint Structure and Function: A Comprehensive Analysis, 3rd ed. Philadelphia, F.A. Davis, 2001.
9. Mallon WJ, Brown HR, Nunley JA: Digital ranges of motion: Normal values in young adults. J Hand Surg 1991;16A:882–887.
10. Moore ML: Clinical Assessment of Joint Motion. In Basmajian JV: Therapeutic Exercise, 3rd ed. Baltimore, Williams & Wilkins, 1978.
11. Norkin CC, White DJ: Measurement of Joint Motion: A Guide to Goniometry, 2nd ed. Philadelphia, F.A. Davis, 1995.
12. Smith LK, Weiss EL, Lehmkuhl LD: Brunnstrom's Clinical Kinesiology, 5th ed. Philadelphia, F.A. Davis, 1996.

MUSCLE LENGTH TESTING of the UPPER EXTREMITY

INTRODUCTION

Unlike the lower extremity, only a few tests exist for examining the length of muscles in the upper extremity. Moreover, very little research has been conducted on the reliability of the tests described in the literature. The purpose of this section is to describe some early tests suggested in the literature for measurement of muscle length of the upper extremity and the rationale for not including these tests in this chapter on upper extremity muscle length measurement techniques. Additionally, nine tests for the examination of upper extremity muscle length are presented.

Apley's Scratch Test

In 1959, a physical education text published by Scott and French[8] introduced a test for upper extremity flexibility called the "opposite arm across the back" test. Hoppenfeld[3] later referred to this test as "Apley's scratch test." In 1960, Myers[7] described these tests to measure the muscle length of the shoulder and elbow, referring to this combination of tests as the "y position of the arms." The test (herein referred to as Apley's scratch test) consists of two parts that, depending on the author, could be performed on one extremity at a time or on two extremities simultaneously. One part involves asking the individual being tested to place the palm of the hand on the back by reaching behind the head and down between the shoulder blades as far as possible (Fig. 6–1). Hoppenfeld[3] suggested that this maneuver was a measurement of shoulder lateral rotation and abduction, and Sullivan and Hawkins[9] suggested that the test was a measurement for shoulder lateral rotation.

The second part of Apley's scratch test consists of asking the subject to place the dorsum of the hand against the back and to reach behind the back and up the spine as far as possible (see Fig. 6–1). Hoppenfeld[3] suggested that this maneuver measured shoulder medial rotation and adduction; Sullivan and Hawkins[9] suggested that the test examined shoulder medial rotation; and Mallon et al.[6] suggested that the test measured shoulder medial rotation and extension, elbow flexion, and scapular movement.

Techniques for documentation of the measurement have varied. Scott and French[8] suggested measuring the distance between the tips of the fingers of both hands when the two parts of the test are performed simultaneously. Goldstein[2] suggested performing the test one upper extremity at a time and recording the distance between the spinous process of C7 and the tip of the fingers. Finally, an alternative measurement presented by Magee[5] is to have the individual perform the test one extremity at a time and to record the levels of the vertebrae that the fingers most closely approximate.

Fig. 6–1. Apley's scratch test (From Magee DJ: Orthopedic Physical Therapy Assessment, 3rd ed. Philadelphia, WB Saunders, 1997, with permission), a composite test measuring multiple motions and muscles that is not included in this chapter.

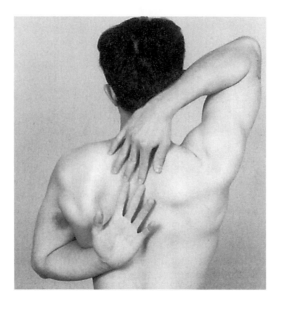

As suggested by the variety of interpretations of Apley's scratch test, the movement that takes place during the testing is poorly defined, and the actual muscles being examined for flexibility are not known. Therefore, the opposite arm across the back test, Apley's scratch test, is not included in the flexibility tests for the upper extremity presented in this chapter.

Shoulder and Wrist Elevation Test

In a text on flexibility written in 1977, Johnson[4] described the shoulder and wrist elevation test to measure shoulder flexibility. The test requires the individual to lift a stick or broom handle until the upper extremities are fully elevated overhead while lying in a prone position with the chin on a stable surface (Fig. 6–2). The individual raises the stick upward as high as possible by flexion at the shoulders.

Two methods have been described for documenting the amount of shoulder elevation achieved in this test. The first is simply to measure the distance from the stable surface to the stick.[1] In the second, which takes into consideration the length of the individual's upper extremity, the length of the upper extremity is measured, and the test score is determined by

Fig. 6–2. Shoulder and wrist elevation test, a composite test measuring multiple motions and muscles that is not included in this chapter.

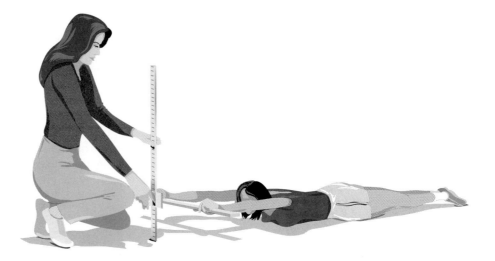

subtracting the height to which the stick is raised from the length of the arm.[4] A score of 0 is considered perfect.

In determining the techniques to include in this chapter, an effort was made to present techniques that can be performed easily, and that give the clinician the option of having the test performed passively or actively. The shoulder and wrist elevation test was not included because of the need for a minimal strength level in the shoulder and trunk musculature of the subject for the test to be performed, the difficulty in controlling back extension by the individual during the testing, and the inability of the test to be performed passively.

TECHNIQUES FOR TESTING MUSCLE LENGTH: UPPER EXTREMITY

Figures 6–3 through 6–29 illustrate the techniques for flexibility testing for the upper extremity that are included in this chapter. These measurement techniques were chosen because they could be performed passively by the clinician or actively by the patient, the tests do not require strength of the patient, and the examination can be performed easily.

Latissimus Dorsi Muscle Length

Fig. 6–3. End ROM for latissimus dorsi muscle length. Bony landmarks (lateral midline of trunk; shoulder, lateral to acromion; lateral epicondyle of humerus) indicated by orange line and dots.

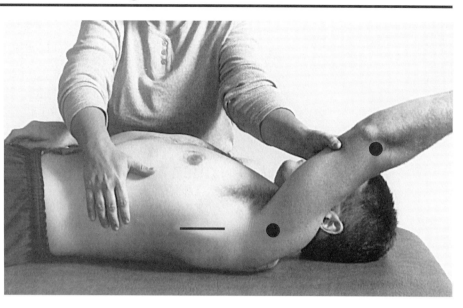

Patient position:	Supine, upper extremities at side with elbows extended; lumbar spine flat against support surface.
Examiner action:	After instructing patient in motion desired, examiner flexes shoulder through available range of motion (ROM) while maintaining elbow in full extension and keeping arms close to head; lumbar spine should remain flat against support surface. (Note: Examiner ordinarily would perform this task standing on same side as extremity being flexed. Examiner is standing on opposite side in photo so landmarks can be seen.) This passive movement allows an estimate of ROM available and demonstrates to patient exact motion required (Fig. 6–3).
Patient/Examiner action:	Patient flexes shoulder through full available ROM, keeping arm close to head. Examiner must ensure that elbow remains extended and lumbar spine remains flat against support surface (see Fig. 6–3).
Goniometer method:	Palpate bony landmarks (shown in Fig. 6–3) and align goniometer accordingly (Fig. 6–4).

Fig. 6–4. Patient position for measurement of latissimus dorsi muscle length using goniometer.

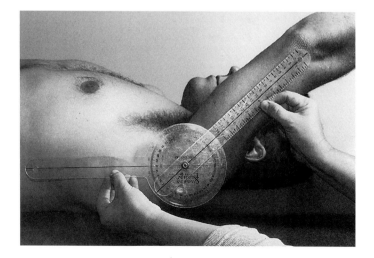

Fig. 6–5. Patient position for measurement of latissimus dorsi muscle length using tape measure.

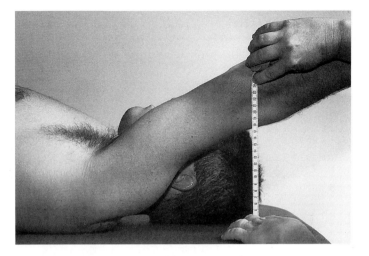

Stationary arm: Aligned with lateral midline of trunk.
Axis: Shoulder, lateral to acromion.
Moving arm: Lateral epicondyle of humerus.

Maintaining proper goniometric alignment, note amount of shoulder flexion (Fig. 6–4).

Tape measure method: Using tape measure or ruler, measure distance (inches or centimeters) between lateral epicondyle of humerus and support surface (Fig. 6–5).

Documentation: Record patient's amount of shoulder flexion or distance from lateral epicondyle of humerus to support surface.

Pectoralis Major Muscle Length: General

Fig. 6-6. Starting position for measurement of pectoralis major muscle length.

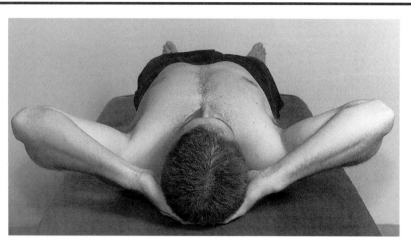

Patient position: Supine, with hands clasped together behind head; cervical spine should not flex any more than necessary to place clasped hands behind head (Fig. 6-6).

Patient/Examiner action: Examiner ensures that patient maintains clasped hands and does not flex cervical spine. Patient relaxes shoulder muscles, allowing elbows to move

Fig. 6–7. Patient position for measurement of pectoralis major muscle length using tape measure.

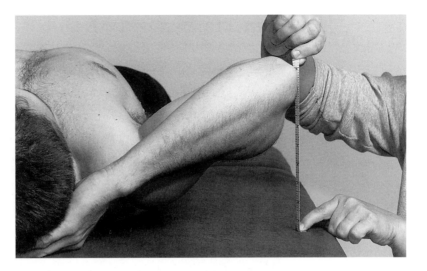

toward support surface; lumbar spine should remain flat against support surface (see Fig. 6–6).

Tape measure alignment:

Using tape measure or ruler, measure distance (inches or centimeters) between olecranon process of humerus and support surface (Fig. 6–7).

Documentation:

Record distance from support surface to olecranon process.

Pectoralis Major Muscle Length: Sternal (Lower) Portion

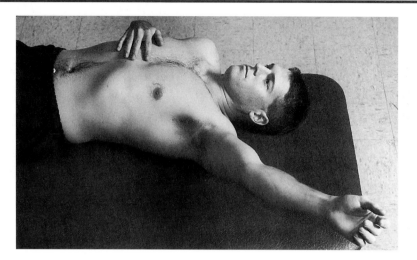

Fig. 6–8. Starting position for measurement of lower portion of pectoralis major muscle length.

Patient position: Supine, with shoulder laterally rotated and abducted to 135 degrees; elbow fully extended, and forearm supinated; lumbar spine flat against support surface (Fig. 6–8).

Patient/Examiner action: Ensuring that patient maintains shoulder in lateral rotation and 135 degrees of abduction, as well as full extension of elbow and supination of forearm, examiner asks patient to relax all shoulder muscles, allowing shoulder move into maximal horizontal abduction. Examiner must ensure that patient maintains lumbar spine flat against support surface and does not allow trunk rotation (especially to side of extremity being measured) (see Fig. 6–8).

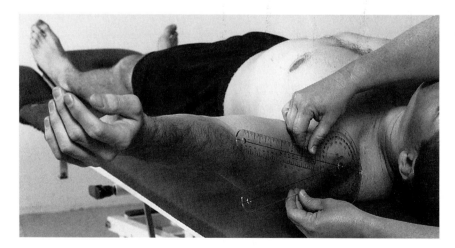

Fig. 6–9. Patient position for measurement of lower portion of pectoralis major muscle length using goniometer. Goniometer aligned with bony landmarks (parallel to support surface, lateral tip of acromion, midline of humerus toward lateral epicondyle).

Fig. 6–10. Patient position for measurement of lower portion of pectoralis major muscle length using tape measure.

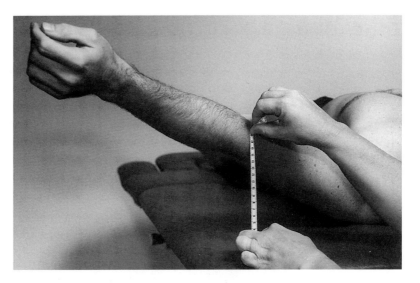

Goniometer method:	Palpate bony landmarks and align goniometer accordingly (Fig. 6–9).
Stationary arm:	Parallel to support surface.
Axis:	Lateral tip of acromion.
Moving arm:	Along midline of humerus toward lateral epicondyle.

Maintaining proper goniometric alignment, note amount of shoulder horizontal abduction (Fig. 6–9).

Tape measure method: Using tape measure or ruler, measure distance (inches or centimeters) between lateral epicondyle of humerus and support surface (Fig. 6–10).

Documentation: Record patient's ROM or distance from support surface and lateral epicondyle of humerus.

Note: Figure 6–11 illustrates patient with excessive length in lower portion of pectoralis major muscle, which is not uncommon.

Fig. 6–11. Example of excessive length in lower portion of pectoralis major muscle.

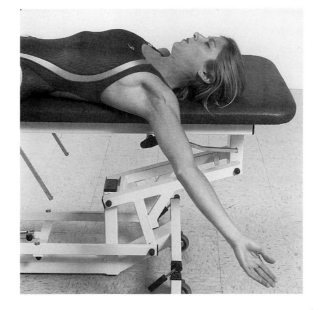

Pectoralis Major Muscle Length: Clavicular (Upper) Portion

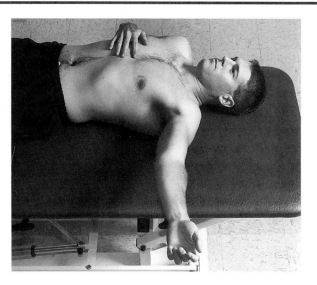

Fig. 6–12. Starting position for measurement of upper portion of pectoralis major muscle length.

Patient position: Supine, with shoulder laterally rotated and abducted to 90 degrees; elbow fully extended; forearm supinated; lumbar spine flat against support surface (Fig. 6–12).

Patient/Examiner action: Ensuring that patient maintains shoulder in lateral rotation and 90 degrees of abduction, as well as full extension of elbow and supination of forearm, examiner asks patient to relax all shoulder muscles, allowing shoulder to move into maximal horizontal abduction. Examiner must ensure that patient maintains lumbar spine flat against support surface and does not allow trunk rotation (especially to side of extremity being measured) (see Fig. 6–12).

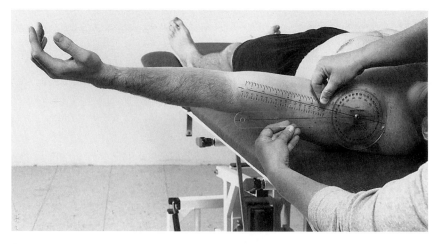

Fig. 6–13. Patient position for measurement of upper portion of pectoralis major muscle length using goniometer. Goniometer aligned with bony landmarks (parallel to support surface, lateral tip of acromion, midline of humerus toward lateral epicondyle).

Fig. 6-14. Patient position for measurement of upper portion of pectoralis major muscle length using tape measure.

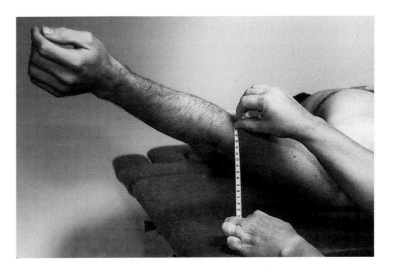

Goniometer method:	Palpate bony landmarks and align goniometer accordingly (Fig. 6–13).
Stationary arm:	Parallel to support surface.
Axis:	Lateral tip of acromion.
Moving arm:	Along midline of humerus toward lateral epicondyle.

Maintaining proper goniometric alignment, note amount of shoulder horizontal abduction (Fig. 6–13).

Tape measure method: Using tape measure, measure distance (inches or centimeters) between lateral epicondyle of humerus and support surface (Fig. 6–14).

Documentation: Record patient's ROM or distance from support surface and lateral epicondyle of humerus.

Note: Figure 6–15 illustrates patient with excessive length in upper portion of pectoralis major muscle, which is not uncommon.

Fig. 6-15. Example of excessive length in upper portion of pectoralis major muscle.

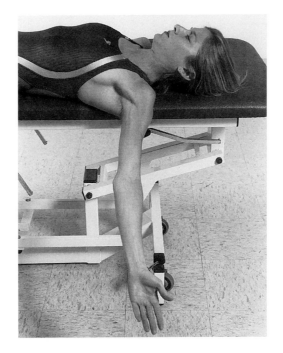

Pectoralis Minor Muscle Length

Fig. 6–16. Starting position for measurement of pectoralis minor muscle length. Bony landmark (posterior acromial border) for tape measure alignment indicated by orange dot.

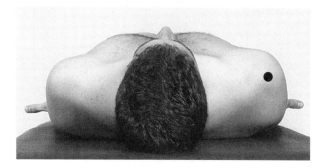

Patient position: Supine, with arms at side; shoulders laterally rotated; forearm supinated (palms up); lumbar spine should be flat against support surface (Fig. 6–16).

Patient/Examiner action: Examiner ensures that patient maintains arms at side with palms up and lumbar spine flat against the support surface. Patient relaxes shoulder muscles, allowing the posterior border of the acromion process to move toward support surface (see Fig. 6–16).

Fig. 6–17. Patient position for measurement of pectoralis minor muscle length using tape measure. Bony landmark (posterior acromial border) indicated by orange dot.

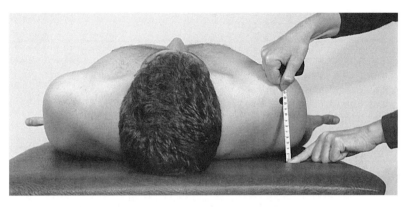

Tape measure alignment:

Palpate posterior acromial border (see Fig. 6–16). Using tape measure or ruler, measure distance (inches or centimeters) between posterior border of acromion process and support surface (Fig. 6–17).

Documentation:

Record distance from posterior border of acromion process and support surface.

Triceps Muscle Length

Fig. 6–18. Starting position for measurement of triceps muscle length. Bony landmarks (humeral head, lateral epicondyle of humerus, radial styloid process) indicated by orange dots.

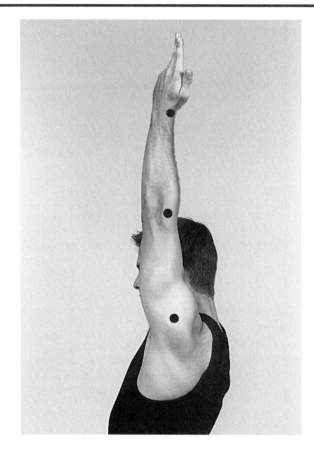

Patient position: Sitting, with shoulder in full flexion; elbow extended; forearm supinated (Fig. 6–18).

Examiner action: After instructing patient in motion desired, examiner flexes elbow through available ROM while maintaining full flexion of shoulder. This passive movement allows an estimate of ROM available and demonstrates to patient exact motion required (Fig. 6–19).

Fig. 6–19. End ROM of triceps muscle length. Bony landmarks (humeral head, lateral epicondyle of humerus, radial styloid process) indicated by orange dots.

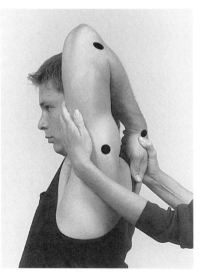

Fig. 6–20. Patient position and goniometer alignment at end of triceps muscle length.

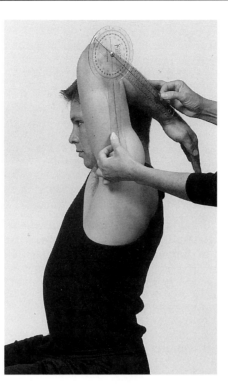

Patient/Examiner action:	Maintaining full shoulder flexion, perform passive, or have patient perform active, flexion of the elbow (Fig. 6–19).
Goniometer alignment:	Palpate following landmarks (shown in Fig. 6–18) and align goniometer accordingly (Fig. 6–20).
Stationary arm:	Lateral midline of humerus toward humeral head.
Axis:	Lateral epicondyle of humerus.
Moving arm:	Lateral midline of radius toward radial styloid.
	Maintaining proper goniometric alignment, read scale of goniometer (Fig. 6–20).
Documentation:	Record patient's maximum amount of elbow flexion.

Biceps Muscle Length

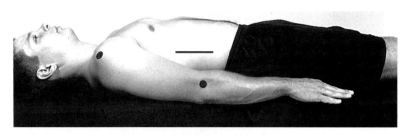

Fig. 6–21. Starting position for measurement of biceps muscle length. Bony landmarks (lateral midline of thorax, lateral aspect of acromion process, lateral epicondyle of humerus) indicated by orange line and dots.

Patient position:	Supine, with shoulder at edge of plinth; elbow extended; forearm pronated (Fig. 6–21).
Examiner action:	After instructing patient in motion desired, examiner extends shoulder through available ROM while maintaining elbow in full extension. This passive movement allows an estimate of ROM available and demonstrates to patient exact motion required (Fig. 6–22).
Patient/Examiner action:	Maintaining full elbow extension, perform passive, or have patient perform active, extension of the shoulder (Fig. 6–22).

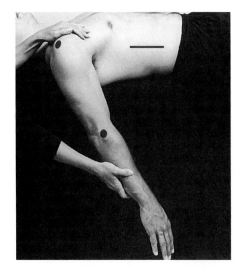

Fig. 6–22. End ROM of biceps muscle length. Bony landmarks (lateral midline of thorax, lateral aspect of acromion process, lateral epicondyle of humerus) indicated by orange line and dots.

Fig. 6–23. Patient position and goniometer alignment at end of biceps muscle length.

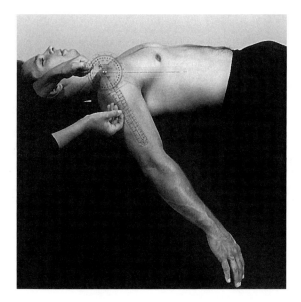

Goniometer alignment:	Palpate following landmarks (shown in Fig. 6–21) and align goniometer accordingly (Fig. 6–23).
Stationary arm:	Lateral midline of thorax.
Axis:	Lateral midline of humerus toward lateral aspect of acromion process.
Moving arm:	Lateral epicondyle of humerus.

Maintaining proper goniometric alignment, read scale of goniometer (Fig. 6–23).

Documentation:	Record patient's maximum amount of shoulder extension.

Flexor Digitorum Superficialis, Flexor Digitorum Profundus, and Flexor Digiti Minimi Muscle Length

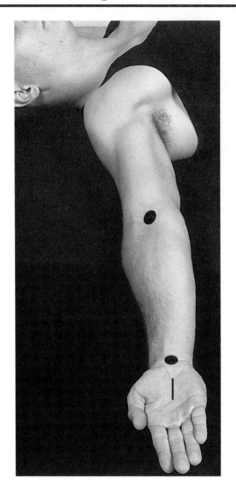

Fig. 6–24. Starting position for measurement of length of forearm flexor muscles. Landmarks (insertion of biceps muscle, lunate, volar midline of 3rd metacarpal) indicated by orange line and dots.

Patient position:	Supine, with shoulder abducted 70 to 90 degrees; elbow extended; forearm supinated; fingers extended (Fig. 6–24).
Examiner action:	After instructing patient in motion desired, examiner extends patient's wrist through available ROM while maintaining elbow and fingers in extension (Fig. 6–25). This passive movement allows an estimate of ROM available and demonstrates to patient exact motion required.
Patient/Examiner action:	Maintaining elbow and fingers in full extension, perform passive, or have patient perform active, extension of the wrist (Fig. 6–25).
Goniometer alignment:	Palpate following landmarks (shown in Fig. 6–25) and align goniometer accordingly (Fig. 6–26).

Fig. 6–25. End ROM of forearm flexor muscle length. Landmarks (insertion of biceps muscle, lunate, volar midline of 3rd metacarpal) indicated by orange line and dots.

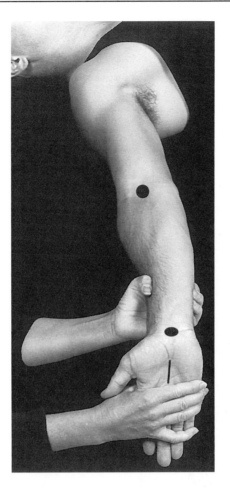

Stationary arm:	Insertion of biceps muscle.
Axis:	Lunate.
Moving arm:	Volar midline of 3rd metacarpal.

Maintaining proper goniometric alignment, read scale of goniometer (see Fig. 6–26). Note: Elbow must be maintained in full extension.

Documentation: Record patient's maximum amount of wrist extension.

Fig. 6–26. Patient position and goniometer alignment at end of forearm flexor muscle length.

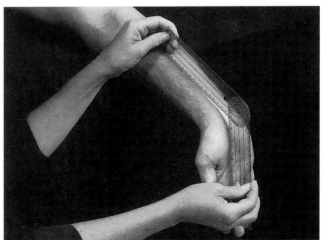

Extensor Digitorum, Extensor Indicis, and Extensor Digiti Minimi Muscle Length

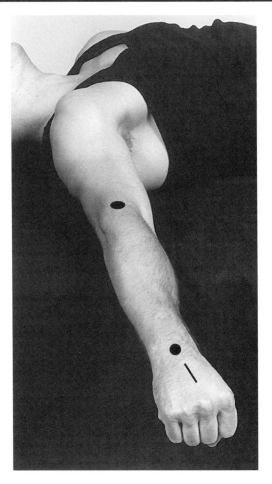

Fig. 6-27. Starting position for measurement of length of forearm extensor muscles. Bony landmarks (lateral epicondyle of humerus, lunate, dorsal midline of 3rd metacarpal) indicated by orange line and dots.

Patient position:	Supine, with shoulder abducted 70 to 90 degrees; elbow extended; forearm pronated; fingers flexed (Fig. 6–27).
Examiner action:	After instructing patient in motion desired, examiner flexes patient's wrist through available ROM while maintaining elbow in extension and fingers in flexion (Fig. 6–28). This passive movement allows an estimate of ROM available and demonstrates to patient exact motion required.
Patient/Examiner action:	Maintaining elbow in extension and fingers in flexion, perform passive, or have patient perform active, flexion of the wrist (Fig. 6–28).

Fig. 6–28. End ROM of forearm extensor muscle length. Bony landmarks (lateral epicondyle of humerus, lunate, dorsal midline of 3rd metacarpal) indicated by orange line and dots.

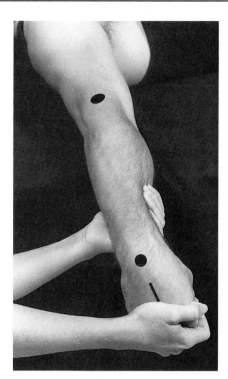

Goniometer alignment:	Palpate following landmarks (shown in Fig. 6–27) and align goniometer accordingly (Fig. 6–29).
Stationary arm:	Lateral epicondyle of humerus.
Axis:	Lunate.
Moving arm:	Dorsal midline of 3rd metacarpal.

Maintaining proper goniometric alignment, read scale of goniometer (see Fig. 6–29). Note: Elbow must be maintained in full extension.

Documentation: Record patient's maximum amount of wrist flexion.

Fig. 6–29. Patient position and goniometer alignment at end of forearm extensor muscle length.

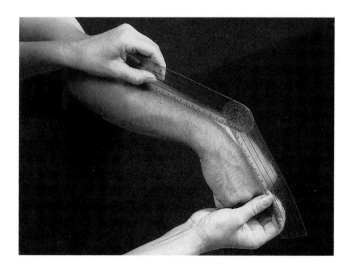

References

1. Corbin CB: Flexibility. Clin Sports Med 1984;3:101–117.
2. Goldstein TS: Functional Rehabilitation in Orthopedics. Gaithersburg, Md, Aspen Publications, 1995.
3. Hoppenfeld S: Physical Examination of the Spine and Extremities. Norwalk, Conn, Appleton & Lange, 1976.
4. Johnson BL: Practical Flexibility Measurement with the Flexomeasure. Portland, Tex, Brown and Littleman, 1977.
5. Magee DJ: Orthopedic Physical Assessment, 3rd ed. Philadelphia, WB Saunders, 1997.
6. Mallon WJ, Herring CL, Sallay PI, et al.: Use of vertebral levels to measure presumed internal rotation of the shoulder: A radiographic analysis. J Shoulder Elbow Surg 1996;5:299–306.
7. Myers H: Range of motion and flexibility. Phys Ther Rev 1960;41:177–182.
8. Scott MG, French E: Flexibility. Measurement and Evaluation in Physical Education. Dubuque, Iowa, Wm. C. Brown, 1959.
9. Sullivan JF, Hawkins RJ: Clinical examination of the shoulder complex. In Andrews JR, Wilk KE: The Athlete's Shoulder. New York: Churchill Livingstone, 1994.

RELIABILITY and VALIDITY of MEASUREMENTS of RANGE of MOTION and MUSCLE LENGTH TESTING of the UPPER EXTREMITY

RELIABILITY AND VALIDITY OF UPPER EXTREMITY GONIOMETRY

Chapters 3 through 6 described techniques for measuring joint range of motion and muscle length of the upper extremity. Research regarding reliability and validity of joint range of motion techniques is presented in this chapter (no studies examining reliability of upper extremity muscle length testing were found). Only those studies providing information as to both relative and absolute reliability or validity are included. More detailed information regarding appropriate analysis of reliability and validity is presented in Chapter 2.

Shoulder Flexion/Extension

Passive

A moderate amount of research has focused on the reliability of shoulder flexion and extension goniometry. The reliability of passive shoulder flexion and extension goniometry was studied by Riddle et al.[14] This group of investigators examined both intrarater and inter-rater reliability of passive shoulder flexion and extension range of motion in a group of 100 adult patients aged 19 to 77 years. The investigators used no standardized goniometric technique or patient positioning in this study. In an effort to determine whether the size of the goniometer used made a difference in the reliability obtained, two different sizes of universal goniometers were employed for the study. Intraclass correlation coefficients (ICCs) were calculated both within and between raters for each type of goniometer used. Intrarater reliability did not vary, and inter-rater reliability varied only slightly with the type of goniometer used to measure both shoulder flexion and extension. However, while intrarater reliabilities for shoulder flexion and extension were good (.98 for flexion and .94 for extension) (Table 7–1), inter-rater reliability for shoulder flexion was not as high (.87 and .89, respectively), and inter-rater reliability for shoulder extension was poor (.26 and .27, respectively) (Table 7–2).

Table 7-1. INTRARATER RELIABILITY: SHOULDER FLEXION/EXTENSION RANGE OF MOTION

SHOULDER FLEXION

Study	Technique	n	Sample	r*	ICC†
Sabari et al.[15]	AROM; sitting; standardized technique	30	Healthy adults (17–92 yr)		.97
	AROM; supine; standardized technique	30			.95
	PROM; sitting; standardized technique	30			.95
	PROM; supine; standardized technique	30			.94
Riddle et al.[14]	PROM; small goniometer; nonstandardized technique	100	Adult patients (19–77 yr)		.98
	PROM; large goniometer; nonstandardized technique	100	Adult patients (19–77 yr)		.98
Walker et al.[16]	AROM; AAOS technique	4	Healthy adults; no ages provided	>.81	
Greene & Wolf[6]	AROM; technique not described	20	Healthy adults (18–55 yr)		.96

SHOULDER EXTENSION

Study	Technique	n	Sample	r	ICC
Riddle et al.[14]	PROM; small goniometer; nonstandardized technique	100	Adult patients (19–77 yr)		.94
	PROM; large goniometer; nonstandardized technique	100	Adult patients (19–77 yr)		.94
Walker et al.[16]	AROM; AAOS technique	4	Healthy adults; no ages provided	>.81	
Greene & Wolf[6]	AROM; technique not described	20	Healthy adults (aged 18–55 yr)		.98

*Pearson's r
† Intraclass correlation
AROM, active range of motion; PROM; passive range of motion; AAOS, American Academy of Orthopaedic Surgeons

Active

A greater number of investigators have examined active shoulder flexion and extension goniometry than have examined passive flexion and extension goniometry. Unfortunately, all these investigators have chosen to focus on intrarater reliability, and no studies providing reliability coefficients between raters for active shoulder flexion or extension were found. In a study designed to compare reliability of the Ortho Ranger (an electronic, computerized goniometer) and the universal goniometer, Greene and Wolf[6] examined intrarater reliability of active shoulder flexion and extension goniometry, in addition to 12 other motions of the upper extremity, in 20 healthy adults. Measurements of shoulder flexion and extension were each taken three times per session across three testing sessions by the same examiner. Intrarater reliability for the measurements was analyzed using an ICC. Results revealed high reliability for the universal goniometer (.96 for flexion, .98 for extension) for both active shoulder flexion and extension (see Table 7–1). The 95% confidence interval (CI) for the universal goniometer was 3.9 degrees for shoulder flexion and 2.4 degrees for shoulder extension.

Table 7–2. INTER-RATER RELIABILITY: SHOULDER FLEXION/EXTENSION RANGE OF MOTION

SHOULDER FLEXION

Study	Technique	n	Sample	ICC*
Riddle et al.[14]	PROM; small goniometer; nonstandardized technique	50	Adult patients (19–77 yr)	.87
	PROM; large goniometer; nonstandardized technique	50	Adult patients (19–77 yr)	.89

SHOULDER EXTENSION

Study	Technique	n	Sample	ICC
Riddle et al.[14]	PROM; small goniometer; nonstandardized technique	50	Adult patients (19–77 yr)	.26
	PROM; large goniometer; nonstandardized technique	50	Adult patients (19–77 yr)	.27

* Intraclass correlation
PROM, passive range of motion

Walker and colleagues[16] also examined intrarater reliability of active shoulder flexion and extension goniometry. In a study designed to determine the normal active range of motion of 26 movements of the upper and lower extremities in older adults, measurements were taken in 60 persons aged 60 to 84 years. Techniques recommended by the American Academy of Orthopaedic Surgeons (AAOS) were used for all measurements. Prior to data collection, intrarater reliability was determined using four subjects. Although the exact number of motions measured to determine reliability was unclear from the authors' description of their methods, they reported Pearson product moment correlation coefficients (Pearson's r) for intrarater reliability "above .81" for active shoulder flexion and extension measurements (see Table 7–1) and a mean error between repeated measures of 5 degrees.

In a report published in 1998, a group of investigators performed a study designed to determine whether intrarater reliability of measurements of active and passive shoulder flexion and abduction changed when the subjects were placed in a seated as compared with a supine position (Sabari et al.[15]). Two measurements were taken of each motion in each position in 30 adult subjects, aged 17 to 92 years. Data were analyzed using ICCs, which ranged from .94 to .97 for intrarater reliability of shoulder flexion, regardless of the type of motion measured (active or passive) or of the patient's position during the measurement (supine or sitting) (see Table 7–1). However, paired t tests between goniometric readings taken in trial 1 compared with trial 2 revealed a significant difference ($p < .05$) in the measurement of passive shoulder flexion taken in a supine position.

Shoulder Abduction

Active

Intrarater reliability of active shoulder abduction has been examined by three groups of investigators whose studies have been described previously (Greene and Wolf,[6] Sabari et al.,[15] and Walker et al.[16]). Techniques

Table 7–3. INTRARATER RELIABILITY: SHOULDER ABDUCTION RANGE OF MOTION

SHOULDER ABDUCTION

Study	Technique	n	Sample	r*	ICC†
Sabari et al.[15]	AROM; sitting; standardized technique	30	Healthy adults (17–92 yr)		.97
	AROM; supine; standardized technique	30			.99
	PROM; sitting; standardized technique	30			.95
	PROM; supine; standardized technique	30			.98
Riddle et al.[14]	PROM; small goniometer; nonstandardized technique	100	Adult patients (19–77 yr)		.98
	PROM; large goniometer; nonstandardized technique	100	Adult patients (19–77 yr)		.98
Pandya et al.[12]	PROM; supine; AAOS technique	150	Patients with Duchenne's muscular dystrophy (<1–20 yr)		.84
Walker et al.[16]	AROM; AAOS technique	4	Healthy adults; no ages provided	>.81	
Greene & Wolf[6]	AROM; technique not described	20	Healthy adults (18–55 yrs)		.96

*Pearson's r
†Intraclass correlation
AROM, active range of motion; PROM, passive range of motion; AAOS, American Academy of Orthopaedic Surgeons

recommended by the AAOS were used in the study by Walker et al.,[16] whereas the other two studies were not specific regarding the measuring techniques employed. All three studies were performed in healthy adult subjects. Greene and Wolf[6] and Sabari et al.[15] analyzed their data using ICCs and performed follow-up measures of concordance on the data. Sabari et al.[15] reported correlations ranging from .97 to .99 for active shoulder abduction goniometry, depending on the patient position used (Table 7–3). Paired t tests revealed no significant difference ($p > .05$) between measures of active shoulder abduction range of motion taken in the two trials, regardless of patient position. Greene and Wolf[6] analyzed their data using the ICC and reported intrarater reliability of .96 (see Table 7–3) and a 95% confidence level of 6.4 degrees. Walker et al.[16] used Pearson's r for data analysis and reported a correlation of greater than .81 (see Table 7–3) and a mean error of 5 degrees (±1 degree).

Passive

Both Sabari et al.[15] and Riddle et al.[14] investigated the reliability of passive shoulder abduction goniometry in adult subjects. These studies, which have been described elsewhere (see the Shoulder Flexion/Extension section), yielded ICCs for intrarater reliability of passive shoulder abduction measurements ranging from .95 to .98 (see Table 7–3).[14, 15] However, follow-up paired t tests between goniometric readings taken in trial 1 compared with trial 2 in the study by Sabari et al.[15] revealed a significant difference ($p < .05$) in the measurement of passive shoulder abduction taken with the

Table 7-4. INTER-RATER RELIABILITY: SHOULDER ABDUCTION RANGE OF MOTION

SHOULDER ABDUCTION

Study	Technique	*n*	Sample	ICC*
Riddle et al.[14]	PROM; small goniometer; nonstandardized technique	50	Adult patients (19–77 yr)	.84
	PROM; large goniometer; nonstandardized technique	50	Adult patients (19–77 yr)	.87
Pandya et al.[12]	PROM; supine; AAOS technique	21	Patients with Duchenne's muscular dystrophy (<1–20 yrs)	.67

* Intraclass correlation
PROM, passive range of motion; AAOS, American Academy of Orthopaedic Surgeons

sub-ject in a sitting position. Riddle et al.[14] also analyzed inter-rater reliability of passive shoulder abduction in adult subjects and reported somewhat lower correlations of .84, using a small goniometer, to .87, using a large goniometer (Table 7–4).

Both intrarater and inter-rater reliabilities have been reported for passive shoulder abduction measurements in children. Pandya et al.[12] examined intrarater reliability of passive shoulder abduction goniometry in 150 children with Duchenne's muscular dystrophy.[12] Intraclass correlation coefficients were used to analyze the data, and reliability was reported as .84 (see Table 7–3). Inter-rater reliability of passive shoulder abduction in a subgroup of 21 children with Duchenne's muscular dystrophy also was examined, and reliability of .67 was reported (see Table 7–4).

Shoulder Medial/Lateral Rotation

Passive

Reliability of passive shoulder rotation goniometry has been studied by only two groups of investigators. Riddle et al.[14] examined both intrarater and inter-rater reliability of measurements of passive shoulder range of motion, including shoulder medial and lateral rotation, using two different sizes of universal goniometers. Range of motion was measured in 100 patients aged 19 to 77 years without the use of standardized measuring or positioning techniques. Intrarater reliability (ICC) for passive shoulder rotation ranged from .93, for medial rotation using a small goniometer, to .99, for lateral rotation using a large goniometer (Table 7–5). Reliability between raters for lateral rotation remained high and was reported as .90 and .88 for a small and a large goniometer, respectively. However, inter-rater reliability for passive shoulder medial rotation was fairly low, equaling .43 with a small goniometer and .55 with a large goniometer (Table 7–6).

MacDermid et al.[10] also examined reliability of passive shoulder rotation goniometry but focused exclusively on passive lateral rotation measurements. In a study of 34 patients older than 55 years with shoulder pathology, MacDermid and colleagues[10] measured passive lateral rotation of the shoulder while the patient was supine with the shoulder abducted 20 to 30 degrees. Both intrarater and inter-rater reliabilities were calculated using ICCs. Intrarater reliability was reported as .89 and .94 (see Table 7–5), and the

Table 7–5. INTRARATER RELIABILITY: SHOULDER MEDIAL/LATERAL ROTATION RANGE OF MOTION

SHOULDER MEDIAL ROTATION

Study	Technique	n	Sample	r*	ICC†
Riddle et al.[14]	PROM; small goniometer; nonstandardized technique	100	Adult patients (19–77 yr)		.93
	PROM; large goniometer; nonstandardized technique	100	Adult patients (19–77 yr)		.94
Walker et al.[16]	AROM; AAOS technique	4	Healthy adults; no ages provided	>.81	
Greene & Wolf[6]	AROM, technique not described	20	Healthy adults (18–55 yr)		.93

SHOULDER LATERAL ROTATION

Study	Technique	n	Sample	r	ICC
Riddle et al.[14]	PROM; small goniometer; nonstandardized technique	100	Adult patients (19–77 yr)		.98
	PROM; large goniometer; nonstandardized technique	100	Adult patients (19–77 yr)		.99
MacDermid et al.[10]	PROM; supine, shoulder abducted 20°–30°	34	Patients with shoulder pathology (over age 55 yr)		.89/.94‡
Boone et al.[2]	AROM; AAOS technique	12	Adult males (26–54 yr)		.96
Walker et al.[16]	AROM; AAOS technique	4	Healthy adults; no ages provided	.78	
Greene & Wolf[6]	AROM; technique not described	20	Healthy adults (18–55 yr)		.91

* Pearson's r
† Intraclass correlation
‡ Two separate examiners
PROM, passive range of motion; AROM, active range of motion; AAOS, American Academy of Orthopaedic Surgeons

standard error of measurement (SEMm) was 7.0 degrees and 4.9 degrees, depending on the examiner performing the measurement. Inter-rater reliability was .85 and .86 (see Table 7–6) with the SEMm reported as 7.5 degrees and 8.0 degrees, depending on whether the first or second measurement was used in the calculation.

Active

More groups have examined active shoulder rotation goniometry than have examined passive rotation goniometry. Greene and Wolf[6] and Walker et al.,[16] whose studies have been described previously, investigated the intrarater reliability of goniometric measurements of active shoulder medial and lateral rotation. The study by Walker et al.[16] included four healthy adults and reported a reliability of greater than .81 for shoulder medial rotation and .78 for lateral rotation (Pearson's r) and a mean error of 5 degrees, whereas Greene and Wolf[6] examined 20 healthy adults and reported a reliability of .91 (ICC) (see Table 7–5) and a 95% confidence level of 14.9 degrees for medial and 17.2 degrees for shoulder lateral rotation.

The reliability of goniometric measurements of active shoulder lateral rotation was examined by Boone and colleagues[2] in a group of 12 adult males aged 26 to 54 years. Four different examiners with varied experience in goniometry performed the measurements using AAOS measurement techniques. Measurements were taken once per week for 4 weeks by each of the four examiners. Average intrarater reliability was .96 (see Table 7–5), and repeated measures analysis of variance (ANOVA) revealed no significant intratester variation for measurements of shoulder lateral rotation. However, although average inter-rater reliability was .97 (see Table 7–6), repeated measures ANOVA demonstrated significant differences between two of the four examiners for measurements of shoulder lateral rotation.

Elbow Flexion/Extension

Active

Several groups of researchers have investigated the reliability of elbow flexion and extension goniometry. The majority of studies regarding the reliability of measuring elbow flexion range of motion involve measurements of active elbow flexion, the exception being a study by Rothstein and colleagues.[13] In contrast, reports of reliability of elbow extension goniometry include about equal numbers of measurements of active and passive joint motion.

Armstrong and colleagues[1] examined intrarater and inter-rater reliability of active elbow and forearm goniometric measurements in a group of 38

Table 7–6. INTER-RATER RELIABILITY: SHOULDER MEDIAL/LATERAL ROTATION RANGE OF MOTION

SHOULDER MEDIAL ROTATION

Study	Technique	n	Sample	ICC*
Riddle et al.[14]	PROM; small goniometer; nonstandardized technique	50	Adult patients (19–77 yr)	.43
	PROM; large goniometer; nonstandardized technique		Adult patients (19–77 yr)	.55

SHOULDER LATERAL ROTATION

Study	Technique	n	Sample	ICC
Riddle et al.[14]	PROM; small goniometer; nonstandardized technique	50	Adult patients (19–77 yr)	.90
	PROM; large goniometer; nonstandardized technique	50	Adult patients (19–77 yr)	.88
MacDermid et al.[10]	PROM; supine, shoulder abducted 20°–30°	34	Patients with shoulder pathology (over age 55 yr)	.85 / .86†
Boone et al.[2]	AROM; AAOS technique	12	Adult males (26–54 yr)	.97

* Intraclass correlation
† See text for further explanation.
PROM, passive range of motion; AROM, active range of motion; AAOS, American Academy of Orthopaedic Surgeons

patients aged 14 to 72 years. Each of the subjects had undergone a surgical procedure for an injury to the elbow, the forearm, or the wrist a minimum of 6 months prior to measurement. Standardized measuring techniques and patient positioning were used during the testing, in which three different instruments were employed to assess range of motion. The instruments used for the study included a universal goniometer, a computerized goniometer, and "a mechanical rotation measuring device."[1] Only the universal goniometer and the computerized goniometer were used to measure elbow flexion and extension, as the rotation measuring device was capable only of measuring forearm rotation. Active elbow flexion and extension range of motion were measured twice for each instrument on all subjects. Five different examiners, who possessed varied amounts of experience in performing goniometry, measured the amount of elbow flexion and extension in each subject. Both intrarater and inter-rater reliability were analyzed using ICCs. Intrarater reliability for active elbow flexion using the universal goniometer ranged from .55 to .98, depending on which examiner performed the measurements (Table 7–7). Similar intrarater reliability levels were obtained for active elbow extension, ranging from .45 to .98 (see Table 7–7). Of interest is the fact that the lowest reliability levels were produced by an experienced

Table 7–7. INTRARATER RELIABILITY: ELBOW FLEXION/EXTENSION RANGE OF MOTION

ELBOW FLEXION

Study	Technique	n	Sample	r*	ICC[†]
Greene & Wolf[6]	AROM; technique not described	20	Healthy adults (18–55 yr)		.94
Goodwin et al.[7]	AROM; standardized technique	23	Healthy females (18–31 yr)	.61–.92[‡]	.56–.91[‡]
Armstrong et al.[1]	AROM; standardized technique	38	Patients (14–72 yr)		.55–.98[§]
Rothstein et al.[13]	PROM; nonstandardized technique	12	Patients; no ages provided	.95–.99[‖]	.86–.96[‖]
Boone et al.[2]	AROM; AAOS technique	12	Healthy adult males (26–54 yr)		.94
Walker et al.[16]	AROM; AAOS technique	4	Healthy adults; no ages provided	>.81	

ELBOW EXTENSION

Study	Technique	n	Sample	r	ICC
Green & Wolf[6]	AROM; technique not described	20	Healthy adults (18–55 yr)		.95
Armstrong et al.[1]	AROM; standardized technique	38	Patients (14–72 yr)		.45–.98[§]
Rothstein et al.[13]	PROM; nonstandardized technique	12	Patients; no ages provided	.95–.98[‖]	.94–.96[‖]
Pandya et al.[12]	PROM; AAOS technique	150	Patients with Duchenne's muscular dystrophy (<1–20 yr)		.87
Walker et al.[16]	AROM; AAOS technique	4	Healthy adults; no ages provided	>.81	

* Pearson's r
[†] Intraclass correlation
[‡] Three separate examiners
[§] Five separate examiners
[‖] Correlation depended on type of goniometer used.
AROM, active range of motion; PROM, passive range of motion; AAOS, American Academy of Orthopaedic Surgeons

Table 7–8. INTER-RATER RELIABILITY: ELBOW FLEXION/EXTENSION RANGE OF MOTION				

ELBOW FLEXION

Study	Technique	*n*	Sample	ICC*
Armstrong et al.[1]	AROM; standardized technique	38	Patients (14–72 yr)	.58/.62[†]
Boone et al.[2]	AROM; AAOS technique	12	Healthy adult males (26–54 yr)	.88
Rothstein et al.[13]	PROM; nonstandardized technique	12	Patients; no ages provided	.85–.97[†]
Petherick et al.[11]	AROM; standardized technique	30	Healthy adults (mean age 24 yr)	.53

ELBOW EXTENSION

Study	Technique	*n*	Sample	ICC
Armstrong et al.[1]	AROM; standardized technique	38	Patients (14–72 yr)	.58/.87[†]
Pandya et al.[12]	PROM; AAOS technique	21	Patients with Duchenne's muscular dystrophy (<1–20 yr)	.91
Rothstein et al.[13]	PROM; nonstandardized technique	12	Patients; no ages provided	.92–.96[†]

* Intraclass correlation
[†] See text for further explanation.
AROM, active range of motion; AAOS, American Academy of Orthopaedic Surgeons; PROM, passive range of motion

hand therapist, while less experienced examiners demonstrated higher reliability. Ninety-five percent CIs within raters averaged 6 degrees for elbow flexion and 7 degrees for elbow extension. Inter-rater reliability for elbow flexion using the universal goniometer was reported as .58 and .62, depending on which set of measurements was used for the analysis. Levels of inter-rater reliability reported by Armstrong et al.[1] were similar to levels of reliability reported previously by Petherick et al.,[11] but were lower than the reliability reported by Boone et al.[2] (discussed subsequently). Elbow extension inter-rater reliability using the universal goniometer was reported as .58 and .87 (Table 7–8), again depending on which set of measurements was used for the analysis. Ninety-five percent CIs between raters averaged 10 degrees for both elbow flexion and extension.

Goodwin and colleagues[7] also used a variety of examiners and instruments in their study of the reliability of measurements of active elbow flexion range of motion. These investigators compared the reliability of the universal goniometer, of a fluid goniometer, and of an electrogoniometer using three experienced examiners measuring a group of 24 healthy females, aged 18 to 31 years. Active elbow flexion was measured in each subject by all three examiners using each of the three instruments on two separate occasions. Standardized measurement techniques and patient positioning were employed by all three examiners in all subjects. Test-retest reliability for each examiner using each type of measuring device was calculated using both Pearson's *r* and the ICC. Reliabilities for the universal goniometer ranged from .61 to .92 using Pearson's *r* and from .56 to .91 using ICCs, depending on which of the three examiners performed the measurements (see Table 7–7).

Several other groups of researchers whose studies have been described previously have investigated the reliability of measurements of active elbow flexion and extension. Greene and Wolf[6] and Walker et al.[16] both examined the intrarater reliability of active elbow flexion and extension goniometry in healthy adults. Reliability was analyzed using either Pearson's r (Walker et al.[16]) or the ICC (Greene and Wolf[6]). Walker et al.[16] reported reliability as greater than .81 (see Table 7–7), with a mean error of 5 degrees. Greene and Wolf[6] reported reliability of .94 for elbow flexion and .95 for elbow extension (see Table 7–7), with 95% confidence levels of 3.0 degrees for elbow flexion and 1.9 degrees for elbow extension.

The reliability (intrarater and inter-rater) of goniometric measurements of active elbow flexion range of motion was examined by Boone and colleagues[2] in a group of 12 healthy males aged 26 to 54 years. Measuring techniques advocated by the AAOS were used in the study. Average intrarater reliability was .94 (see Table 7–7), and repeated measures of ANOVA revealed no significant intra-tester variation for measurements of elbow flexion. Although average inter-rater reliability was .88 (see Table 7–8), repeated measures ANOVA demonstrated significant differences between all four of the examiners for measurements of elbow flexion.

One other group of researchers examined the reliability of active elbow flexion goniometry, but this group confined their investigation to inter-rater reliability of this motion. Petherick and colleagues[11] compared the inter-rater reliability of active elbow flexion measurements taken with the universal goniometer with those taken with the fluid-based goniometer in a group of 30 healthy subjects with a mean age of 24 years. Two examiners measured active elbow flexion three times with both instruments on each subject. Standardized measuring techniques and patient positioning were used during the testing procedure. The mean of the three measurements was used to calculate the ICC for each instrument. Intrarater reliability was not reported for either of the two examiners. Inter-rater reliability using the universal goniometer to measure active elbow flexion was reported as .53 (see Table 7–8), whereas reliability using the fluid-based goniometer was .92. The reliability level using the universal goniometer was similar to that reported by Armstrong et al.[1] but lower than that reported by Boone et al.[2] (see Table 7–8).

Passive

While the majority of the studies examining the reliability of measurements of passive elbow motion have focused on passive elbow extension, one group of researchers investigated the intrarater and inter-rater reliability of goniometric measurements of passive elbow flexion as well as extension. Rothstein and colleagues[13] measured passive elbow flexion and extension in 12 patients of unstated age using three different, commonly used, goniometers. Twelve different examiners performed the measurements, although any one patient was measured by only two different examiners. Data were analyzed using both Pearson's r and the ICC. Intrarater reliability ranged from .86 to .99 for elbow flexion and from .94 to .98 for elbow extension (see Table 7–7). Inter-rater reliability ranged from .85 to .97 for elbow flexion and from .92 to .96 for elbow extension (see Table 7–8). In the case of both intrarater and inter-rater reliability levels, values obtained were dependent on the type of goniometer used and the type of statistical analysis performed. Additionally, inter-rater reliability levels were dependent on which measurement was used for comparison purposes (first measurement, second measurement, or mean).

Reliability of passive elbow extension, but not of flexion, was investigated in a pediatric population by Pandya and colleagues.[12] American Academy of Orthopaedic Surgeons' techniques were used to measure passive elbow extension with the universal goniometer. Intrarater reliability of passive elbow extension measurements was analyzed on 150 subjects with Duchenne's muscular dystrophy, and inter-rater reliability was analyzed on a subgroup of 21 of those subjects. In this group of children with muscular dystrophy, intrarater reliability was .87 (see Table 7–7), while inter-rater reliability was .91 (see Table 7–8).

Forearm Pronation/Supination

Some investigators who examined the reliability of goniometric measurements of elbow flexion and extension also examined the reliability of goniometric measurements of forearm pronation and supination. Although no studies were discovered that examined the reliability of measurements of passive forearm motion, three separate groups have investigated the reliability of measurements of active forearm motion. Both Greene and Wolf[6] and Walker et al.[16] examined the intrarater reliability of active forearm pronation and supination in healthy adults. In their study comparing the reliability of the universal goniometer and the Ortho Ranger (see the more complete description of the study in the preceding Shoulder Flexion/Extension section), Greene and Wolf[6] measured active forearm pronation and supination in 20 healthy subjects aged 18 to 55 years. Data were analyzed using the ICC, and intrarater reliability was .90 for forearm pronation and .98 for forearm supination (Table 7–9). Ninety-five percent CIs were reported for forearm pronation and supination, and were 9.1 degrees and 8.2 degrees, respectively. Walker et al.[16] measured active forearm pronation and supination in a group of four healthy adults and obtained intrarater reliability levels of greater than .81, and a mean error of 5 degrees, for both measurements using Pearson's r (see Table 7–9).

Both intrarater and inter-rater reliability of active forearm pronation and supination were investigated by Armstrong and her colleagues[1] in a group of 38 subjects aged 14 to 72 years. Each subject had undergone a surgical procedure to the upper extremity a minimum of six months prior to measurement. Three separate instruments and five separate examiners were used in the study (see the full description in the preceding Elbow Flexion/

Table 7–9. INTRARATER RELIABILITY: FOREARM PRONATION/SUPINATION RANGE OF MOTION

FOREARM PRONATION

Study	Technique	n	Sample	r*	ICC†
Green & Wolf[6]	AROM; technique not described	20	Healthy adults (18–55 yr)		.90
Armstrong et al.[1]	AROM; standardized technique	38	Patients (14–72 yr)		.96–.99‡
Walker et al.[16]	AROM; AAOS technique	4	Healthy adults; no ages provided	>.81	

FOREARM SUPINATION

Study	Technique	n	Sample	r	ICC
Green & Wolf[6]	AROM; technique not described	20	Healthy adults (18–55 yr)		.98
Armstrong et al.[1]	AROM; standardized technique	38	Patients (14–72 yr)		.96–.99‡
Walker et al.[16]	AROM; AAOS technique	4	Healthy adults; no ages provided	>.81	

* Pearson's r
† Intraclass correlation
‡ Five separate examiners
AROM, active range of motion; AAOS, American Academy of Orthopaedic Surgeons

Table 7–10. INTER-RATER RELIABILITY: FOREARM PRONATION/SUPINATION RANGE OF MOTION

FOREARM PRONATION

Study	Technique	*n*	Sample	ICC*
Armstrong et al.[1]	AROM; standardized technique	38	Patients (14–72 yr)	.83/.86[†]

FOREARM SUPINATION

Study	Technique	*n*	Sample	ICC
Armstrong et al.[1]	AROM; standardized technique	38	Patients (14–72 yr)	.90/.93[†]

* Intraclass correlation
[†] See text for further information.
AROM, active range of motion

Extension section). Intrarater reliability for the universal goniometer ranged from .96 to .99 for both active forearm pronation and supination motions, depending on the examiner performing the measurement (see Table 7–9). Inter-rater reliability was slightly lower for the two measurements, with reliability coefficients reported as .83 and .86 for forearm pronation and .90 and .93 for forearm supination, depending on which set of measurements was used for the analysis (Table 7–10). Ninety-five percent CIs within raters averaged 8 degrees for both forearm pronation and supination, whereas CIs between raters averaged 10 degrees for pronation and 11 degrees for supination.

Wrist Flexion/Extension

Passive

LaStayo and Wheeler[9] coordinated a multicenter study that focused on the reliability of three different methods of performing goniometric measurement of passive wrist flexion and extension. One hundred forty patients, aged 6 to 81 years, from eight different clinical sites around the United States, were recruited for the study. Thirty-two examiners from the eight clinics performed the goniometric measurements. In each of the clinics participating in the study, examiners were randomly paired for purposes of determining inter-rater reliability. Passive wrist flexion and extension were measured twice in each subject by each member of the randomly chosen pair of examiners, using three different measuring techniques. The three techniques used for measuring passive wrist motion included positioning the goniometer: 1) along the radial side of the forearm, with the stationary arm aligned with the "radial midline of the forearm" and the moving arm aligned with the "longitudinal axis of the second metacarpal"; 2) along the ulnar side of the forearm, with the stationary arm aligned with the "longitudinal midline of the ulna toward the olecranon" and the moving arm aligned with the "longitudinal axis of the third metacarpal"; and 3) along the dorsal (for flexion) or volar (for extension) surface of the wrist, with the stationary arm aligned with the dorsal or volar surface of the forearm and the moving arm aligned with the "longitudinal axis of the third metacarpal."[9] The ICC was used to analyze the data for both intrarater and inter-rater reliability. Intrarater reliability ranged from .80 for measurements of passive wrist extension using ulnar or radial alignment to .92 for measurements of passive wrist flexion using dorsal alignment (Table 7–11). The SEMm for wrist flexion within examiners ranged from 5.48 to 9.68 degrees for the radial alignment technique, from 5.52 to 9.10 degrees for the ulnar alignment technique, and from 4.11 to 7.12 degrees for the dorsal alignment technique, depending on the clinic in which the measurements were taken. For wrist extension, the SEMm within examiners ranged from 6.60 to 9.98 degrees using the radial alignment technique, from 6.29 to 10.58 degrees using the ulnar alignment technique, and from 3.87 to 9.20 degrees using the volar alignment technique, again depending on the clinic in which the measurements were taken. Inter-rater reliability ranged from .80 for measurements of passive wrist extension using radial or ulnar alignment to .93 for measurements of passive wrist flexion using dorsal alignment. The SEMm for wrist flexion between examiners ranged from 4.74 to 9.28 degrees for the radial alignment technique, from 4.67 to 8.85 degrees for the ulnar alignment technique, and from 4.59 to 6.50 degrees for the dorsal alignment technique. For wrist extension, the SEMm between examiners ranged from 6.36 to 11.16 degrees using the radial alignment technique, from 6.29 to 11.33 degrees

Table 7–11. INTRARATER RELIABILITY: WRIST FLEXION/EXTENSION RANGE OF MOTION

WRIST FLEXION

Study	Technique	n	Sample	r*	ICC†
LaStayo & Wheeler[9]	PROM; radial alignment	140	Patients (6–81 yr)		.86
	PROM; ulnar alignment	140	Patients (6–81 yr)		.87
	PROM; dorsal alignment	140	Patients (6–81 yr)		.92
Horger[8]	AROM; nonstandardized technique	48	Patients (18–71 yr)		.96
	PROM; nonstandardized technique	48	Patients (18–71 yr)		.96
Walker et al.[16]	AROM; AAOS technique	4	Healthy adults; no ages provided	>.81	
Greene & Wolf[6]	AROM; technique not described	20	Healthy adults (18–55 yr)		.96

WRIST EXTENSION

Study	Technique	n	Sample	r	ICC
LaStayo & Wheeler[9]	PROM; radial alignment	140	Patients (6–81 yr)		.80
	PROM; ulnar alignment	140	Patients (6–81 yr)		.80
	PROM; volar alignment	140	Patients (6–81 yr)		.84
Horger[8]	AROM; nonstandardized technique	48	Patients (18–71 yr)		.96
	PROM; nonstandardized technique	48	Patients (18–71 yr)		.96
Pandya et al.[12]	PROM; AAOS technique	150	Patients with Duchenne's muscular dystrophy (<1–20 yr)		.87
Walker et al.[16]	AROM; AAOS technique	4	Healthy adults; no ages provided	>.81	
Greene & Wolf[6]	AROM; technique not described	20	Healthy adults (18–55 yr)		.94

* Pearson's r
† Intraclass correlation
PROM, passive range of motion; AROM, active range of motion; AAOS, American Academy of Orthopaedic Surgeons

using the ulnar alignment technique, and from 3.53 to 9.20 degrees using the volar alignment technique. As was the case for the SEMm within examiners, variations in the SEMm were dependent on the clinic in which the measurements were taken. The authors concluded that the dorsal/volar alignment technique was "the most reliable method both within and between testers for measurements of passive wrist flexion and extension."[9]

In an earlier study, Horger[8] compared intrarater and inter-rater reliability of goniometric measurements of active compared with passive wrist motion. Thirteen examiners, with a range of experience of 2 months to 17 years, participated in the study. Forty-eight patients, whose ages ranged from 18 to 71 years, had both active and passive wrist motions measured twice each by two randomly paired examiners. No specific method of patient positioning or measuring technique was used during the study. The ICC was used to analyze the data, and results are reported in Tables 7–11 and 7–12. Intrarater reliability was high (.96) and did not vary, regardless of the motion (flexion compared with extension) or type of motion (active compared with passive) measured. The SEMm within raters was 3.5 and 4.4 degrees for passive wrist extension and flexion, respectively, whereas the SEMm for active motions was 3.7 degrees for extension and 4.5 degrees for flexion. Levels of inter-rater reliability were slightly lower (.84 to .91) and tended to be slightly higher for wrist flexion than for wrist extension. The SEMm between raters for passive wrist motions was 7.0 degrees for extension and 8.2 degrees for flexion. For active motion, the SEMm between raters was 7.0 degrees for extension and 6.6 degrees for flexion.

A third group of investigators, whose work has been described previously (see the preceding Shoulder Abduction section), examined the reliability of goniometric measurements of passive wrist motion, but this group measured wrist extension and not flexion (Pandya et al.[12]). Both intrarater and inter-rater reliability of goniometric measurements of passive wrist extension were investigated in groups of 150 and 21 patients, respectively, with Duchenne's muscular dystrophy. Techniques advocated by the AAOS were used in the study, and intrarater reliability was .87 (see Table 7–11), while inter-rater reliability was .83 (Table 7–12).

Active

While only Horger[8] has reported inter-rater reliability of goniometric measurements of active wrist motion, two other groups of investigators, in addition to Horger, have reported intrarater reliability of active wrist motion measurements. Both Walker et al.[16] and Greene and Wolf[6] have examined the intrarater reliability of goniometric measurements of active wrist flexion and extension. Healthy adults were used as the subjects in both studies, which have been described previously (see the preceding Shoulder Flexion/Extension section). Greene and Wolf[6] reported intrarater reliability levels that were quite similar to those reported by Horger[8] (see Table 7–11), with 95% CIs of 9.0 degrees for wrist flexion and 9.3 degrees for wrist extension. Intrarater reliability levels reported by Walker et al.[16] could not be precisely determined, being cited only as greater than .81 (see Table 7–11), with a mean error of 5 degrees.

Wrist Abduction/Adduction

Both intrarater and inter-rater reliability of wrist abduction (radial deviation) and adduction (ulnar deviation) motions have been investigated by Horger,[8] and Boone et al.[2] have investigated intrarater and inter-rater reliability of

Table 7–12. INTER-RATER RELIABILITY: WRIST FLEXION/EXTENSION RANGE OF MOTION

WRIST FLEXION

Study	Technique	n	Sample	ICC*
Horger[8]	AROM; nonstandardized technique	48	Patients (18–71 yr)	.91
	PROM; nonstandardized technique	48	Patients (18–71 yr)	.86
LaStayo & Wheeler[9]	PROM; radial alignment	140	Patients (6–81 yr)	.88
	PROM; ulnar alignment	140	Patients (6–81 yr)	.89
	PROM; dorsal alignment	140	Patients (6–81 yr)	.93

WRIST EXTENSION

Study	Technique	n	Sample	ICC
Horger[8]	AROM; nonstandardized technique	48	Patients (18–71 yr)	.85
	PROM; nonstandardized technique	48	Patients (18–71 yr)	.84
LaStayo & Wheeler[9]	PROM; radial alignment	140	Patients (6–81 yr)	.80
	PROM; ulnar alignment	140	Patients (6–81 yr)	.80
	PROM; volar alignment	140	Patients (6–81 yr)	.84
Pandya et al.[12]	PROM; AAOS technique	21	Patients with Duchenne's muscular dystrophy (<1–20 yr)	.83

* Intraclass correlation
AROM, active range of motion; PROM, passive range of motion; AAOS, American Academy of Orthopaedic Surgeons

wrist adduction measurements. These studies have been described previously (see the Wrist Flexion/Extension section for Horger[8] and the Shoulder Medial/Lateral Rotation section for Boone et al.[2]) and involved the use of different research protocols. Horger[8] used patients as subjects in her study and employed 13 examiners who measured both active and passive wrist motions without the use of a standardized technique. On the other hand, Boone et al.[2] used healthy adults as subjects and employed four examiners who measured only active wrist motions using AAOS techniques. Horger[8] reported intrarater reliability coefficients greater than or equal to .90 for goniometric measurements of active and passive wrist motions, with the exception of passive wrist adduction, where intrarater reliability was reported as .78 (Table 7–13). The SEMm within raters reported in the Horger[8] study ranged from 2.6 degrees, for active wrist abduction, to 3.5 degrees, for active wrist adduction. Intrarater reliability for goniometric measurements of active wrist adduction were higher in the Horger[8] study than in the study by Boone et al.[2] (.92 and .76, respectively) (see Table 7–13), and ANOVA reported in the Boone et al.[2] study revealed significant intratester variation for one examiner in measurements of active wrist adduction. While inter-rater reliability for measurements of active wrist adduction was similar between the two studies (Table 7–14), the ANOVA reported by Boone et al.[2] revealed significant intertester variation in measurements of wrist adduction between two of the examiners. The SEMm between examiners reported by Horger[8] ranged from 3.0 to 5.8 degrees for wrist abduction and adduction motions.

Table 7–13. INTRARATER RELIABILITY: WRIST ABDUCTION (RADIAL DEVIATION)/WRIST ADDUCTION (ULNAR DEVIATION) RANGE OF MOTION

WRIST ABDUCTION (RADIAL DEVIATION)

Study	Technique	n	Sample	r*	ICC[†]
Greene & Wolf[6]	AROM; technique not described	20	Healthy adults (18–55 yr)		.91
Horger[8]	AROM; nonstandardized technique	48	Patients (18–71 yr)		.90
	PROM; nonstandardized technique	48	Patients (18–71 yr)		.91
Walker et al.[16]	AROM; AAOS technique	4	Healthy adults; ages not provided	>.81	

WRIST ADDUCTION (ULNAR DEVIATION)

Study	Technique	n	Sample	r	ICC
Greene & Wolf[6]	AROM; technique not described	20	Healthy adults (18–55 yr)		.94
Horger[8]	AROM; nonstandardized technique	48	Patients (18–71 yr)		.92
	PROM; technique not standardized	48	Patients (18–71 yr)		.78
Walker et al.[16]	AROM; AAOS technique	4	Healthy adults; ages not provided	>.81	
Boone et al.[2]	AROM; AAOS technique	12	Adult males (26–54 yr)		.76

* Pearson's r
† Intraclass correlation
AROM, active range of motion; PROM, passive range of motion; AAOS, American Academy of Orthopaedic Surgeons

Table 7–14. INTER-RATER RELIABILITY: WRIST ABDUCTION (RADIAL DEVIATION)/WRIST ADDUCTION (ULNAR DEVIATION) RANGE OF MOTION

WRIST ABDUCTION (RADIAL DEVIATION)

Study	Technique	n	Sample	ICC*
Horger[8]	AROM; nonstandardized technique	48	Patients (18–71 yr)	.86
	PROM; nonstandardized technique	48	Patients (18–71 yr)	.66

WRIST ADDUCTION (ULNAR DEVIATION)

Study	Technique	n	Sample	ICC
Horger[8]	AROM; nonstandardized technique	48	Patients (18–71 yr)	.78
	PROM; nonstandardized technique	48	Patients (18–71 yr)	.83
Boone et al.[2]	AROM; AAOS technique	12	Adult males (26–54 yr)	.73

* Intraclass correlation
AROM, active range of motion; PROM, passive range of motion; AAOS, American Academy of Orthopaedic Surgeons

As they did for wrist flexion and extension motions, Greene and Wolf[6] and Walker et al.[16] used healthy adults to examine intrarater reliability of goniometric measurements of active wrist abduction and adduction range of motion. Greene and Wolf[6] reported intrarater reliability of .91 and a 95% CI of 7.6 degrees for active wrist abduction and a reliability of .94 and 95% CI of 8.4 degrees for active wrist adduction. Walker et al.[16] (1984) reported reliability only as greater than .81, with a mean error of 5 degrees for both measurements (see Table 7–13).

Finger Motion

So few studies were found in which statistical analysis of reliability levels were reported for goniometric measurements of finger range of motion that all such studies are discussed in this single section. No studies that used inferential statistics to analyze the reliability of goniometric measurements of the thumb were evident in the literature.

Only a single group of investigators has used the correlation coefficient to report reliability of discrete motion of any digit. Flowers and LaStayo[5] examined the intrarater reliability of goniometric measurements of passive extension of the proximal interphalangeal (PIP) joint in 20 fused PIP joints from seven patients. This examination of reliability was part of a larger study that investigated the correlation between the time spent in serial casting and the change in range of motion in PIP joints of the fingers. The measurement of passive motion in both studies involved placement of the goniometer over the dorsal surface of the joint while a predetermined, controlled extension torque was applied across the PIP joint. After the torque had been applied for 20 seconds, the goniometer was read, and the range of motion was recorded. Intrarater reliability of this so-called "torque passive range of motion test"[3, 5] was reported as .98 (ICC) (Table 7–15). Breger-Lee et al.[3] reported poor intrarater and inter-rater reliability using a technique that was similar, but with a dial rather than a universal goniometer.

In a study published in 2000, Brown et al.[4] investigated intrarater and inter-rater reliability of the finger goniometer compared with the Dexter hand evaluation and therapy system goniometer in the measurement of total active digit motion. Thirty patients, aged 21 to 66 years, with orthopaedic injuries of the upper extremity of at least 3 months' duration, were recruited for the study. Three examiners performed the goniometric measurements, which consisted of measuring the total active flexion and the total active extension of one injured finger and of the corresponding contralateral uninjured finger (not the thumb) of each subject. Each measurement was repeated three times by each examiner using standardized patient positioning and techniques for goniometer placement. Goniometer readings were rounded to the nearest 5 degrees. Both intrarater and inter-rater reliability were calculated using the ICC.

Table 7–15. INTRARATER RELIABILITY: FINGER ROM				
Study	**Technique**	**n**	**Sample**	**ICC***
Flowers & LaStayo[5]	PROM; PIP extension	20	Patients with fused PIP joints; 18–84 yr	.98
Brown et al.[4]	AROM; total active motion for digit	30	Patients with UE orthopaedic injuries; 21–66 yr	.97–.98[†]

* Intraclass correlation
[†] Three separate examiners
PROM, passive range of motion; PIP, proximal interphalangeal; AROM, active range of motion; UE, upper extremity

Table 7-16. INTER-RATER RELIABILITY: FINGER ROM				
Study	**Technique**	***n***	**Sample**	**ICC***
Brown et al.[4]	AROM; total active motions for digit	30	Patients with UE orthopaedic injuries; 21–66 yr	.98

* Intraclass correlation
AROM, active range of motion; UE, upper extremity

Intrarater reliability using the finger goniometer ranged from .97 to .98, depending on the examiner performing the measurement (see Table 7–15), whereas inter-rater reliability was .98 (Table 7–16).

RELIABILITY OF MUSCLE LENGTH TESTING

No research exists as to the reliability of measurements of muscle length of the upper extremity. Such research would be quite valuable for the clinician attempting to provide an upper extremity flexibility examination. The reader is encouraged to use the information on each technique presented in Chapter 6 and to perform reliability studies to enhance the knowledge base of muscle length testing.

References

1. Armstrong AD, MacDermid JC, Chinchalkar S, et al.: Reliability of range-of-motion measurement in the elbow and forearm. J Shoulder Elbow Surg 1998;7:573–580.
2. Boone DC, Azen SP, Lin C, et al.: Reliability of goniometric measurements. Phys Ther 1978;58:1355–1360.
3. Breger-Lee D, Voelker ET, Giurintano D, et al.: Reliability of torque range of motion. J Hand Ther 1993;6:29–34.
4. Brown A, Cramer LD, Eckhaus D, et al.: Validity and reliability of the Dexter hand evaluation and therapy system in hand-injured patients. J Hand Ther 2000;13:37–45.
5. Flowers KR, LaStayo P: Effect of total end range time on improving passive range of motion. J Hand Ther 1994;7:150–157.
6. Greene BL, Wolf SL: Upper extremity joint movement: Comparison of two measurement devices. Arch Phys Med Rehabil 1989;70:288–290.
7. Goodwin J, Clark C, Deakes J, et al.: Clinical methods of goniometry: A comparative study. Disabil Rehabil 1992;14:10–15.
8. Horger MM: The reliability of goniometric measurements of active and passive wrist motions. Am J Occ Ther 1990;44:342–348.
9. LaStayo PC, Wheeler DL: Reliability of passive wrist flexion and extension goniometric measurements: A multicenter study. Phys Ther 1994;74:162–176.
10. MacDermid JC, Chesworth BM, Patterson S, et al.: Intratester and intertester reliability of goniometric measurement of passive lateral shoulder rotation. J Hand Ther 1999;12:187–192.
11. Petherick M, Rheault W, Kimble S, et al.: Concurrent validity and intertester reliability of universal and fluid-based goniometers for active elbow range of motion. Phys Ther 1988;68:966–969.
12. Pandya S, Florence JM, King WM, et al.: Reliability of goniometric measurements in patients with Duchenne muscular dystrophy. Phys Ther 1985;65:1339–1342.
13. Rothstein JM, Miller PJ, Roettger RF: Goniometric reliability in a clinical setting: Elbow and knee measurements. Phys Ther 1983;63:1611–1615.
14. Riddle DL, Rothstein JM, Lamb RL: Goniometric reliability in a clinical setting: Shoulder measurements. Phys Ther 1987;67:668–673.
15. Sabari JS, Maltzev I, Lubarsky D, et al.: Goniometric assessment of shoulder range of motion: Comparison of testing in supine and sitting position. Arch Phys Med Rehabil 1998;79:647–651.
16. Walker JM, Sue D, Miles-Elkousy N, et al.: Active mobility of the extremities in older subjects. Phys Ther 1984;64:919–923.

HEAD, NECK, AND TRUNK

8

MEASUREMENT of RANGE of MOTION of the THORACIC and LUMBAR SPINE

ANATOMY AND OSTEOKINEMATICS

The intervertebral joints of the spine are composed of the superior and inferior vertebral facets, the vertebral bodies, and the discs that are interposed between the vertebral bodies. Ten (five pairs) facet joints make up the lumbar spine, and 24 (12 pairs) facet joints are in the thoracic spine. Motion at the intervertebral joints is relatively small and consists of gliding of the inferior facet of the vertebra above on the superior facet of the vertebra below. The combined effect of small motions at each facet and series of vertebrae produces a large range of motion (ROM) for the entire vertebral column.

The orientation of each facet joint determines the amount and direction of movement at the intervertebral joints. The spine can move anteriorly and posteriorly around the medial-lateral axis (flexion and extension), sidebend right and left around the anterior-posterior axis in the frontal plane (lateral flexion), and rotate right and left around the longitudinal axis of the spine in the transverse plane.

LIMITATIONS OF MOTION: THORACIC AND LUMBAR SPINE

Six main ligaments, which provide stability and limit motion, are associated with the intervertebral joints. The anterior longitudinal ligament prevents excessive spinal extension, while the posterior longitudinal, ligamentum flavum, interspinous, and supraspinous ligaments limit flexion of the spine. In addition, the spinous processes of the thoracic spine also limit extension. The intertransverse ligaments limit lateral flexion. Rotation of the spine is limited by facet orientation. Information on normal range of motion for the thoracic and lumbar spine may be found in Appendix C.

TECHNIQUES OF MEASUREMENT: THORACIC AND LUMBAR SPINE

Tape Measure

The least expensive instrument for measuring spinal movement, and perhaps the easiest to use, is a tape measure. Additionally, a tape measure has probably been used in the clinic for measuring range of motion of the spine longer than any other measurement technique.[5]

Flexion and Extension

SCHOBER METHOD

One of the most common tape measure procedures used to measure lumbar flexion relates to a technique originated by Schober and subsequently modified for measurement of spinal flexion. According to Macrae and Wright,[5] in 1937 Schober described the original two-mark method for measuring spinal flexion, in which one mark is made at the lumbosacral junction, and a second mark is made 10 cm above the first mark while the subject stands with the spine in a neutral position. After the standing subject bends forward as far as possible, the increase in distance between the first and second marks provides an estimate of the amount of flexion of the spine. Because the tape measure technique relies on stretching or distraction of the skin overlying the spine, the technique (and modifications of the technique) is sometimes referred to as the skin distraction method.

Macrae and Wright[5] modified the original Schober method by introducing a third mark, a measurement mark placed 5 cm below the lumbosacral junction. This modification uses a mark at the lumbosacral junction and other marks 5 cm inferior and 10 cm superior to the lumbosacral junction. The rationale offered by Macrae and Wright[5] for making the modification of the original Schober technique is that when using the Schober technique in their pilot work, the authors observed that the skin above and below the lumbosacral spine was distracted during flexion of the lumbar spine, leading to inaccuracies in measurement. Therefore, the technique that Macrae and Wright[5] referred to as the "modified" Schober technique, included three marks: 1) the lumbosacral junction; 2) 5 cm inferior to the lumbosacral junction; and 3) 10 cm superior to the lumbosacral junction.

Van Adrichen and van der Korst[9] suggested that using the lumbosacral junction (the base mark used for the Schober technique), which had to be identified by palpation, added difficulty to this method of measurement. Given this information, Williams et al.[10] suggested the use of the "modified-modified Schober," rather than either the Schober or the modified Schober. The modified-modified Schober uses two skin landmarks (as opposed to the three skin landmarks used with the modified Schober). The two landmarks include a point bisecting a line that connects the two posterior superior iliac spines (PSIS) (base line) and a mark 15 cm superior to the base line landmark. Given the ease of palpating the PSIS and the difficulty in determining the lumbosacral junction, the base line for measuring lumbar flexion and thoracolumbar flexion used in this chapter is the bisection of the line connecting the two PSIS described by Williams et al.[10] (See Figs. 8–2 to 8–9.)

Moll and Wright[7] suggested that modifications of the Schober technique might be appropriate for the examination of lumbar extension. These authors suggested measuring the change in skin marks as the marks move closer together during the extension movement. Again, for reasons previously described, the base line for measuring lumbar extension used in this chapter is the bisection of the line connecting the two PSIS described by Williams et al. (See Figs. 8–22 to 8–25.)

FINGERTIP-TO-FLOOR METHOD

In an attempt to examine flexion of the spine quickly and reproducibly, some authors have advocated the fingertip-to-floor method.[3, 4] The fingertip-to-floor method differs from the Schober method and its modifications in that

Fig. 8-1. Illustration of fingertip-to-floor test, a composite test measuring multiple motions and muscles.

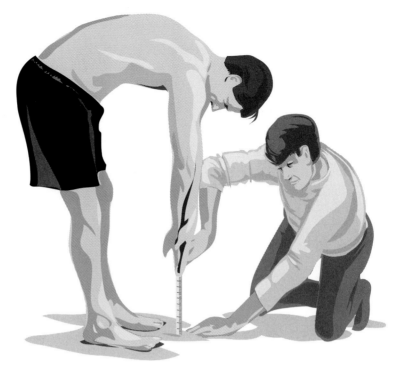

these measurements are not taken directly over the lumbar spine. The patient simply bends forward, and the distance between the tip of the middle finger and the floor is measured with a tape measure (Fig. 8-1).

Lateral Flexion

Two methods for using a tape measure to examine lateral flexion of the spine have been introduced in the literature, with neither method becoming predominant in clinical use. These two methods are placing marks at the lateral thigh and the fingertip-to-floor method.

Measuring lateral flexion by placing a mark at the location on the lateral thigh that the third fingertip can touch during erect standing and after lateral flexion (see Figs. 8-42 to 8-44) was first introduced by Mellin.[6] The distance between the two marks represents the range of lateral flexion to that side.

Using the fingertip-to-floor method, the distance from the third fingertip to the floor is measured, first with the patient standing erect, and then after the subject laterally flexes the spine.[2] The change in the distance from erect standing to lateral flexion is considered the range of lateral flexion (see Fig. 8-45).

Rotation

Using the lateral tip of the ipsilateral acromium and the greater trochanter of the contralateral femur, Frost et al.[2] described a method for measuring rotation in the thoracolumbar spine using a tape measure. See Figures 8-58 to 8-61, which describe this technique in detail.

Goniometer

The standard goniometer, consisting of two hinged rulers rotating on a protractor (described in detail in Chapter 1), is commonly used for measuring range of motion of the spine. Techniques for measurement of flexion (see Figs. 8–10 to 8–13), extension (see Figs. 8–30 to 8–33), and lateral flexion (see Figs. 8–46 to 8–49) are described later in this chapter. A goniometer is not commonly used to measure rotation of the thoracolumbar spine.

Inclinometer

The American Medical Association (AMA) published the *Guides to the Evaluation of Permanent Impairment,*[1] in which the use of inclinometers has been stipulated as "a feasible and potentially accurate method of measuring spine mobility." Therefore, it can be suggested that the use of the inclinometer for appropriate measurement of spinal mobility appears to have gained acceptance.

Several options exist in the use of the inclinometer for measurement of spinal movement. Two inclinometers can be used simultaneously to measure spinal movement (referred to as the double inclinometer method). Or, one inclinometer can be used to measure the same spinal movement (referred to as the single inclinometer method). In addition, the inclinometer can be held against the subject during the examination of range of motion, or the inclinometer can be strapped on and attached to the individual (back range of motion device). All these techniques have been accepted by the AMA[1] as appropriate methods for measurement of spinal mobility. This chapter describes use of the dual inclinometer technique to measure movement of the lumbar and thoracic spine for flexion (see Figs. 8–14 to 8–17), extension (see Figs. 8–34 to 8–37), lateral flexion (see Figs. 8–50 to 8–53), and rotation (see Figs. 8–62 to 8–64).

However, Saunders[8] suggests that the protocol for measurement of flexion and extension of the lumbar spine proposed by the AMA[1] is "seriously flawed" because the erect standing position is used as the reference, or zero, point. He advocates that the actual measurement at the end of the range of flexion or extension is the important parameter, and not the range of motion from the erect standing position (in which the individual may be in a lordotic, neutral, or kyphotic posture for this initial measurement) to full range of motion advocated by the AMA.[1] Saunders[8] recommends the use of what he refers to as the "curve angle method," which is presented as an alternative technique in the descriptions of measurement of lumbar flexion and extension using the inclinometer later in this chapter.

The "back range of motion" (BROM) (Performance Attainment Associates, Roseville, Minnesota) device was developed using mechanisms based on the inclinometer technique. The BROM device consists of two plastic frames that are secured to the lumbar spine of the subject by two elastic straps. One frame consists of an L-shaped slide arm that is free to move within a notch on the fixed base unit during flexion and extension; ROM is read from a protractor scale. The second frame has two measurement devices attached to it. One attachment is a vertically mounted gravity-dependent inclinometer that measures lateral flexion. The second attachment is a horizontally mounted compass to measure rotation. During the measurement of trunk rotation, the device requires that a magnetic yoke be secured to the pelvis. Description and figures for using the BROM device to measure flexion (see

Figs. 8–18 to 8–21), extension (see Figs. 8–38 to 8–41), lateral flexion (see Figs. 8–54 to 8–57), and rotation (see Figs. 8–65 to 8–69) are presented later in this chapter. From a clinical perspective, it remains to be seen whether the BROM will be readily accepted as a device of choice by the AMA in the new revision of its publication, the *Guides to the Evaluation of Permanent Impairment.*[1]

Flexion—Lumbar Spine: Tape Measure Method

Fig. 8–2. Starting position for measurement of lumbar flexion using tape measure method. Bony landmarks for tape measure align-ment (midline of spine in line with PSIS, 15 cm above base line mark) indi-cated by orange line and dots.

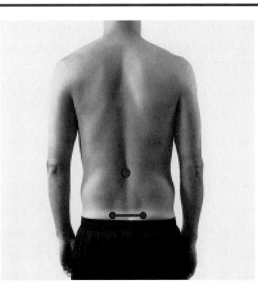

Patient position:	Standing, feet shoulders' width apart (Fig. 8–2).
Patient action:	Patient is instructed in desired motion. Running both hands down front of both legs, patient flexes spine as far as possible while keeping knees extended. Patient then returns to starting position. This movement provides an estimate of range of motion (ROM) and demonstrates to patient exact motion desired (Fig. 8–3).

Fig. 8–3. End ROM of lum-bar flexion. Bony land-marks for tape measure alignment (midline of spine in line with PSIS, 15 cm above base line mark) indi-cated by orange line and dots.

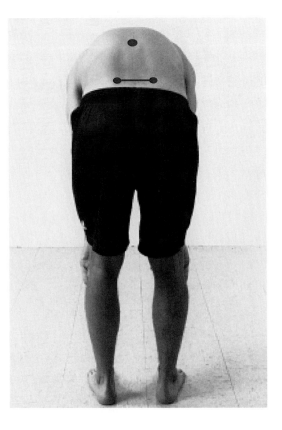

Fig. 8–4. Initial tape measure alignment for measurement of lumbar flexion. Bony landmarks for tape measure alignment (midline of spine in line with PSIS, 15 cm above base line mark) indicated by orange line and dots.

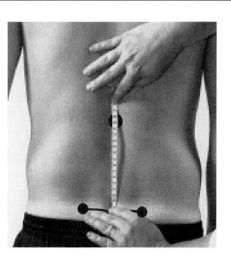

Tape measure alignment:	Palpate following bony landmarks (shown in Fig 8–2) and align tape measure accordingly (Fig. 8–4).
Base line:	Midline of spine in line with posterior superior iliac spines (PSIS).
Superior:	15 cm above base line landmark.

Tape measure is aligned with 0 cm at base line landmark and maintained against subject's spine (see Fig. 8–4).

Patient/Examiner action: As patient flexes spine through available ROM, examiner allows tape measure to unwind from tape measure case. Tape measure should be held firmly against patient's skin during movement. Examiner records distance between superior and base line landmarks (Fig. 8–5).

Documentation: Flexion ROM recorded is difference between original 15 cm measurement and length measured at end of flexion motion. Example: 16.5 cm (measurement at full flexion) − 15 cm (initial measurement) = 1.5 cm of lumbar flexion. Record patient's ROM.

Alternative Technique

Patient/Examiner action: At maximal flexion, distance from tip of the middle finger to the floor is measured (see Fig. 8–1).

Documentation: Distance between tip of middle finger and floor is recorded.

Fig. 8–5. Tape measure alignment at end ROM of lumbar flexion. Bony landmarks for tape measure alignment (midline of spine in line with PSIS, 15 cm above base line mark) indicated by orange line and dots.

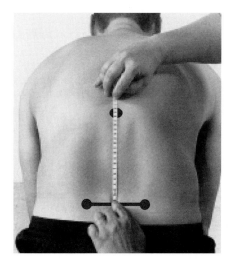

Flexion—Thoracolumbar Spine: Tape Measure Method

Fig. 8-6. Starting position for measurment of thoracolumbar flexion using tape measure method. Bony landmarks for tape measure alignment (midline of spine in line with PSIS, spinous process of C7 vertebra) indicated by orange line and dots.

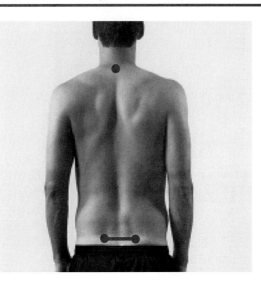

Patient position:	Standing, feet shoulders' width apart (Fig. 8-6).
Patient action:	Patient is instructed in desired motion. Running both hands down front of both legs, patient flexes spine as far as possible while keeping knees extended. Patient then returns to starting position. This movement provides an estimate of ROM and demonstrates to patient exact motion desired (Fig. 8-7).
Tape measure alignment:	Palpate following bony landmarks (shown in Fig. 8-6) and align tape measure accordingly (Fig. 8-8).
Base line:	Midline of spine in line with PSIS.
Superior:	Spinous process of C7 vertebra.

Fig. 8-7. End ROM of thoracolumbar flexion. Bony landmarks for tape measure alignment (midline of spine in line with PSIS, C7 vertebra) indicated by orange line and dots.

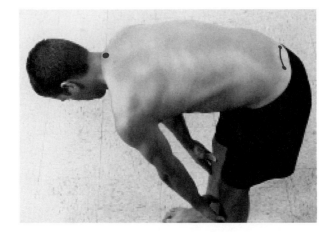

Fig. 8–8. Initial tape measure alignment for measurement of thoracolumbar flexion. Bony landmarks for tape measure alignment (midline of spine in line with PSIS, spinous process of C7 vertebra) indicated by orange line and dots.

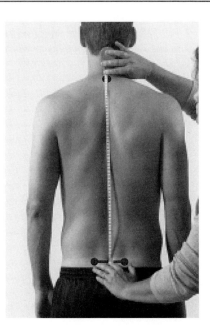

Tape measure is aligned with 0 cm at base line landmark. Maintaining tape measure against subject's spine, measure distance between base line and superior landmark; referred to as initial measurement (Fig. 8–8).

Patient/Examiner action:

As patient flexes spine through available ROM, examiner allows tape measure to unwind from tape measure case. Tape measure should be held firmly against patient's skin during movement. Examiner records distance between superior and base line landmarks; referred to as final measurement (Fig. 8–9).

Documentation:

Flexion ROM recorded is difference between initial and final measurement. Example: 57 cm (final measurement) − 50 cm (initial measurement) = 7 cm of thoracolumbar flexion. Record patient's ROM.

Fig. 8–9. Tape measure alignment at end ROM of thoracolumbar flexion. Bony landmarks for tape measure alignment (midline of spine in line with PSIS, spinous process of C7 vertebra) indicated by orange line and dots.

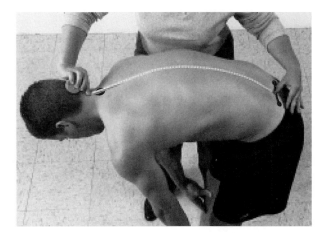

Flexion—Lumbar Spine: Goniometer Technique

Fig. 8–10. Starting position for measurement of lumbar flexion using goniometer technique. Landmarks for goniometric alignment (mid-axillary line at level of lowest rib, mid-axillary line) indicated by orange line and dot.

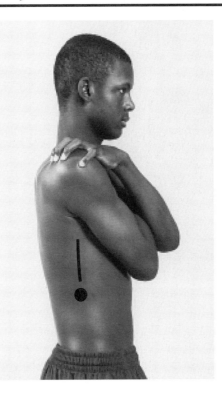

Patient position: Standing; feet shoulders' width apart (Fig. 8–10).

Patient action: Patient is instructed in desired motion. Running both hands down front of both legs, patient flexes spine as far as possible while keeping knees extended. Patient then returns to starting position. This movement provides an estimate of ROM and demonstrates to patient exact motion required (Fig. 8–11).

Fig. 8–11. End ROM of lumbar flexion. Landmarks for goniometric alignment (mid-axillary line at level of lowest rib, mid-axillary line) indicated by orange line and dot.

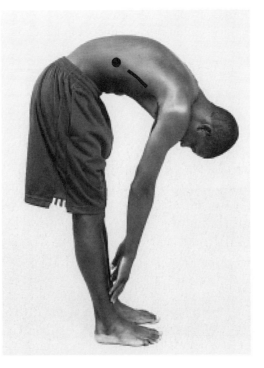

Fig. 8–12. Goniometer alignment at beginning range of lumbar flexion.

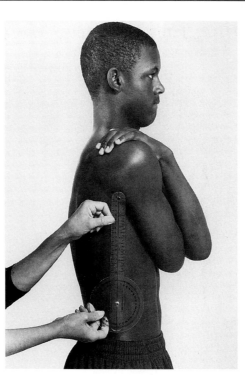

Goniometer alignment:	Palpate following landmarks (shown in Fig. 8–10) and align goniometer accordingly (Fig. 8–12).
Stationary arm:	Vertical to floor.
Axis:	Midaxillary line at level of lowest rib.
Moving arm:	Along midaxillary line.
	Read scale of goniometer.
Patient/Examiner action:	Running both hands down front of legs, patient flexes spine as far as possible while keeping knees extended (see Fig. 8–11).
Confirmation of alignment:	Repalpate landmarks and confirm proper goniometer alignment at end ROM, correcting alignment as necessary (Fig. 8–13). Read scale of goniometer.
Documentation:	Record patient's ROM.

Fig. 8–13. Goniometer alignment at end ROM of lumbar flexion.

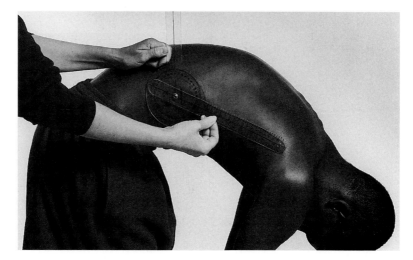

Flexion—Lumbar Spine: Inclinometer Method

Fig. 8–14. Starting position for measurement of lumbar flexion using dual inclinometer (AMA) technique. Bony landmarks for inclinometer alignment (midline of spine in line with PSIS, 15 cm above base line mark) indicated by orange line and dots.

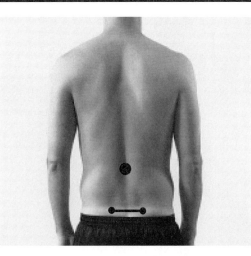

Patient position:	Standing; feet shoulders' width apart (Fig. 8–14).
Patient action:	Patient is instructed in desired motion. Running both hands down front of both legs, patient flexes spine as far as possible while keeping knees extended. Patient then returns to starting position. This movement provides an estimate of ROM and demonstrates to patient exact motion desired (Fig. 8–15).
Inclinometer alignment:	Palpate following bony landmarks (shown in Fig. 8–14) and align inclinometers accordingly (Fig. 8–16). Ensure that inclinometers are set at 0 degrees.
Base line:	Midline of spine in line with PSIS.
Superior:	15 cm above base line landmark.

Fig. 8–15. End ROM of lumbar flexion. Bony landmarks for inclinometer alignment (midline of spine in line with PSIS, 15 cm above base line mark) indicated by orange line and dots.

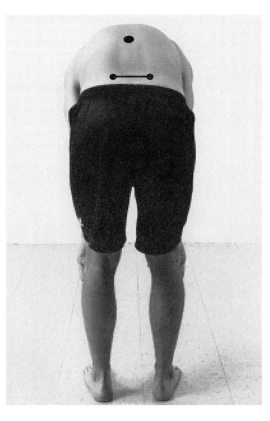

Fig. 8–16. Initial inclinometer alignment for measurement of lumbar flexion using dual inclinometer (AMA) technique. Inclinometers set at 0 degrees.

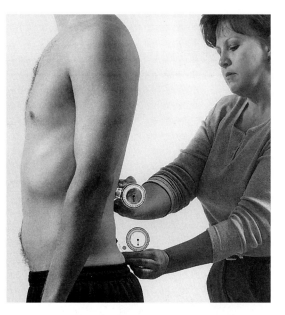

Patient/Examiner action:	Holding inclinometers in place as patient flexes spine through available ROM, examiner reads angle on each device (Fig. 8–17). Inclinometer at superior landmark indicates flexion of lumbar spine and hips. Inclinometer at base line landmark indicates flexion of the hips alone.
Documentation:	Flexion ROM recorded is measurement at base line landmark (after full flexion) subtracted from measurement at superior landmark (after full flexion). Example: 105 degrees (reading at superior landmark) − 45 degrees (reading at base line landmark) = 60 degrees of lumbar flexion. Record patient's ROM.
Note:	Thoracolumbar flexion can be measured using the spinous process of C7 vertebra as the superior landmark. Figure 8–6 indicates this superior landmark.

Alternative Technique: The Curve Angle Method

Patient/Examiner action:	Patient flexes spine through available ROM. Examiner places *single* inclinometer at base line landmark at midline of spine in line with PSIS (see Fig. 8–14) and sets the inclinometer at 0 degrees. With patient maintaining full lumbar flexion, examiner then moves *single* inclinometer to superior landmark (Fig. 8–14).
Documentation:	Flexion ROM recorded is the measurement at the superior landmark.

Fig. 8–17. Inclinometer alignment at end ROM of lumbar flexion.

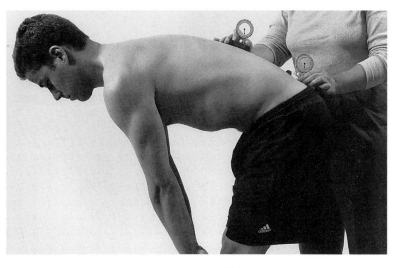

Flexion—Lumbar Spine: BROM Device

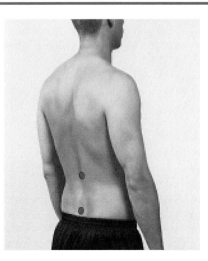

Fig. 8–18. Starting position for measurement of lumbar flexion using BROM. Bony landmarks for BROM alignment (spinous process of S1 vertebra, spinous process of T12 vertebra) indicated by orange dots.

Patient position:	Standing erect; feet shoulders' width apart (Fig. 8–18).
Patient action:	Patient is instructed in desired motion. Running both hands down front of both legs, patient flexes spine as far as possible while keeping knees extended. Patient then returns to starting position. This movement provides an estimate of ROM and demonstrates to patient exact motion desired (Fig. 8–19).

BROM alignment:
  Base line:
  Superior:
	Palpate following bony landmarks (Fig. 8–18).
	Spinous process of S1 vertebra.
	Spinous process of T12 vertebra.

Fig. 8–19. End ROM of lumbar flexion. Bony landmarks for BROM alignment (spinous process of S1 vertebra, spinous process of T12 vertebra) indicated by orange dots.

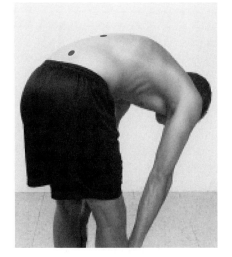

Fig. 8–20. Alignment of BROM flexion/extension unit at beginning range of lumbar flexion. Bony landmark for alignment of moveable arm of BROM (spinous process of T12 vertebra) indicated by orange dot.

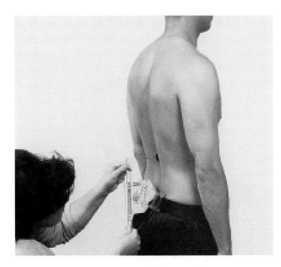

Examiner action:

Place BROM flexion/extension unit (consisting of base and movable arm) with pivot point on spinous process of S1 vertebra. Hold in place by attaching with Velcro straps to lower abdomen (down-pull of strap is essential to maintain unit against sacrum during flexion and extension) (Fig. 8–20).

With patient standing erect, examiner places tip of moving arm at level of T12 spinous process. Record reading from unit as initial measurement (see Fig. 8–20).

Patient/Examiner action:

Running both hands down front of legs, patient flexes spine through available ROM. Examiner places tip of moving arm at level of T12 spinous process. Record reading from unit as full flexion measurement (Fig. 8–21).

Documentation:

Flexion ROM is the measurement of initial reading (in erect standing) subtracted from the full flexion reading. Example: 115 degrees (reading at full flexion) − 80 degrees (reading in standing) = 35 degrees of lumbar flexion. Record patient's ROM.

Fig. 8–21. BROM alignment at end ROM of lumbar flexion. Bony landmark for alignment of moveable arm of BROM (spinous process of T12 vertebra) indicated by orange dot.

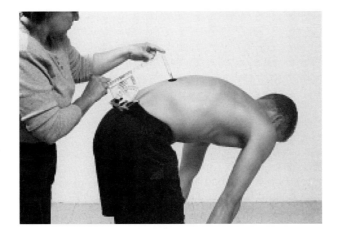

Extension—Lumbar Spine: Tape Measure Method

Fig. 8–22. Starting position for measurement of lumbar extension using tape measure method. Bony landmarks for tape measure alignment (midline of spine in line with PSIS, 15 cm above base line mark) indicated by orange line and dots.

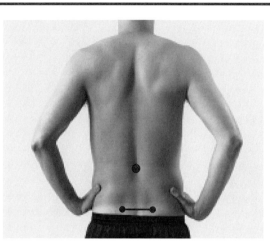

Patient position:	Standing, feet shoulders' width apart; hands on hips (Fig. 8–22).
Patient action:	Patient is instructed in desired motion. Placing hands on waist, patient bends backward as far as possible while keeping knees extended. Patient then returns to starting position. This movement provides an estimate of ROM and demonstrates to patient exact motion desired (Fig. 8–23).
Tape measure alignment:	Palpate following bony landmarks (shown in Fig. 8–22) and align tape measure accordingly (Fig. 8–24).
Base line:	Midline of spine in line with PSIS.
Superior:	15 cm above base line landmark.

Tape measure is aligned with 0 cm at base line landmark and maintained against subject's spine (see Fig. 8–24).

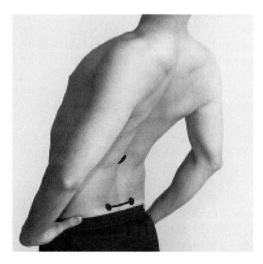

Fig. 8–23. End ROM of lumbar extension. Bony landmarks for tape measure alignment (midline of spine in line with PSIS, 15 cm above base line mark) indicated by orange line and dots.

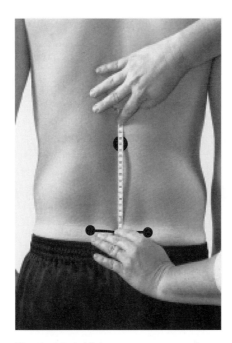

Fig. 8–24. Initial tape measure alignment for measurement of lumbar extension. Bony landmarks for tape measure alignment (midline of spine in line with PSIS, 15 cm above base line mark) indicated by orange line and dots.

Patient/Examiner action: As patient extends spine through available ROM, examiner allows tape measure to retract into tape measure case. Tape measure should be held firmly against patient's skin during movement. Examiner records distance between superior and base line landmarks (Fig. 8–25).

Documentation: Extension ROM recorded is difference between original 15 cm measurement and length measured at end of extension motion. Example: 15 cm (initial measurement) − 13.0 cm (measurement at full extension) = 2 cm of extension. Record patient's ROM.

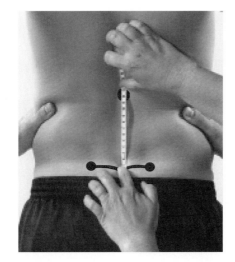

Fig. 8–25. Tape measure alignment at end ROM of lumbar extension. Bony landmarks for tape measure alignment (midline of spine in line with PSIS, 15 cm above base line mark) indicated by orange line and dots.

Extension—Lumbar Spine: Tape Measure Method—Prone

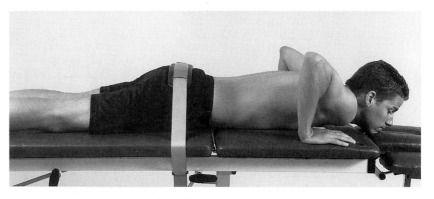

Fig. 8–26. Starting position for measurement of lumbar extension in prone using tape measure method. Note stabilization belt across pelvis.

Patient position: Prone; hands under shoulders. Stabilization belt placed across pelvis at buttocks (Fig. 8–26).

Patient action: Patient is instructed in desired motion. Patient extends elbows and raises trunk as far as possible. Although increased muscle activity will appropriately occur across upper back, patient should relax muscles of lumbar spine. Patient then returns to starting position. This movement provides an estimate of ROM and demonstrates to patient exact motion desired (Fig. 8–27).

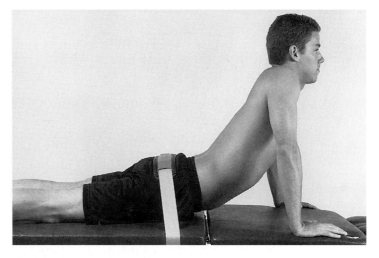

Fig. 8–27. End ROM of lumbar extension in prone.

Fig. 8–28. Tape measure alignment at end ROM of lumbar extension in prone.

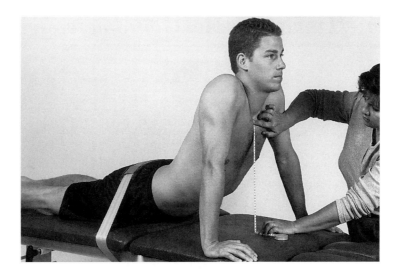

Tape measure alignment:	Palpate following landmarks and align tape measure accordingly (Fig. 8–28).
Superior:	Sternal notch.
Inferior:	Perpendicular to, and in contact with, support surface.
Patient/Examiner action:	At end of ROM in prone extension, examiner measures distance from sternal notch to support surface (see Fig. 8–28).
Documentation:	Distance between sternal notch and support surface is recorded.
Precaution:	Lifting of pelvis from support surface (shown in Fig. 8–29) should be prevented.

Fig. 8–29. Lifting pelvis from support surface during lumbar extension in prone due to lack of pelvic stabilization.

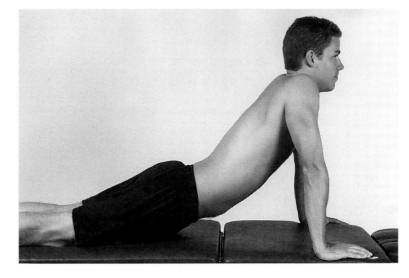

Extension—Lumbar Spine: Goniometer Technique

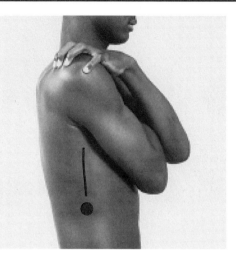

Fig. 8–30. Starting position for measurement of lumbar extension using goniometer technique. Landmarks (mid-axillary line at level of lowest rib, mid-axillary line) indicated by orange line and dot.

Starting position:	Standing; feet shoulders' width apart (Fig. 8–30).
Patient action:	Patient is instructed in desired motion. Patient crosses arms, placing hands on opposite shoulders and bends backward as far as possible while keeping knees extended. Patient then returns to starting position. This movement provides an estimate of ROM and demonstrates to patient exact motion desired (Fig. 8–31).
Goniometer alignment:	Palpate following landmarks (shown in Fig. 8–30) and align goniometer accordingly (Fig. 8–32).
Stationary arm:	Vertical to floor.
Axis:	Midaxillary line at level of lowest rib.
Moving arm:	Along midaxillary line.

Read scale of goniometer.

Fig. 8–31. End ROM of lumbar extension. Landmarks (mid-axillary line at level of lowest rib, mid-axillary line) indicated by orange line and dot.

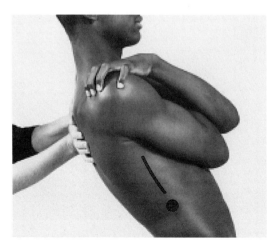

Fig. 8–32. Goniometer alignment at beginning range of lumbar extension.

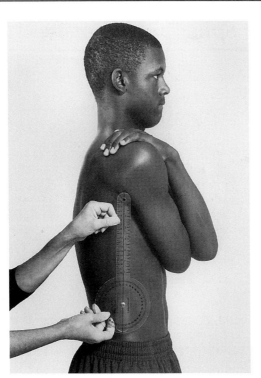

Patient/Examiner action: Patient crosses arms, placing hands on opposite shoulders and bends backward as far as possible; full extension of knees should be maintained (see Fig. 8–31).

Confirmation of alignment: Repalpate landmarks and confirm proper goniometer alignment at end ROM, correcting alignment as necessary (Fig. 8–33). Read scale of goniometer.

Documentation: Record patient's ROM.

Fig. 8–33. Goniometer alignment at end ROM of lumbar extension.

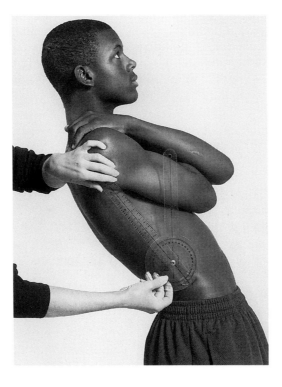

Extension—Lumbar Spine: Inclinometer Method

Fig. 8–34. Starting position for measurement of lumbar extension using dual inclinometer (AMA) technique. Bony landmarks for inclinometer alignment (midline of spine in line with PSIS, 15 cm above base line mark) indicated by orange line and dots.

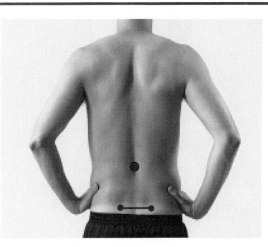

Patient position:	Standing; feet shoulders' width apart; hands on hips (Fig. 8–34).
Patient action:	Patient is instructed in desired motion. Placing hands on hips, patient bends backward as far as possible while keeping knees extended. Patient then returns to starting position. This movement provides an estimate of ROM and demonstrates to patient exact movement desired (Fig. 8–35).
Inclinometer alignment:	Palpate following bony landmarks (shown in Fig. 8–34) and align inclinometers accordingly (Fig. 8–36). Ensure that inclinometers are set at 0 degrees.
Base line:	Midline of spine in line with PSIS.
Superior:	15 cm above base line landmark.
Patient/Examiner action:	Holding inclinometers in place as patient extends spine through available ROM, examiner reads angle on each device (Fig. 8–37). Inclinometer at superior landmark indicates extension of lumbar spine and hips. Inclinometer at base line landmark indicates extension of hips alone.
Documentation:	Extension ROM recorded is measurement at base line landmark (after full extension) subtracted from measurement at superior landmark (after full extension). Example: 45 degrees (reading at superior landmark) − 20 degrees (reading at base line landmark) = 25 degrees of extension. Record patient's ROM.

Fig. 8–35. End ROM of lumbar extension. Bony landmarks for inclinometer alignment (midline of spine in line with PSIS, 15 cm above base line mark) indicated by orange line and dots.

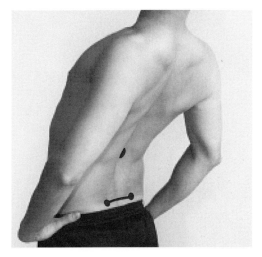

Fig. 8–36. Initial inclinometer alignment for measurement of lumbar extension using dual inclinometer (AMA) technique. Inclinometers set at 0 degrees.

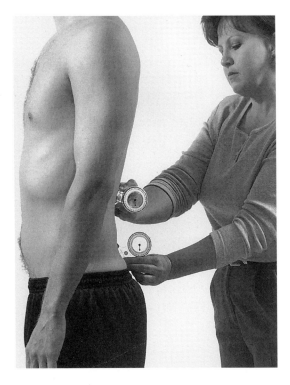

Note:

Thoracolumbar extension can be measured using the spinous process of C7 vertebra as the superior landmark. Figure 8–6 indicates this superior landmark.

Alternative Technique: The Curve Angle Method

Patient/Examiner action:

Patient extends spine through available ROM. Examiner places *single* inclinometer at base landmark at midline of spine in line with PSIS (see Fig. 8–34) and sets the inclinometer at 0 degrees. With patient maintaining full lumbar extension, examiner then moves *single* inclinometer to superior landmark (see Fig. 8–34).

Documentation:

Extension ROM recorded is the measurement at the superior landmark.

Fig. 8–37. Inclinometer alignment at end ROM of lumbar extension.

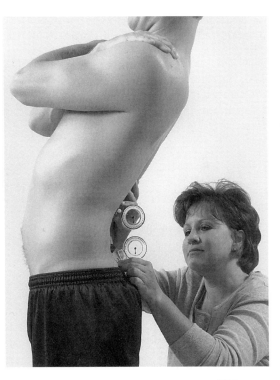

Extension—Lumbar Spine: BROM Device

Fig. 8–38. Starting position for measurement of lumbar extension using BROM. Bony landmarks for BROM alignment (spinous process of S1 vertebra, spinous process of T12 vertebra) indicated by orange dots.

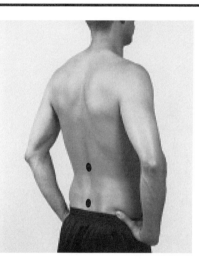

Patient position:	Standing erect; feet shoulders' width apart (Fig. 8–38).
Patient action:	Patient is instructed in desired motion. Placing hands on waist, patient bends backward as far as possible while keeping knees extended. Patient then returns to starting position. This movement provides an estimate of ROM and demonstrates to patient exact motion desired (Fig. 8–39).
BROM alignment: **Base line:** **Superior:**	Palpate following bony landmarks (Fig. 8–38). Spinous process of S1 vertebra. Spinous process of T12 vertebra.
Examiner action:	Place BROM flexion/extension unit (consisting of base and movable arm) with pivot point on spinous process of S1 vertebra. Hold in place by attaching with Velcro straps to lower abdomen (down-pull of strap is essential to maintain unit against sacrum during flexion and extension) (Fig. 8–40).

Fig. 8–39. End ROM of lumbar extension. Bony landmarks for BROM alignment (spinous process of S1 vertebra, spinous process of T12 vertebra) indicated by orange dots.

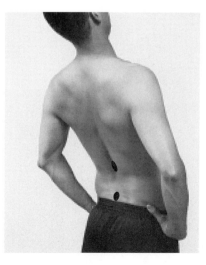

Fig. 8–40. Alignment of BROM flexion/extension unit at beginning of range of lumbar extension. Bony landmark for alignment of moveable arm of BROM (spinous process of T12 vertebra) indicated by orange dot.

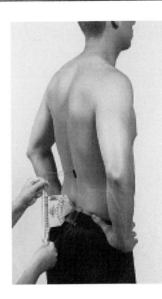

With patient standing erect, examiner places tip of moving arm at level of T12 spinous process (see Fig. 8–40). Record reading from unit as initial measurement.

Patient/Examiner action: Placing hands on waist, patient extends spine through available ROM. Examiner places tip of moving arm at level of T12 spinous process (Fig. 8–41). Record reading from full extension measurement.

Documentation: Extension ROM is the measurement of full extension reading subtracted from initial reading (in erect standing). Example: 85 degrees (initial reading) − 75 degrees (reading in full extension) = 10 degrees of lumbar extension. Record patient's ROM.

Fig. 8–41. BROM alignment at end ROM of lumbar extension.

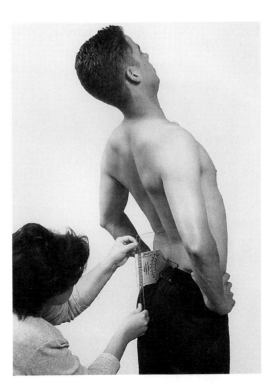

Lateral Flexion—Thoracolumbar Spine: Tape Measure Method

Fig. 8–42. Starting position for measurement of thoracolumbar lateral flexion using the tape measure method. Landmark indicated by orange dot at level of tip of middle finger.

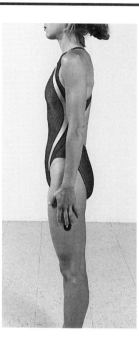

Patient position: Standing, feet shoulders' width apart; palm of hand against thigh (Fig. 8–42).

Patient action: Patient is instructed in desired motion. Running hand down side of leg, patient laterally flexes spine as far as possible. Patient keeps knees extended and does not bend trunk forward or backward while performing movement. Patient then returns to starting position. This movement provides an estimate of ROM and demonstrates to patient exact motion desired (Fig. 8–43).

Landmark: With patient positioned in erect standing, mark is placed on thigh level with tip of middle finger (see Fig. 8–42).

Fig. 8–43. End ROM of thoracolumbar lateral flexion. Landmark indicated by orange dot at level of tip of middle finger at end ROM.

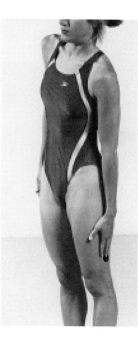

Fig. 8–44. Measurement of difference between skin marks on thigh (indicated by orange dots) using tape measure.

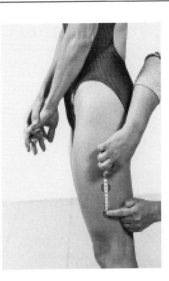

Patient/Examiner action: Patient laterally flexes spine, running hand down side of leg as far as possible. At maximal lateral flexion, position of the middle fingertip against thigh is marked again (see Fig. 8–43).

Documentation: Lateral flexion ROM is difference between skin mark on thigh in erect standing and skin mark on thigh in full lateral flexion (Fig. 8–44). Record patient's ROM.

Alternative Technique

Patient/Examiner action: At maximal lateral flexion, distance from tip of middle finger to floor is measured (Fig. 8–45).

Documentation: Distance between tip of middle finger and floor is recorded.

Fig. 8–45. Tape measure alignment at end ROM of lateral flexion using alternative (distance-to-floor) technique.

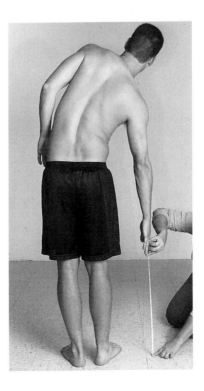

Lateral Flexion—Lumbar Spine: Goniometer Technique

Fig. 8–46. Starting position for measurement of lumbar lateral flexion using goniometer technique. Landmarks for goniometer alignment (spinous process of S1 vertebra, spinous process of C7 vertebra) indicated by orange dots.

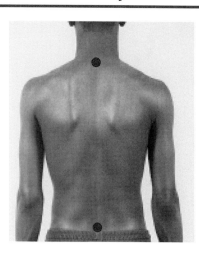

Patient position:	Standing; feet shoulders' width apart (Fig. 8–46).
Patient action:	Patient is instructed in desired motion. Running hand down side of leg, patient laterally flexes spine as far as possible. Patient keeps knees extended and does not bend trunk forward or backward while performing movement. Patient then returns to starting position. This movement provides an estimate of ROM and demonstrates to patient exact motion desired (Fig. 8–47).
Goniometer alignment:	Palpate following bony landmarks (shown in Fig. 8–46) and align goniometer accordingly (Fig. 8–48).
Stationary arm:	Vertical to floor.
Axis:	Spinous process of S1 vertebra.
Moving arm:	Spinous process of C7 vertebra.

Read scale of goniometer.

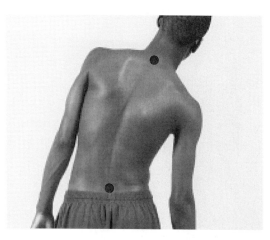

Fig. 8–47. End ROM of lumbar lateral flexion. Landmarks for goniometer alignment (spinous process of S1 vertebra, spinous process of C7 vertebra) indicated by orange dots.

Fig. 8–48. Goniometer alignment at beginning range of lumbar lateral flexion.

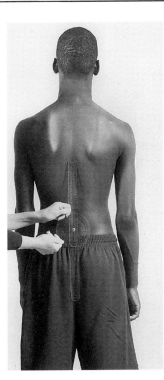

Patient/Examiner action: Running hand down side of leg, patient laterally flexes spine as far as possible (see Fig. 8–47).

Confirmation of alignment: Repalpate landmarks and confirm proper goniometer alignment at end ROM, correcting alignment as necessary (Fig. 8–49). Read scale of goniometer.

Documentation: Record patient's ROM.

Fig. 8–49. Goniometer alignment at end ROM of lumbar lateral flexion.

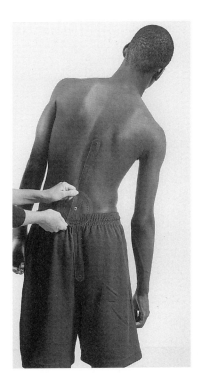

Lateral Flexion—Lumbar Spine: Inclinometer Method

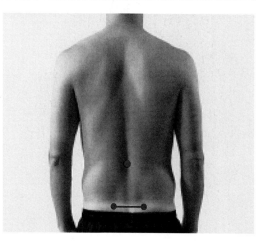

Fig. 8–50. Starting position for measurement of lumbar lateral flexion using inclinometer method. Bony landmarks for inclinometer alignment (midline of spine at level of PSIS, 15 cm above base line landmark) indicated by orange line and dots.

Patient position:	Standing, feet shoulders' width apart; arms at side (Fig. 8–50).
Patient action:	Patient is instructed in desired motion. Running hand down side of leg, patient laterally flexes spine as far as possible. Patient keeps knees extended and does not bend trunk forward or backward while performing movement. Patient then returns to starting position. This movement provides an estimate of ROM and demonstrates to patient exact motion desired (Fig. 8–51).
Inclinometer alignment:	Palpate following bony landmarks (shown in Fig. 8–50) and align inclinometers accordingly (Fig. 8–52). Ensure that inclinometers are set at 0 degrees.
Inferior:	Midline of spine in line with PSIS.
Superior:	15 cm above base line landmark.

Fig. 8–51. End ROM of lumbar lateral flexion. Bony landmarks for inclinometer alignment (midline of spine at level of PSIS, 15 cm above base line landmark) indicated by orange line and dots.

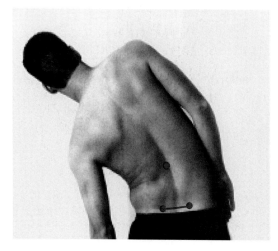

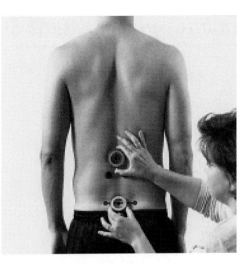

Fig. 8–52. Initial inclinometer alignment for measurement of lumbar lateral flexion. Bony landmarks for inclinometer alignment (midline of spine at level of PSIS, 15 cm above base line landmark) indicated by orange line and dots.

Patient/Examiner action: Patient laterally flexes spine through available ROM while examiner holds both inclinometers in place. When patient reaches end ROM, examiner reads angle on each device (Fig. 8–53).

Documentation: Lateral flexion ROM recorded is measurement at base line landmark (after full lateral flexion) subtracted from measurement at superior landmark (after full lateral flexion). Example: 20 degrees (reading at superior landmark) − 0 degrees (reading at base line landmark) = 20 degrees of lateral flexion. Record patient's ROM.

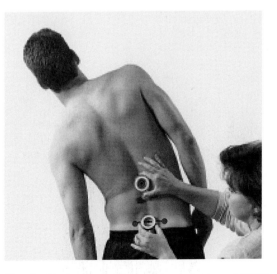

Fig. 8–53. Inclinometer alignment at end ROM of lumbar lateral flexion. Bony landmarks for inclinometer alignment (midline of spine at level of PSIS, 15 cm above base line landmark) indicated by orange line and dots.

Lateral Flexion—Lumbar Spine: BROM Device

Fig. 8–54. Starting position for measurement of lumbar lateral flexion using the BROM. Bony landmark (spinous process of T12 vertebra) indicated by orange dot.

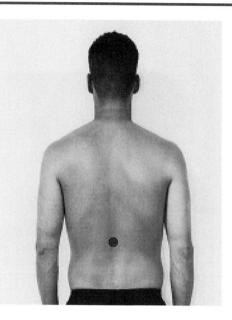

Patient position:	Standing erect; feet shoulders' width apart (Fig. 8–54).
Patient action:	Patient is instructed in desired motion. Running hand down side of leg, patient laterally flexes spine as far as possible. Patient keeps knees extended and does not bend trunk forward or backward while performing movement. Patient then returns to starting position. This movement provides an estimate of ROM and demonstrates to patient exact motion desired (Fig. 8–55).
BROM alignment:	Palpate spinous process of T12 vertebra (see Fig. 8–54).
	Examiner places center of BROM lateral flexion/rotation unit firmly against patient's back so that feet of unit are in line with spinous process of T12. Examiner places thumbs over feet of unit and grasps patient's rib cage with fingers. Position of unit is adjusted on patient's back until inclinometer reads 0 degrees (Fig. 8–56).

Fig. 8–55. End ROM of lumbar lateral flexion. Bony landmark (spinous process of T12 vertebra) indicated by orange dot.

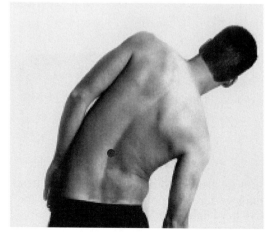

Fig. 8–56. BROM alignment at beginning range of lumbar lateral flexion.

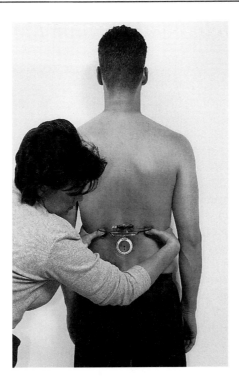

Patient/Examiner action: Patient laterally flexes spine through available ROM while examiner holds lateral flexion/rotation unit in place. When patient reaches end ROM, examiner reads inclinometer (Fig. 8–57).

Documentation: Record patient's ROM.

Fig. 8–57. BROM alignment at end ROM of lumbar lateral flexion.

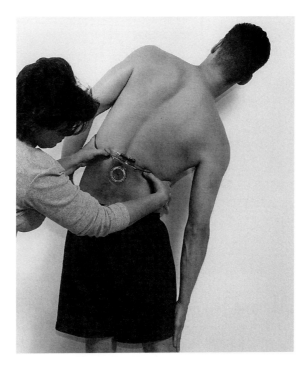

Rotation—Thoracolumbar Spine: Tape Measure Method

Patient position:	Sitting erect, arms crossed and hands on opposite shoulders (Fig. 8–58).
Patient action:	Patient is instructed in desired motion. Maintaining neutral position of spine and arms crossed with hands on opposite shoulders, patient rotates spine as far as possible. No lateral flexion should occur during rotation. Patient then returns to starting position. This movement provides an estimate of ROM and demonstrates to patient exact motion desired (Fig. 8–59).
Tape measure alignment:	Palpate following bony landmarks and align tape measure accordingly (Fig. 8–60).
Superior:	Lateral tip of ipsilateral acromion.
Inferior:	Greater trochanter of contralateral femur.
Examiner action:	Tape measure is aligned with 0 cm at superior landmark and maintained against subject's back. After placing tape measure at acromion, examiner asks patient to maintain tape measure at that position. Distance between superior and inferior landmark is measured; referred to as initial measurement (see Fig. 8–60).
Patient/Examiner action:	As patient rotates spine through available ROM while holding tape measure on superior landmark, examiner allows tape measure to unwind from tape

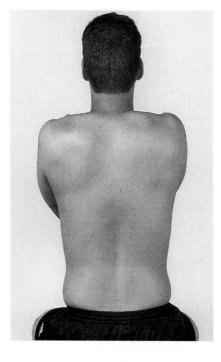

Fig. 8–58. Starting position for measurement of thoracolumbar rotation using tape measure method.

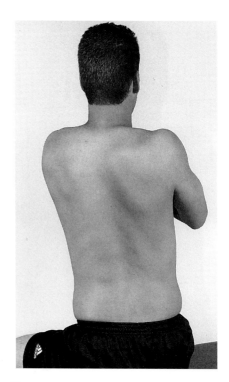

Fig. 8–59. End ROM of thoracolumbar rotation.

Fig. 8–60. Initial tape measure alignment for measurement of thoracolumbar rotation in sitting. Note: Patient holds tape measure against superior landmark (lateral tip of ipsilateral acromion).

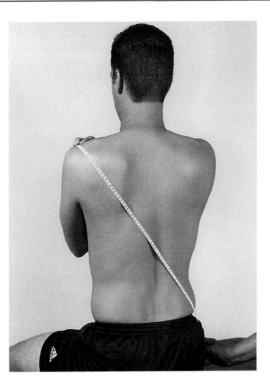

measure case. Examiner records distance between superior and inferior landmarks; referred to as final measurement (Fig. 8–61).

Documentation:

Rotation ROM is difference between length measured at beginning of rotation motion (initial measurement) and length measured at end of rotation motion (final measurement). Example: 86 cm (final measurement) − 80 cm (initial measurement) = 6 cm of rotation. Record patient's ROM.

Fig. 8–61. Tape measure alignment at end ROM of thoracolumbar rotation.

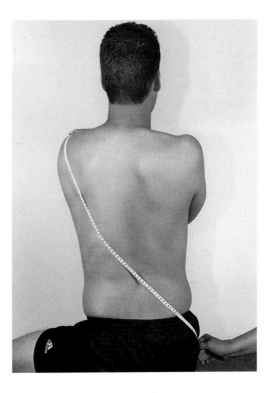

Rotation—Thoracic Spine: Inclinometer Method

Fig. 8–62. Starting position for measurement of thoracic rotation using inclinometer method. Bony landmarks (spinous process of T12 vertebra, spinous process of T1 vertebra) indicated by orange dots.

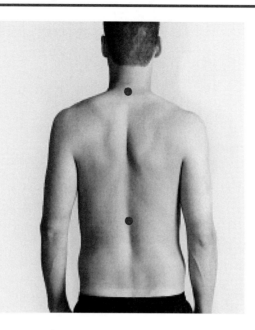

Patient position:	Standing; feet shoulders' width apart (Fig. 8–62).
Patient action:	Patient is instructed in desired motion. Patient forward flexes until thoracic spine is as parallel to floor as possible. In this position, ask subject to rotate the trunk maximally. This movement provides an estimate of ROM and demonstrates to patient exact motion desired.
Inclinometer alignment:	Palpate following bony landmarks (shown in Fig. 8–62) and align inclinometers accordingly. With patient flexed so that thoracic spine is as close to horizontal as possible, one inclinometer is held at base line landmark and one held at superior landmark (Fig. 8–63). Ensure that inclinometers are set at 0 degrees.
Base line:	Spinous process of T12 vertebra.
Superior:	Spinous process of T1 vertebra.

Fig. 8–63. Initial inclinometer alignment for measurement of thoracic rotation with patient flexed to horizontal. Bony landmarks (spinous process of T12 vertebra, spinous process of T1 vertebra) indicated by orange dots.

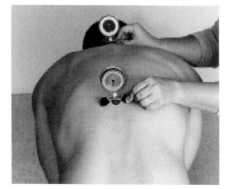

Fig. 8–64. Inclinometer alignment at end ROM of thoracic rotation. Bony landmarks (spinous process of T12 vertebra, spinous process of T1 vertebra) indicated by orange dots.

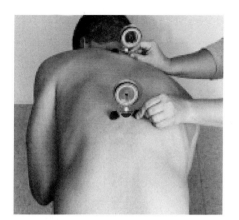

Patient/Examiner action:	Holding inclinometers in place as patient rotates spine through available ROM, examiner reads angle on each device (Fig. 8–64).
Documentation:	Rotation ROM recorded is the measurement of angle at T12 vertebra (after full rotation) subtracted from angle at T1 vertebra (after full rotation). Example: 70 degrees (reading at T1) − 50 degrees (reading at T12) = 20 degrees of rotation. Record patient's ROM.
Bony landmarks:	

Rotation—Lumbar Spine: BROM

Fig. 8-65. Starting position for measurement of lumbar rotation using BROM. Bony landmarks (spinous process of S1 vertebra, spinous process of T12 vertebra) indicated by orange dots.

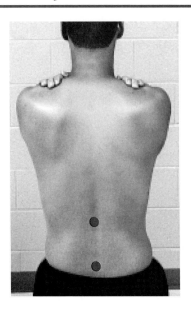

Patient position:	Sitting erect on nonrotating stool facing west; feet flat on floor. Patient crosses arms, placing hands on opposite shoulders (Fig. 8-65).
Patient action:	Patient is instructed in desired motion. Maintaining neutral position of spine and arms crossed with hands on opposite shoulders, patient rotates spine as far as possible. No lateral flexion should occur during rotation. Patient then returns to starting position. This movement provides an estimate of ROM and demonstrates to patient exact motion desired (Fig. 8-66).

BROM alignment:
   Base line:
   Superior:
	Palpate following bony landmarks (shown in Fig. 8-65).
	Spinous process of S1 vertebra.
	Spinous process of T12 vertebra.

To measure rotation, a magnetic reference is used in conjunction with a horizontally placed magnetic inclinometer. Magnetic reference is placed over S1 vertebra and held in place with Velcro straps (Fig. 8-67).

Fig. 8-66. End ROM of lumbar rotation. Bony landmarks (spinous process of S1 vertebra, spinous process of T12 vertebra) indicated by orange dots.

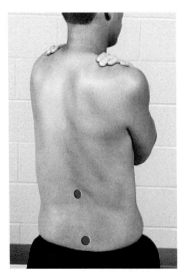

Fig. 8–67. Addition of magnetic reference.

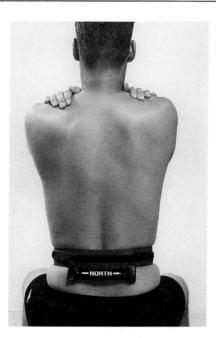

Examiner places center of BROM lateral flexion/rotation unit firmly against patient's back so that feet of unit are in line with spinous process of T12 and sets the horizontal inclinometer at 0 degrees. Examiner then changes hand position, holding rotation unit so examiner's thumbs grasp feet of unit and examiner's fingers grasp patient's rib cage (Fig. 8–68).

Patient/Examiner action: Holding rotation unit in place as patient rotates spine through available ROM, examiner reads number of degrees on inclinometer (Fig. 8–69).

Documentation: Record patient's ROM.

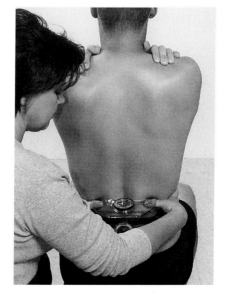

Fig. 8–68. BROM alignment at beginning range of lumbar rotation.

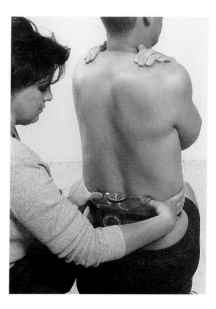

Fig. 8–69. BROM alignment at end ROM of lumbar rotation.

References

1. American Medical Association: Guides to the Evaluation of Permanent Impairment, 4th ed. Chicago, 1993.
2. Frost M, Stuckey S, Smalley LA, Dorman G: Reliability of measuring trunk motions in centimeters. Phys Ther 1982;62:1431–1437.
3. Gauvin MG, Riddle DL, Rothstein JM: Reliability of clinical measurements of forward bending using the modified fingertip-to-floor method. Phys Ther 1990;70:443–447.
4. Hyytiainen K, Salminen JJ, Suvitie T, et al.: Reproducibility of nine tests to measure spinal mobility and trunk muscle strength. Scand J Rehabil Med 1991;23:3–10.
5. Macrae IF, Wright V: Measurement of back movement. Ann Rheum Dis 1969;28:584–589.
6. Mellin GP: Accuracy of measuring lateral flexion of the spine with a tape. Clin Biomech (Bristol, Avon) 1986;1:85–89.
7. Moll JMV, Wright V: Normal range of motion: An objective clinical study. Ann Rheum Dis 1971;30:381–386.
8. Saunders HD: Saunders Digital Inclinometer. The Saunders Group, Chaska, MN, 1998.
9. van Adrichem JAM, van der Korst JK: Assessment of the flexibility of the lumbar spine. Scand J Rheumatol 1973;2:87–91.
10. Williams R, Binkley J, Bloch R, et al.: Reliability of the modified-modified Schober and double inclinometer methods for measuring lumbar flexion and extension. Phys Ther 1993;73:26–37.

9

MEASUREMENT of RANGE of MOTION of the CERVICAL SPINE and TEMPOROMANDIBULAR JOINT

CERVICAL SPINE

ANATOMY AND OSTEOKINEMATICS

Fourteen facet joints (seven pairs) on seven vertebrae make up the cervical spine. The first two cervical vertebrae are unique. The atlas (C1) has no body or spinous process and is shaped like a ring. Articulation between the two superior facets of the atlas and the two condyles on the occiput of the skull forms the atlanto-occipital joint. Movement between the atlas and the occiput (atlanto-occipital joint) is primarily a nodding motion in the sagittal plane about a medial-lateral axis. The axis (C2) has a vertical projection called the dens (also known as the odontoid process) that arises from the superior surface of the body. The dens of the axis fits into a ring formed by the anterior arches of the atlas and the transverse (cruciform) ligament so that the atlas pivots around the dens of the axis. Fifty percent of rotation in the cervical spine occurs at the atlantoaxial joint.

The facet joint surfaces change from horizontal to a 45-degree angle from the horizontal plane in the typical cervical articulations of C3 through C7. The cervical spine is designed for great mobility, with gliding of the inferior facets of the vertebrae above on the superior facets of the vertebrae below. The motions available at the cervical spine consist of flexion and extension in the sagittal plane, lateral flexion in the frontal plane, and rotation in the transverse plane.

LIMITATIONS OF MOTION: CERVICAL SPINE

Limitation of motion in the first two cervical vertebrae is due to a ligamentous support system specific to this area of the spine. This support structure at the atlanto-occipital and atlantoaxial joints includes the tectorial membrane and the atlantoaxial (anterior and posterior), alar, and transverse at lantal ligaments. From C2 to C7, the anterior longitudinal ligament and contact of the spinous processes limit excessive extension. Flexion is limited by the same ligaments that limit flexion in the lumbar spine (the posterior longitudinal, ligamentum flavum, and interspinous ligaments), with the addition of the ligamentum nuchae in the cervical spine. Running along the tips of the spinous processes of the cervical spine, the ligamentum nuchae is actually a continuation of the supraspinous ligament. Lateral flexion is limited

209

by the bony configuration of the saddle-shaped surface of the vertebral body, and rotation is limited by the fibers of the annulus fibrosis of the disk. Appendix C provides information regarding normal range of motion (ROM) of the cervical spine.

TECHNIQUES OF MEASUREMENT: CERVICAL SPINE

Tape Measure and Goniometer

Measurement of range of motion of the cervical spine using both the tape measure and the goniometer is commonplace. These measurement devices are easy to use, as well as relatively inexpensive.

Inclinometer

In Chapter 8, describing measurement of the thoracic and lumbar spine, it is noted that the American Medical Association (AMA) has accepted the inclinometer as "a feasible and potentially accurate method of measuring spine mobility."[2] This statement was directed not only at the examination of the thoracic and lumbar spine but also at measurement of the cervical spine. Specifically included in the *Guides to the Evaluation of Permanent Impairment*[2] is the use of single and double inclinometers that are held in place manually.

Attachment of Inclinometer to the Head

The process of attaching an inclinometer to the head to measure cervical range of motion has undergone a sort of evolution, beginning with the inclinometer attached to the ears and worn as headphones in the early 1960s and progressing, with increasing sophistication, to the cervical range of motion (CROM) device (Performance Attainment Associates, 958 Lydia Drive, Roseville, MN 55113) in the late 1990s. This evolution included the "bubble goniometer,"[4] attachment of the inclinometer to the head with elastic straps,[3] a "cloth helmet,"[1] the use of rigid headgear with three scales calibrated in degrees mounted on a skull cap,[7] the use of an inclinometer mounted on a wood block and placed on the head,[10] the "rangiometer,"[12] and finally the CROM device.[11] Although not included in the *Guides to the Evaluation of Permanent Impairment*,[2] the CROM device has been widely adopted by clinicians.

TEMPOROMANDIBULAR JOINT

ANATOMY AND OSTEOKINEMATICS

The temporomandibular joint (TMJ) is unique in that the mandible has two articulations with the temporal bone forming two separate but solidly connected joints. Both joints must be considered together in any examination. In addition, each TMJ has a disc that completely divides each joint into two cavities. Movement that occurs in the upper cavity (the joint formed by the temporal bone and the superior surface of the disc) is a gliding or translatory motion, while the movement that occurs in the lower cavity (the joint formed by the mandibular condyle and the inferior surface of the disc) is a rotatory or hinge movement.

Mandibular depression involves opening the mouth in the sagittal plane. Kraus[8] described *functional* mandibular depression as the "patient's ability to actively open his or her mouth to 40 mm." Magee[9] suggested that "only 25 to 35 mm of opening is needed for everyday activity," and that maximal mouth opening ranges from 35 to 50 mm. Freidman and Weisberg[5] suggested that the amount of functional opening varies according to the individual's size, and that on average an individual should be able to place two to two-and-a-half knuckles between the upper and lower incisors.

Protrusion involves anterior movement of the mandible in the horizontal plane. Magee[9] describes normal protrusion as 3 to 6 mm; Kraus[8] suggests that the mandibular central incisors should move past the maxillary central incisors "by several millimeters."

Lateral deviation, or excursion, describes lateral movement of the mandible in the horizontal plane. Magee[9] describes normal lateral deviation as 10 to 15 mm; Iglarsh and Snyder-Mackler[6] suggest that lateral deviation in each direction should be one-fourth the width of the mouth opening.

LIMITATIONS OF MOTION: TEMPOROMANDIBULAR JOINT

The temporomandibular, or lateral, ligament is a strong ligament that limits mandibular depression, protrusion, and lateral deviation. The limitation of protrusion is assisted by the stylomandibular ligament.

TECHNIQUES OF MEASUREMENT: TEMPOROMANDIBULAR JOINT

The most frequently used device for measuring range of motion of the TMJ is a small ruler. A unique tool that can be used to measure motion at the TMJ is the Therabite (Therabite Corporation, 3415 West Chester Pike; Newtown Square, PA, 19073). Procedures for using both of these devices are described later in this chapter.

Flexion—Cervical Spine: Tape Measure Method

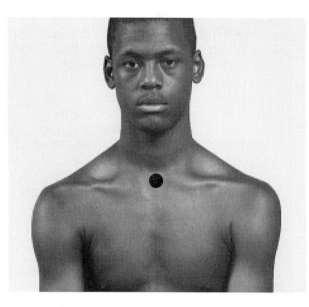

Fig. 9–1. Starting position for measurement of cervical flexion using tape measure method. Bony landmark (sternal notch) indicated by orange dot.

Patient position: Sitting erect (Fig. 9–1).

Patient action: After being instructed in motion desired, patient flexes neck maximally. Patient then returns to starting position. This movement provides an estimate of range of motion (ROM) and demonstrates to patient exact motion desired (Fig. 9–2). If patient is able to touch chin to chest, full flexion ROM is indicated. No further measurement is needed.

Fig. 9–2. End ROM of cervical flexion. Bony landmark (sternal notch) indicated by orange dot.

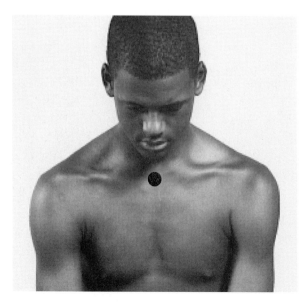

Fig. 9–3. Initial tape measure alignment for measurement of cervical flexion. Bony landmark (sternal notch) indicated by orange dot.

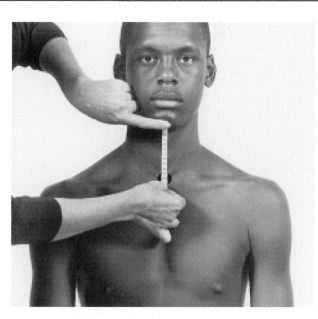

Tape measure alignment:

Palpate following bony landmarks (shown in Fig. 9–1) and align tape measure accordingly (Fig. 9–3). Tape measure should be aligned with 0 cm at tip of mandible.

Superior: Tip of mandible (chin).

Inferior: Sternal notch.

Measure distance between sternal notch to tip of mandible; referred to as the initial measurement (see Fig. 9–3).

Patient/Examiner action: Patient flexes cervical spine through available ROM. Examiner measures distance between sternal notch and chin; referred to as the final measurement (Fig. 9–4).

Documentation: Difference between initial and final measurements is the ROM. Record patient's ROM in centimeters.

Fig. 9–4. Tape measure alignment at end ROM of cervical flexion. Bony landmark (sternal notch) indicated by orange dot.

Flexion—Cervical Spine: Goniometer Technique

Fig. 9–5. Starting position for measurement of cervical flexion using goniometer technique.

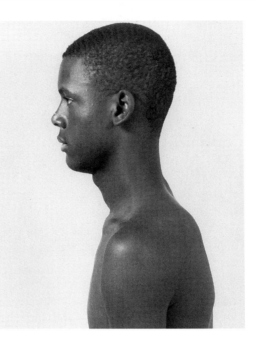

Patient position:	Sitting erect (Fig. 9–5).
Patient action:	After being instructed in motion desired, patient actively flexes cervical spine. Patient then returns to starting position. This movement provides an estimate of ROM and demonstrates to patient exact motion desired (Fig. 9–6). Patient returns to starting position and is manually positioned so that a line between the ear lobe and base of nares is parallel to floor.

Fig. 9–6. End ROM of cervical flexion.

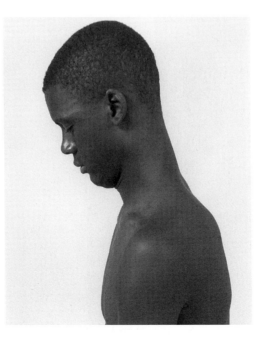

Fig. 9–7. Goniometer alignment at beginning range of cervical flexion.

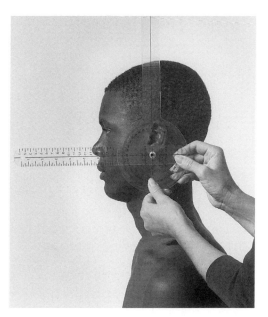

Goniometer alignment:	Palpate following landmarks and align goniometer accordingly (Fig. 9–7).
Stationary arm:	Perpendicular to floor.
Axis:	Ear lobe.
Moving arm:	Base of nares.

Read scale of goniometer.

Patient/Examiner action: Patient performs active cervical flexion (see Fig. 9–6).

Confirmation of alignment: Repalpate landmarks and confirm proper goniometer alignment at end ROM, correcting alignment as necessary (Fig. 9–8). Read scale of goniometer.

Documentation: Record patient's ROM.

Fig. 9–8. Goniometer alignment at end ROM of cervical flexion.

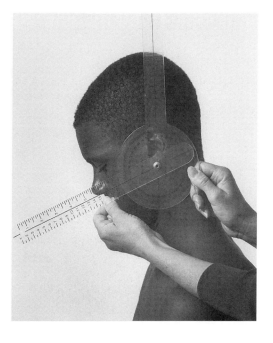

Flexion—Cervical Spine: Inclinometer Method

Fig. 9–9. Starting position for measurement of cervical flexion using inclinometer method. Bony landmark (spinous process of T1 vertebra) indicated by orange dot.

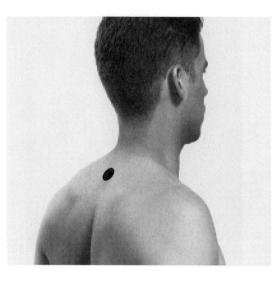

Patient position:	Sitting erect (Fig. 9–9).
Patient action:	After being instructed in motion desired, patient flexes neck maximally. Patient then returns to starting position. This movement provides an estimate of ROM and demonstrates to patient exact motion desired (Fig. 9–10).
Inclinometer alignment:	Palpate following bony landmarks (shown in Fig. 9–9) and align inclinometers accordingly (Fig. 9–11). Ensure that inclinometers are set at 0 degrees once they are positioned on patient.
Inferior:	Spinous process of T1 vertebra.
Superior:	*Vertex of skull.

---

* Defined as ½ distance between glabella (flattened triangular area on forehead, also known as "bridge of nose") and inion (palpable "bump" at base of occiput).

Fig. 9–10. End ROM of cervical flexion. Bony landmark (spinous process of T1 vertebra) indicated by orange dot.

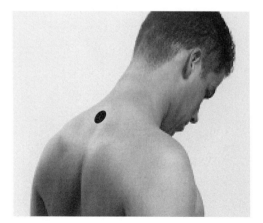

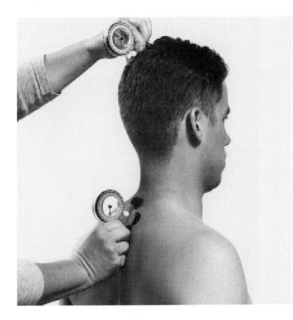

Fig. 9–11. Initial inclinometer alignment for measurement of cervical flexion. Bony landmark (spinous process of T1 vertebra) indicated by orange dot. Inclinometers set at 0 degrees.

Patient/Examiner action: Patient flexes cervical spine through available ROM as examiner holds inclinometers in place. Examiner reads angle on inclinometers at end of flexion ROM (Fig. 9–12).

Documentation: Flexion ROM recorded is measurement at inferior landmark subtracted from measurement at superior landmark. Example: 45 degrees (reading at superior landmark) − 5 degrees (reading at inferior landmark) = 40 degrees of flexion. Record patient's ROM.

Fig. 9–12. Inclinometer alignment at end ROM of cervical flexion. Bony landmark (spinous process of T1 vertebra) indicated by orange dot.

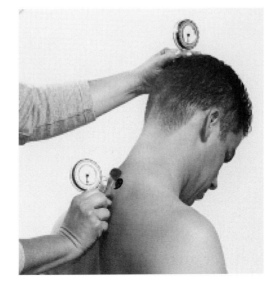

Flexion—Cervical Spine: CROM Device

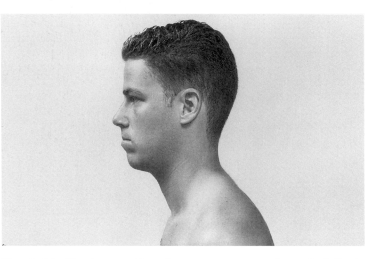

Fig. 9–13. Starting position for measurement of cervical flexion using CROM device.

Patient position: Sitting erect (Fig. 9–13).

Patient action: After being instructed in motion desired, patient actively flexes cervical spine. Patient then returns to starting position. This movement provides an estimate of ROM and demonstrates to patient exact motion desired (Fig. 9–14).

CROM alignment: Examiner positions CROM device on bridge of patient's nose and on ears as one would put on a pair of eyeglasses. Velcro straps are fastened firmly behind head to hold CROM device in place (Fig. 9–15). Record scale of inclinometer on side of patient's head; referred to as initial measurement.

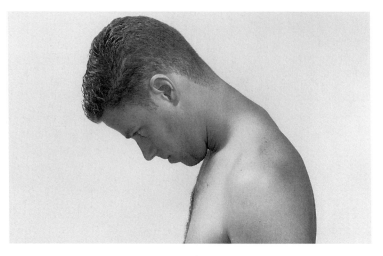

Fig. 9–14. End ROM of cervical flexion.

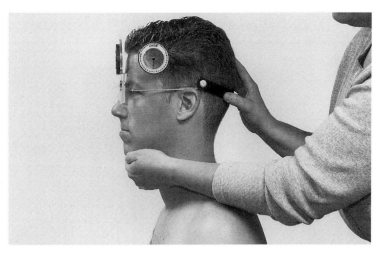

Fig. 9–15. CROM alignment at beginning range of cervical flexion.

Patient/Examiner action:	Patient performs active cervical flexion while maintaining thoracic spine against back of chair (see Fig. 9–14).
Confirmation of alignment:	Ensure that CROM device has remained in place at end ROM. Read scale of inclinometer on side of patient's head; referred to as final measurement (Fig. 9–16).
Documentation:	Flexion ROM recorded is initial measurement subtracted from final measurement. Example: 45 degrees (final measurement) − 0 degrees (initial measurement) = 45 degrees of flexion. Record patient's ROM.

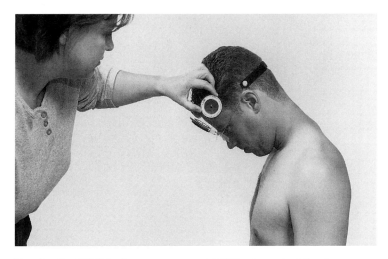

Fig. 9–16. CROM alignment at end ROM of cervical flexion.

Extension—Cervical Spine: Tape Measure Method

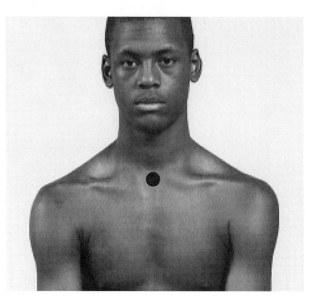

Fig. 9-17. Starting position for measurement of cervical extension using tape measure method. Bony landmark (sternal notch) indicated by orange dot.

Patient position: Sitting erect (Fig. 9–17).

Patient action: After being instructed in motion desired, patient extends neck as far as possible. Patient then returns to starting position. This movement provides an estimate of ROM and demonstrates to patient exact motion desired (Fig. 9–18).

Fig. 9-18. End ROM of cervical extension. Bony landmark (sternal notch) indicated by orange dot.

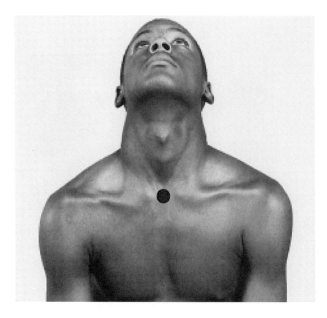

Fig. 9–19. Initial tape measure alignment for measurement of cervical flexion. Bony landmark (sternal notch) indicated by orange dot.

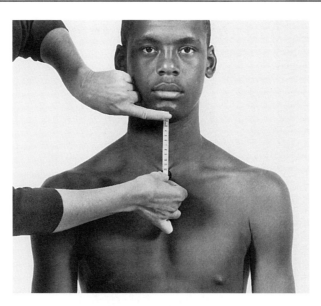

Tape measure alignment:

Palpate following bony landmarks (shown in Fig. 9–17) and align tape measure accordingly (Fig. 9–19). Tape measure should be aligned with 0 cm at tip of mandible.

  Superior: Tip of mandible (chin).

  Inferior: Sternal notch.

Measure distance between sternal notch to tip of mandible; referred to as the initial measurement (see Fig. 9–19).

Patient/Examiner action:

Patient extends cervical spine through available ROM. Examiner measures distance between sternal notch and chin; referred to as the final measurement (Fig. 9–20).

Documentation:

Difference between initial and final measurements is the ROM. Record patient's ROM in centimeters.

Fig. 9–20. Tape measure alignment at end ROM of cervical extension. Bony landmark (sternal notch) indicated by orange dot.

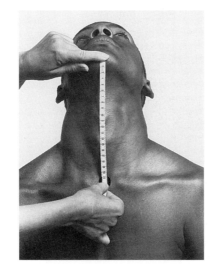

Extension—Cervical Spine: Goniometer Technique

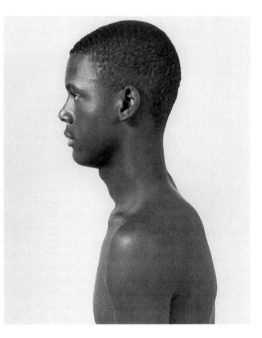

Fig. 9–21. Starting position for measurement of cervical flexion using goniometer technique.

Patient position: Sitting erect (Fig. 9–21).

Patient action: After being instructed in motion desired, patient actively extends cervical spine. This movement provides an estimate of ROM and demonstrates to patient exact motion desired (Fig. 9–22). Patient returns to starting position and is manually positioned so that a line between the ear lobe and base of nares is parallel to floor.

Fig. 9–22. End ROM for cervical extension.

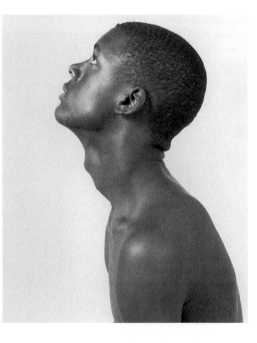

Fig. 9–23. Goniometer alignment at beginning range of cervical extension.

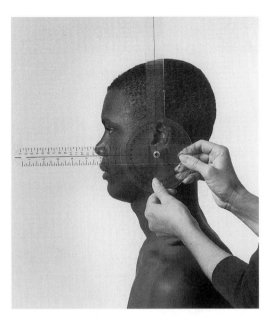

Goniometer alignment:	Palpate following landmarks and align goniometer accordingly (Fig. 9–23).
Stationary arm:	Perpendicular to floor.
Axis:	Ear lobe.
Moving arm:	Base of nares.
	Read scale of goniometer.
Patient/Examiner action:	Patient performs active cervical extension (see Fig. 9–22).
Confirmation of alignment:	Repalpate landmarks and confirm proper goniometer alignment at end ROM, correcting alignment as necessary (Fig. 9–24). Read scale of goniometer.
Documentation:	Record patient's ROM.

Fig. 9–24. Goniometer alignment at end ROM of cervical extension.

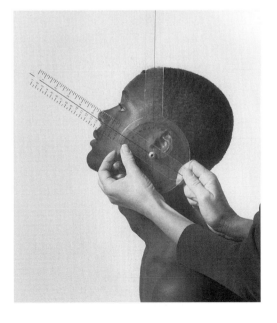

Extension—Cervical Spine: Inclinometer Method

Fig. 9–25. Starting position for measurement of cervical extension using inclinometer method. Bony landmark (spinous process of T1 vertebra) indicated by orange dot.

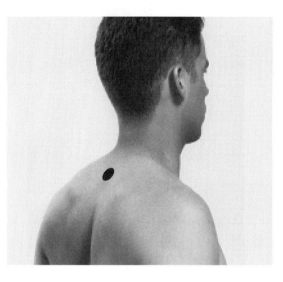

Patient position:	Sitting erect (Fig. 9–25).
Patient action:	After being instructed in motion desired, patient extends neck as far as possible. Patient then returns to starting position. This movement provides an estimate of ROM and demonstrates to patient exact motion desired (Fig. 9–26).
Inclinometer alignment:	Palpate following bony landmarks (shown in Fig. 9–25) and align inclinometers accordingly (Fig. 9–27). Ensure that inclinometers are set at 0 degrees once they are positioned on patient.
Inferior:	Spinous process of T1 vertebra.
Superior:	*Vertex of skull.

---

* Defined as $\frac{1}{2}$ distance between glabella (flattened triangular area on the forehead, also known as "bridge of nose") and inion (palpable "bump" at base of occiput).

Fig. 9–26. End ROM of cervical extension. Bony landmark (spinous process of T1 vertebra) indicated by orange dot.

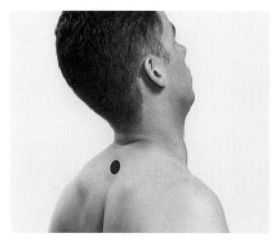

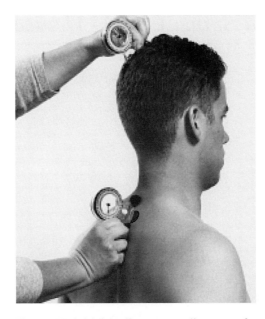

Fig. 9–27. Initial inclinometer alignment for measurement of cervical extension. Bony landmark (spinous process of T1 vertebra) indicated by orange dot. Inclinometers set at 0 degrees.

Patient/Examiner action:

Patient extends cervical spine through available ROM as examiner holds inclinometers in place. Examiner reads angle on inclinometers at end of extension ROM (Fig. 9–28).

Documentation:

Extension ROM recorded is measurement at the inferior landmark subtracted from measurement at superior landmark. Example: 30 degrees (reading at superior landmark) − 0 degrees (reading at inferior landmark) = 30 degrees of extension. Record patient's ROM.

Fig. 9–28. Inclinometer alignment at end ROM of cervical extension. Bony landmark (spinous process of T1 vertebra) indicated by orange dot.

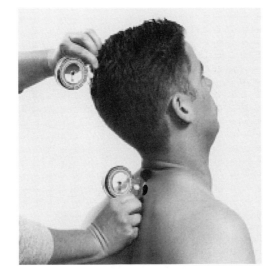

Extension—Cervical Spine: CROM Device

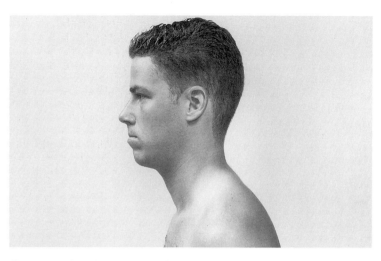

Fig. 9–29. Starting position for measurement of cervical extension using CROM device.

Patient position: Sitting erect (Fig. 9–29).

Patient action: After being instructed in motion desired, patient actively extends cervical spine. Patient then returns to starting position. This movement provides an estimate of ROM and demonstrates to patient exact motion desired (Fig. 9–30).

CROM alignment: Examiner positions CROM device on bridge of patient's nose and on the ears as one would put on a pair of eyeglasses. Velcro straps are fastened firmly behind head to hold CROM device in place (Fig. 9–31). Read scale of inclinometer on side of patient's head; referred to as initial measurement.

Fig. 9–30. End ROM of cervical extension.

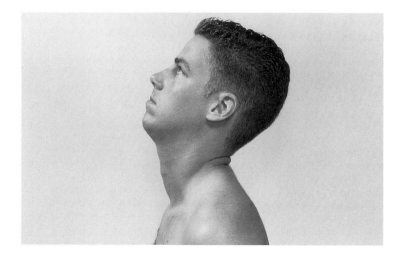

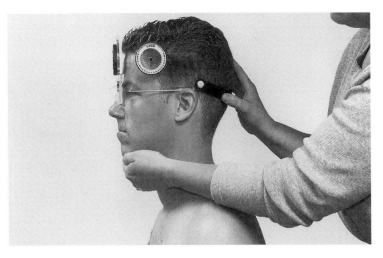

Fig. 9–31. CROM alignment at beginning range of cervical extension.

Patient/Examiner action: Patient performs active cervical extension while maintaining thoracic spine against back of chair (see Fig. 9–30).

Confirmation of alignment: Ensure that CROM device has remained in place at end ROM. Read scale of inclinometer on side of patient's head; referred to as final measurement (Fig. 9–32).

Documentation: Extension ROM recorded is initial measurement subtracted from final measurement. Example: 25 degrees (final measurement) − 0 degrees (initial measurement) = 25 degrees of extension. Record patient's ROM,

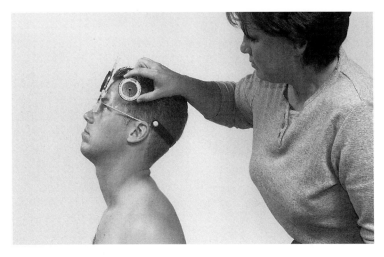

Fig. 9–32. CROM alignment at end ROM of cervical extension.

Lateral Flexion—Cervical Spine: Tape Measure Method

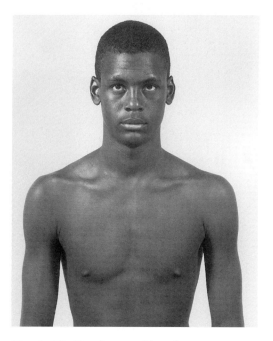

Fig. 9–33. Starting position for measurement of cervical lateral flexion using tape measure method.

Patient position:	Sitting erect (Fig. 9–33).
Patient action:	After being instructed in motion desired, patient actively laterally flexes cervical spine, bringing ear as close as possible to shoulder; no rotation, flexion, or extension of cervical spine is allowed. Examiner must ensure patient does not elevate shoulders during movement. Patient then returns to starting position. This movement provides an estimate of ROM and demonstrates to patient exact motion desired (Fig. 9–34).

Fig. 9–34. End ROM of cervical lateral flexion.

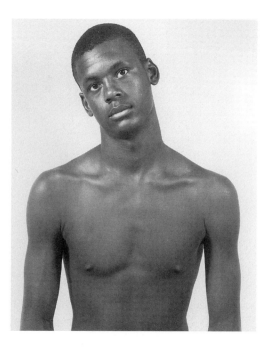

Fig. 9–35. Initial tape measure alignment for measurement of cervical lateral flexion.

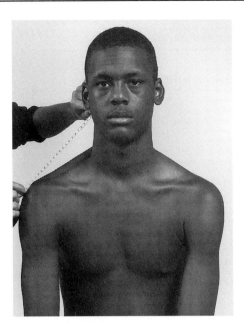

Tape measure alignment:	Palpate following landmarks and align tape measure accordingly (Fig. 9–35). Tape measure should be aligned with 0 cm at tip of mastoid process.
Superior:	Tip of mastoid process (behind ear).
Inferior:	Lateral tip of acromion process.

Measure distance between lateral tip of acromion process and tip of mastoid process; referred to as the initial measurement (see Fig. 9–35).

Patient/Examiner action: Patient laterally flexes cervical spine toward side of tape measure through available ROM. Examiner measures distance from acromion process to mastoid process; referred to as final measurement (Fig. 9–36).

Documentation: Difference between initial and final measurements is the ROM. Record patient's ROM in centimeters.

Fig. 9–36. Tape measure alignment at end ROM of cervical lateral flexion.

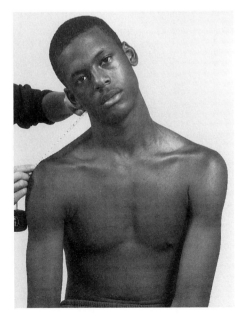

Lateral Flexion—Cervical Spine: Goniometer Technique

Fig. 9-37. Starting position for measurement of cervical lateral flexion using goniometer technique. Bony landmark (spinous process of C7 vertebra) indicated by orange dot.

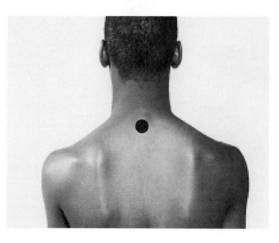

Patient position:	Sitting erect (Fig. 9-37).
Patient action:	After being instructed in motion desired, patient actively laterally flexes cervical spine, bringing ear as close as possible to shoulder; no rotation, flexion, or extension of cervical spine is allowed. Examiner must ensure patient does not elevate shoulders during movement. Patient then returns to starting position. This movement provides an estimate of ROM and demonstrates to patient exact motion desired (Fig. 9-38).
Goniometer alignment:	Palpate following bony landmarks (shown in Fig. 9-37) and align goniometer accordingly (Fig. 9-39).
Stationary arm:	Perpendicular to floor.
Axis:	Spinous process of C7 vertebra.
Moving arm:	Posterior midline of skull.

Read scale of goniometer.

Fig. 9-38. End ROM of cervical lateral flexion. Bony landmark (spinous process of C7 vertebra) indicated by orange dot.

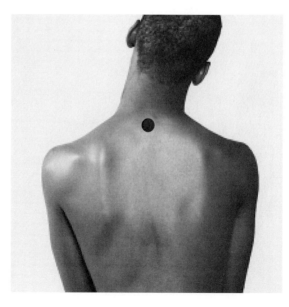

Fig. 9–39. Goniometer alignment at beginning range of cervical lateral flexion.

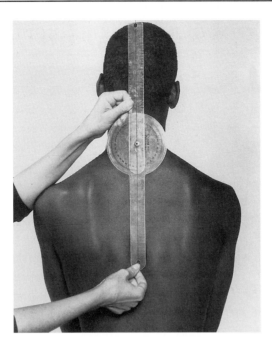

Patient/Examiner action:	Patient performs active lateral cervical flexion. Examiner ensures that patient's shoulders do not elevate during movement (see Fig. 9–38).
Confirmation of alignment:	Repalpate landmarks and confirm proper goniometer alignment at end ROM, correcting alignment as necessary (Fig. 9–40). Read scale of goniometer.
Documentation:	Record patient's ROM.

Fig. 9–40. Goniometer alignment at end ROM of cervical lateral flexion.

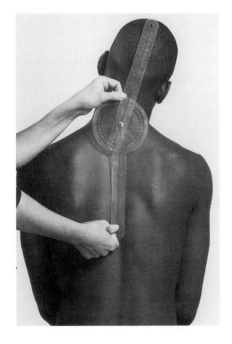

Lateral Flexion—Cervical Spine: Inclinometer Method

Fig. 9–41. Starting position for measurement of cervical lateral flexion using inclinometer method. Bony landmark (spinous process of T1 vertebra) indicated by orange dot.

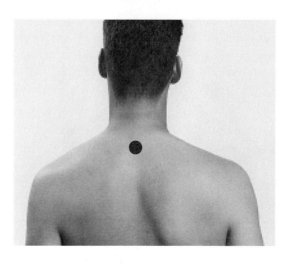

Patient position:	Sitting erect (Fig. 9–41).
Patient action:	After being instructed in motion desired, patient actively laterally flexes cervical spine, bringing ear as close as possible to shoulder; no rotation, flexion, or extension of cervical spine is allowed. Examiner must ensure patient does not elevate shoulders during movement. Patient then returns to starting position. This movement provides an estimate of ROM and demonstrates to patient exact motion desired (Fig. 9–42).
Inclinometer alignment:	Palpate following bony landmarks (shown in Fig. 9–41) and align inclinometers accordingly (Fig. 9–43). Ensure that inclinometers are set at 0 degrees once they are positioned on patient.
Inferior:	Spinous process of T1 vertebra.
Superior:	*Vertex of skull.

---

*Defined as $\frac{1}{2}$ distance between glabella (flattened triangular area on forehead, also known as "bridge of nose") and inion (palpable "bump" at base of occiput).

Fig. 9–42. End ROM of cervical lateral flexion. Bony landmark (spinous process of T1 vertebra) indicated by orange dot.

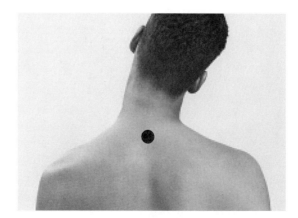

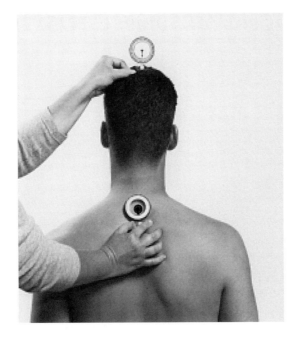

Fig. 9–43. Initial inclinometer alignment for measurement of cervical lateral flexion. Bony landmark (spinous process of T1 vertebra) indicated by orange dot. Inclinometers set at 0 degrees.

Patient/Examiner action: Patient laterally flexes cervical spine through available ROM as examiner holds inclinometers in place. Examiner reads angle on inclinometers at end of lateral flexion ROM (Fig. 9–44).

Documentation: Lateral flexion ROM recorded is measurement at the inferior landmark subtracted from measurement at superior landmark. Example: 30 degrees (reading at superior landmark) − 5 degrees (reading at inferior landmark) = 25 degrees of lateral flexion. Record patient's ROM.

Fig. 9–44. Inclinometer alignment at end ROM of cervical lateral flexion. Bony landmark (spinous process of T1 vertebra) indicated by orange dot.

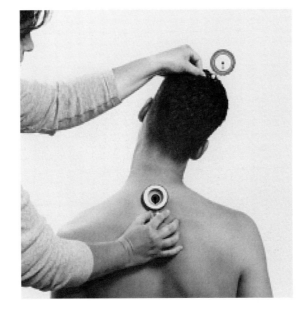

Lateral Flexion—Cervical Spine: CROM Device

Fig. 9–45. Starting position for measurement of cervical lateral flexion using CROM device.

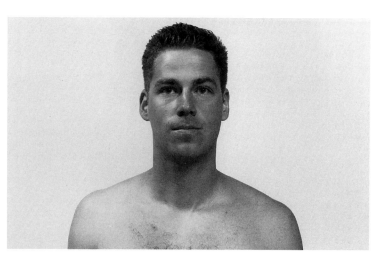

Patient position: Sitting erect (Fig. 9–45).

Patient action: After being instructed in motion desired, patient actively laterally flexes cervical spine, bringing ear as close as possible to shoulder; no rotation, flexion, or extension of cervical spine is allowed. Examiner must ensure patient does not elevate shoulders during movement. Patient then returns to starting position. This movement provides an estimate of ROM and demonstrates to patient exact motion desired (Fig. 9–46).

CROM alignment: Examiner positions CROM device on bridge of patient's nose and on the ears as one would put on a pair of eyeglasses. Velcro straps are fastened firmly behind head to hold CROM device in place (Fig. 9–47). Read scale of inclinometer on patient's forehead; referred to as initial measurement.

Fig. 9–46. End ROM of cervical lateral flexion.

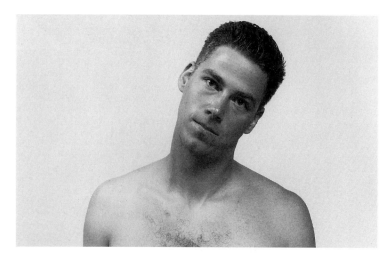

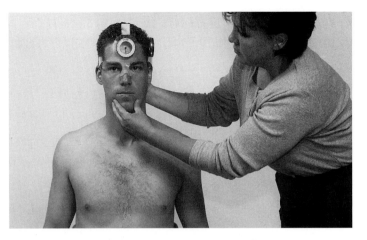

Fig. 9–47. CROM alignment at beginning range of cervical lateral flexion.

Patient/Examiner action:	Patient performs active lateral cervical flexion. Examiner ensures that patient's shoulders do not elevate during movement.
Confirmation of alignment:	Ensure that CROM device has remained in place at end ROM. Read scale of inclinometer on patient's forehead; referred to as final measurement (Fig. 9–48).
Documentation:	Lateral flexion ROM recorded is initial measurement subtracted from final measurement. Example: 40 degrees (final measurement) − 0 degrees (initial measurement) = 40 degrees of lateral flexion. Record patient's ROM.

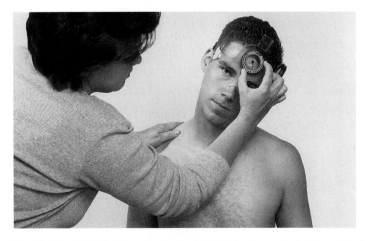

Fig. 9–48. CROM alignment at end ROM of cervical lateral flexion.

Rotation—Cervical Spine: Tape Measure Method

Fig. 9–49. Starting position for measurement of cervical rotation using tape measure method.

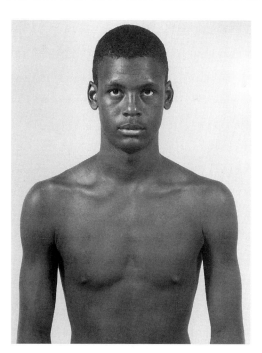

Patient position:	Sitting erect (Fig. 9–49).
Patient action:	After being instructed in motion desired, patient actively rotates cervical spine; no flexion, extension, or lateral flexion of cervical spine is allowed. Examiner must ensure patient does not rotate trunk during movement. Patient then returns to starting position. This movement provides an estimate of ROM and demonstrates to patient exact motion desired (Fig. 9–50).
Tape measure alignment:	Palpate following landmarks and align tape measure accordingly (Fig. 9–51). Tape measure should be aligned with 0 cm at tip of mandible.

Fig. 9–50. End ROM of cervical rotation.

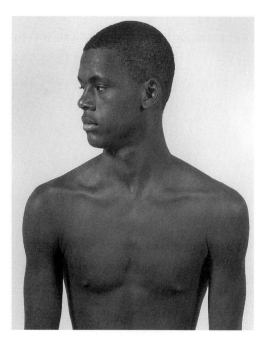

Fig. 9–51. Initial tape measure alignment for measurement of cervical rotation.

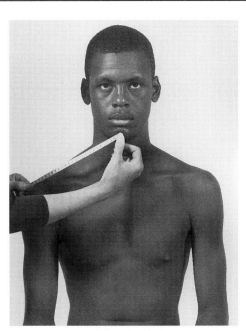

Superior:	Tip of mandible (chin).
Inferior:	Lateral tip of acromion process.

Measure distance between lateral tip of acromion process and tip of mandible; referred to as initial measurement (see Fig. 9–51).

Patient/Examiner action: Patient rotates cervical spine through available ROM toward side of tape measure. Examiner ensures that patient's trunk does not rotate during movement and measures distance from lateral tip of acromion process to tip of mandible; referred to as final measurement (Fig. 9–52).

Documentation: Difference between initial and final measurements is the ROM. Record patient's ROM in centimeters.

Fig. 9–52. Tape measure alignment at end ROM of cervical rotation.

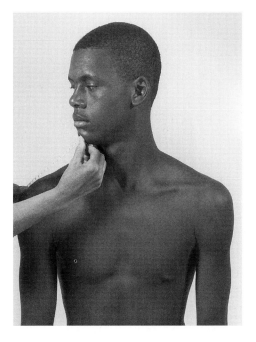

Rotation—Cervical Spine: Goniometer Technique

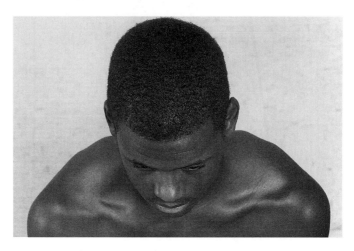

Fig. 9–53. Starting position for measurement of cervical rotation using goniometer technique.

Patient position:	Sitting erect (Fig. 9–53).
Patient action:	After being instructed in motion desired, patient actively rotates cervical spine; no flexion, extension, or lateral flexion of cervical spine is allowed. Examiner must ensure patient does not rotate trunk during movement. Patient then returns to starting position. This movement provides an estimate of ROM and demonstrates to patient exact motion desired (Fig. 9–54).

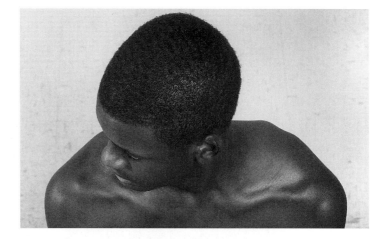

Fig. 9–54. End ROM of cervical rotation.

Fig. 9–55. Goniometer alignment at beginning range of cervical rotation.

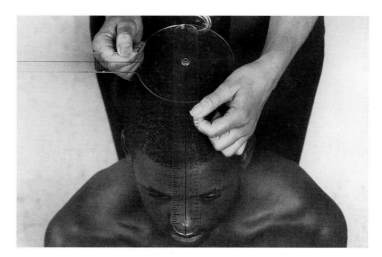

Goniometer alignment:	Palpate following landmarks and align goniometer accordingly (Fig. 9–55). (Note: Measurement occurs from the top of patient's head.)
Stationary arm:	Imaginary line connecting patient's two acromion processes.
Axis:	Top of subject's head.
Moving arm:	Nose.
	Read scale of goniometer.
Patient/Examiner action:	Patient rotates cervical spine through available ROM. Examiner ensures that patient's trunk does not rotate (see Fig. 9–54).
Confirmation of alignment:	Repalpate landmarks and confirm proper goniometer alignment at end ROM, correcting alignment as necessary (Fig. 9–56). Read scale of goniometer.
Documentation:	Record patient's ROM.

Fig. 9–56. Goniometer alignment at end ROM of cervical rotation.

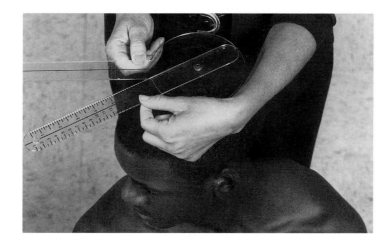

Rotation—Cervical Spine: Inclinometer Method

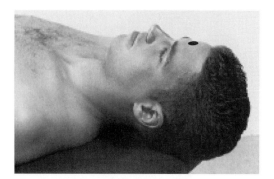

Fig. 9-57. Starting position for measurement of cervical rotation using inclinometer method. Bony landmark (base of forehead) indicated by orange dot.

Patient position:	Lying supine, with top of patient's head slightly over end of table; nose pointing to ceiling (Fig. 9-57).
Patient action:	After being instructed in motion desired, patient actively rotates cervical spine as far as possible; no flexion, extension, or lateral flexion of cervical spine is allowed. Examiner must ensure patient does not rotate trunk during movement. Patient then returns to starting position. This movement provides an estimate of ROM and demonstrates to patient exact motion desired (Fig. 9-58).

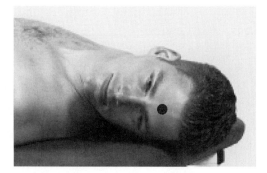

Fig. 9-58. End ROM of cervical rotation. Bony landmark (base of forehead) indicated by orange dot.

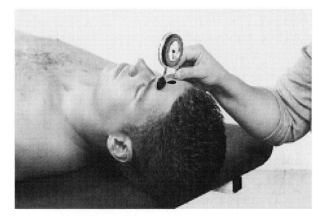

Fig. 9–59. Initial inclinometer alignment for measurement of cervical rotation. Bony landmark (base of forehead) indicated by orange dot. Inclinometer set at 0 degrees.

Inclinometer alignment: Palpate base of forehead (see Fig. 9–57) and align inclinometer accordingly (Fig. 9–59). Ensure inclinometer is set at 0 degrees.

Patient/Examiner action: Patient rotates cervical spine through available ROM as examiner holds inclinometer in place. Examiner reads angle on inclinometer at end of rotation ROM (Fig. 9–60).

Documentation: Record patient's ROM.

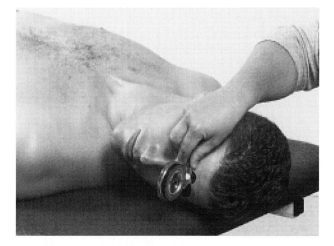

Fig. 9–60. Inclinometer alignment at end ROM of cervical rotation. Bony landmark (base of forehead) indicated by orange dot.

Rotation—Cervical Spine: CROM Device

Fig. 9–61. Starting position for measurement of cervical rotation using CROM device.

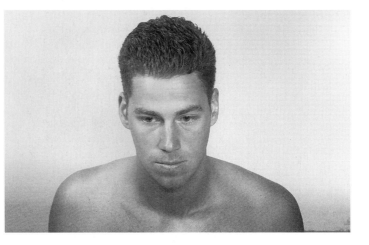

Patient position: Sitting erect, facing west (Fig. 9–61).

Patient action: After being instructed in motion desired, patient actively rotates cervical spine as far as possible; no flexion, extension, or lateral flexion of cervical spine is allowed. Examiner must ensure patient does not rotate trunk during movement. Patient then returns to starting position. This movement provides an estimate of ROM and demonstrates to patient exact motion desired (Fig. 9–62).

CROM alignment: To obtain accurate measurement, determine which direction is north. Place magnetic yoke on subject's shoulders with arrow pointing north (Fig. 9–63).

Examiner should add rotation arm to the CROM device. Examiner positions CROM device on bridge of patient's nose and on ears as one would put on a pair of eyeglasses. Velcro straps are fastened firmly behind head to hold CROM device in place (see Fig. 9–63). As subject faces straight ahead, meter on top of subject's head is set to 0 degrees.

Fig. 9–62. End ROM of cervical rotation.

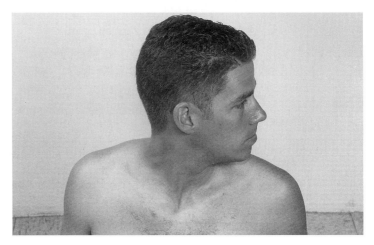

Fig. 9–63. CROM alignment at beginning range of cervical rotation; note placement of magnetic yoke pointing north. Inclinometer over vertex of skull set at 0 degrees.

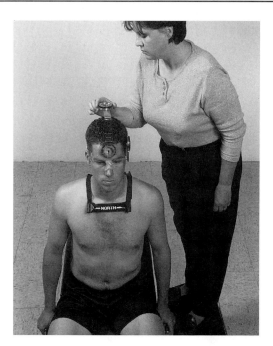

Patient/Examiner action:	Patient performs active cervical rotation (see Fig. 9–62).
Confirmation of alignment:	Ensure that CROM device has remained in place at end ROM. Read scale of inclinometer at top of head (Fig. 9–64).
Documentation:	Record patient's ROM.

Fig. 9–64. CROM alignment at end ROM of cervical rotation.

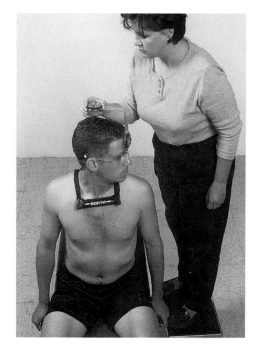

Mandibular Depression (Opening)—Temporomandibular Joint: Ruler Method

Fig. 9–65. End ROM of mandibular depression.

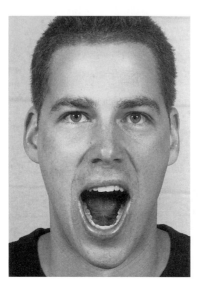

Patient position:	Sitting erect.
Patient action:	Patient opens mouth as wide as possible. This movement provides an estimate of ROM and demonstrates to patient exact motion desired (Fig. 9–65).
Patient/Examiner action:	Tips of right (or left) maxillary and mandibular central incisors are used as reference points. As patient maximally opens mouth, distance between tips of right (or left) maxillary and mandibular central incisors are measured with ruler (Fig. 9–66).
Documentation:	Distance between tips of central incisors is recorded.

Fig. 9–66. Ruler alignment at end ROM of mandibular depression.

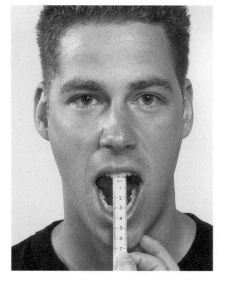

Mandibular Depression (Opening)—Temporomandibular Joint: Therabite Range of Motion Scale

Fig. 9–67. End ROM of mandibular depression.

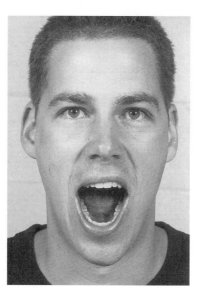

Patient position:	Sitting erect.
Patient action:	Patient opens mouth as wide as possible. This movement provides an estimate of ROM and demonstrates to patient exact motion desired (Fig. 9–67).
Patient/Examiner action:	Tips of right (or left) maxillary and mandibular central incisors are used as reference points. As patient maximally opens mouth, Therabite device (Therabite Corporation, 3415 West Chester Pike, Newtown Square, PA, 19073) is used. Notch of Therabite rests on tip of right (or left) mandibular central incisor and scale is rotated until Therabite contacts top of right (or left) maxillary central incisor (Fig. 9–68).
Documentation:	Measurement at point of contact on tip of maxillary central incisor is recorded.

Fig. 9–68. Therabite alignment at end ROM of mandibular depression.

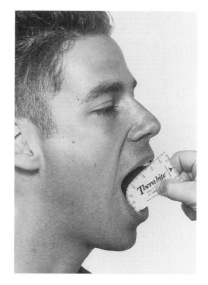

Protrusion—Temporomandibular Joint

Fig. 9–69. End ROM of mandibular protrusion.

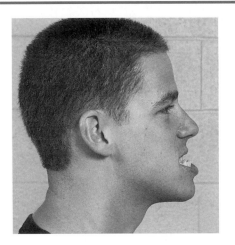

Patient position:	Sitting erect.
Patient action:	Patient slightly disoccludes mouth (slight opening of mouth, just enough to eliminate tooth contact) and protrudes or juts the lower jaw anteriorly past the upper teeth. This movement provides an estimate of ROM and demonstrates to patient exact motion desired (Fig. 9–69).

Fig. 9–70. Ruler alignment at end ROM of mandibular protrusion.

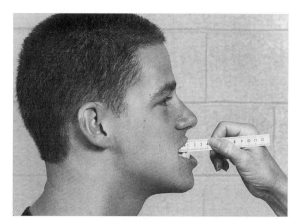

Patient/Examiner action:	Tips of right (or left) maxillary and mandibular central incisors are used as reference points. As patient protrudes lower jaw, distance that tip of right (or left) mandibular central incisor moves horizontally past tip of right (or left) maxillary central incisor is measured with ruler (Fig. 9–70).
Documentation:	Distance between tips of central incisors is recorded.
Note:	One edge of Therabite device contains a ruler that can be used for measurement of protrusion.

Lateral Deviation (Excursion)—Temporomandibular Joint

Fig. 9–71. End ROM of mandibular lateral deviation.

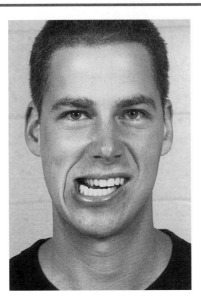

Patient position:	Sitting erect.
Patient action:	Patient slightly disoccludes mouth (slight opening of mouth just enough to eliminate tooth contact) and moves mandible laterally in horizontal plane, first to one side and then to other side. This movement provides an estimate of ROM and demonstrates to patient exact motion desired (Fig. 9–71).

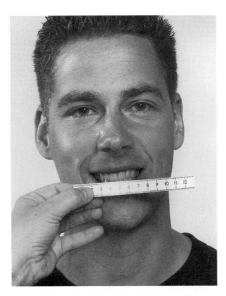

Fig. 9–72. Ruler alignment at beginning range of mandibular lateral deviation. (Note that space between mandibular central incisors is aligned with 5 cm mark of ruler.)

Fig. 9–73. Ruler alignment at end ROM of mandibular lateral deviation. (Note that space between mandibular central incisors lines up with 4.3 cm, indicating 0.7 cm of mandibular lateral deviation.)

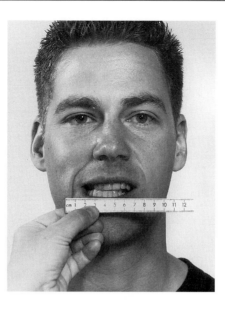

Patient/Examiner action: Space between maxillary central incisors and space between mandibular central incisors (interproximal space) are used as reference points for initial measurement with ruler (Fig. 9–72). At beginning of ROM, ruler is placed in front of central incisors, and distance from space between maxillary central incisors and space between mandibular central incisors is measured; referred to as initial measurement. In Figure 9–72, the spaces between both the maxillary and the mandibular central incisors line up with the 5 cm mark on the ruler, so the initial measurement equals 0 cm. As patient laterally deviates the jaw, distance from space between maxillary central incisors and space between mandibular central incisors is measured with ruler; referred to as final measurement (Fig. 9–73).

Documentation: Difference between initial and final measurements is the ROM. Record patient's ROM in centimeters.

Note: One edge of Therabite device contains a ruler that can be used for measurement of lateral deviation.

References

1. Alaranta H, Hurri H, Heliovaara M, et al.: Flexibility of the spine: Normative values of goniometric and tape measurements. Scand J Rehabil Med 1994;26:147–154.
2. American Medical Association: Guides to the Evaluation of Permanent Impairment, 4th ed. Chicago, 1993.
3. Balogun JA, Abereoje OK, Olaogun MO, Obajuluwa VA: Inter- and intratester reliability of measuring neck motions with tape measure and Myrin gravity-reference goniometer. J Orthop Sports Phys Ther 1989;10:248–253.
4. Bennett JG, Bergmanis LE, Carpenter JK, Skowlund HV: Range of motion of the neck. Phys Ther 1963;43:45–47.
5. Freidman MH, Weisberg J. Application of orthopedic principles in evaluation of the temporomandibular joint. Phys Ther 1982;62:597–603.
6. Iglarsh A, Snyder-Mackler L. Temporomandibular joint and the cervical spine. In Richardson JK, Iglarsh ZA. Clinical Orthopaedic Physical Therapy. Philadelphia: WB Saunders, 1994, pp 1–72.
7. Kadir N, Grayson MF, Goldberg AAJ, Swain M: A new neck goniometer. Rheumatol Rehabil 1981;20:219–226.
8. Kraus SL. Evaluation and management of temporomandibular disorders. In Saunders HD, Saunders R. Evaluation, Treatment and Prevention of Musculoskeletal Disorders, 3rd ed. Philadelphia: WB Saunders, 1993.
9. Magee DJ. Orthopedic Physical Assessment. 3rd ed. Philadelphia: W.B. Saunders, 1997.
10. Tucci SM, Hicks JE, Gross EG, et al.: Cervical motion assessment: A new, simple and accurate method. Arch Phys Med Rehabil 1986;67:225–230.
11. Youdas JW, Garrett TR, Suman VJ, et al.: Normal range of motion of the cervical spine: An initial goniometric study. Phys Ther 1992;72:770–780.
12. Zachman ZJ, Traina AD, Keating JC, et al.: Interexaminer reliability and concurrent validity of two instruments for the measurement of cervical ranges of motion. J Manipulative Physiol Ther 1989;12:205–210.

10

RELIABILITY and VALIDITY of MEASUREMENT of RANGE of MOTION for the SPINE and TEMPOROMANDIBULAR JOINT

Chapters 8 and 9 described the techniques for measurement of the spine and the temporomandibular joint. The purpose of this chapter is to present information on the reliability and validity of these techniques of measurement of the spine. Following an extensive review of published literature, each study related to reliability and validity was screened. Inclusion in this chapter was dependent on the study comprising appropriate statistical analysis that included the use of an intraclass correlation (ICC) or Pearson product moment correlation coefficient (Pearson's r) with appropriate follow-up procedures (refer to Chapter 2 for further discussion of reliability and validity). In a few instances, where only one study was performed using a specific technique, an article that did not meet the established criteria was nevertheless included in this chapter, but these exceptions to the criteria were rare and are specifically noted in the text.

No attempt was made to rate one measurement technique as better or worse than another technique. As indicated previously, the purpose of this chapter is to present information on the accuracy and reproducibility of the measurement techniques of the spine. This information, with the accompanying tables, will enable the reader to make an educated decision as to the most appropriate measurement technique for a particular clinical situation.

THORACIC AND LUMBAR SPINE

TAPE MEASURE

Flexion

Schober Method

Methods for using the tape measure for measuring range of motion of the lumbar spine are numerous. The earliest technique used was the Schober method, in which the distance between the lumbosacral junction and a point 10 cm above the lumbosacral junction was measured before and after the patient flexed and extended his or her spine.[22, 29] The original Schober method has been modified by changing the landmarks used when measuring the range of motion of the spine. These changes in landmarks include measuring the distance between points 5 cm inferior and 10 cm superior to the lumbosacral junction (known as the modified Schober[22]) and measuring from a point in the center of a line connecting the two posterior superior iliac spines to a mark 15 cm superior to this baseline landmark (the modified-modified Schober[40]). Chapter 8 provides detailed descriptions of these measurement techniques.

In a study examining lumbar range of motion of 172 individuals, Fitzgerald et al.[11] used the original Schober method. Prior to data collection, reliability of the Schober technique was determined by two independent testers using as subjects 17 college-age students not involved in the larger study. Inter-rater reliability of the original Schober technique was reported to be 1.0 (Pearson's r). Although no follow-up statistical test was performed after the Pearson correlation analysis, as is appropriate (refer to Chapter 2), this study was included in this chapter because it is the only reliability study performed using the original Schober technique.

Prior to collecting values of back mobility in 282 children without disability, Haley et al.[15] established reliability in a pilot study. In one of the few studies to examine intrarater reliability of the modified Schober test, one tester measured six children between the ages of 5 and 9 years. The intrarater reliability was statistically analyzed using an ICC, yielding results of .83. The authors reported that the test was not only accurate but also "relatively easy and quick to perform on young children."

Inter-rater reliability of the modified Schober technique for measuring lumbar flexion was reported by Burdett et al.,[7] who measured 23 individuals between the ages of 20 and 40 years. The authors reported inter-rater reliability of .72 using an ICC and .71 using Pearson's r. Follow-up testing using an analysis of variance (ANOVA) indicated no significant difference between testers.

A comprehensive study by Hyytiainen et al.[18] provided intrarater and inter-rater reliability on the modified Schober test to measure lumbar flexion. Examining 30 males using the modified Schober method, the authors reported intrarater reliability of .88 and inter-rater reliability of .87 (Pearson's r). Follow-up testing using a paired t test indicated no significant difference related to the intrarater or inter-rater reliability. The authors concluded that the tape measure "was easy to use and required no expensive equipment."

Williams et al.[40] examined the intrarater and inter-rater reliability of the modified-modified Schober method for measuring lumbar flexion using three clinicians whose clinical experience ranged from 3 to 12 years. Examination of 15 patients with low back pain resulted in intrarater reliability using Pearson correlation coefficients of .89 for clinician #1, .78 for clinician #2, and .83 for clinician #3. Performing an ICC across all three clinicians resulted in an overall inter-tester reliability coefficient of .72.

Macrae and Wright[22] tested their contention that the modified Schober was a better test than the original Schober by comparing the correlations of lumbar flexion measurements obtained by both methods to measurements obtained radiographically (x-rays). The correlation coefficient (Pearson's r) between the original Schober and the x-ray (validity) was .90 (standard error = 6.2 degrees), and between the modified Schober technique and the x-ray (validity) it was .97 (standard error = 3.3 degrees). Although data on test-retest reliability were not obtained, the authors concluded that "the proposed modification was an improvement over the original Schober's."

In a second study comparing the modified Schober to radiographic examination of lumbar flexion in an attempt to determine validity, Portek et al.[35] evaluated 11 subjects. The reliability correlation between the modified Schober technique and x-ray (validity) was reported as .43 (Pearson's r). However, a t test revealed no significant difference between the measures obtained with the modified Schober and with x-rays. In contrast to the study by Macrae and Wright,[22] this study demonstrated little correlation between the clinical and the radiographic techniques. The authors concluded that the

Table 10–1. TAPE MEASURE: INTRATESTER RELIABILITY FOR LUMBAR FLEXION					
STUDY	**TECHNIQUE**	***n***	**SAMPLE**	**CORRELATION**	
				ICC*	***r*†**
Haley et al.[15]	Modified Schober	6	Healthy children (5–9 yr)	.83	
Hyytiainen et al.[18]	Modified Schober	30	Healthy adults (35–44 yr)		.88
Williams et al.[40]	Modified–Modified Schober	15	Low back pain adults (25–53 yr; $\bar{x} = 35.7$)		.89, .78, .83‡

* Intraclass correlation
† Pearson's *r*
‡ Three testers performed measurements.

modified Schober "only gave indices of back movement which did not reflect true intervertebral movement."

Summary: Tape Measure for Measurement of Lumbar Flexion

Tables 10–1 to 10–3 provide a summary of studies reviewed related to the reliability and validity of using a tape measure for measuring lumbar flexion. As indicated in the tables, intrarater reliability ranged from .72 to .89 (Table 10–1) and inter-rater reliability ranged from .71 to 1.0 (Table 10–2) for all techniques using a tape measure. Correlation between measurement with a tape measure using either the Schober or the modified Schober technique and radiographic examination yielded reliability coefficients of greater than .90 for one study and .43 for a second study (Table 10–3).

Extension

Using a modification of the Schober technique to measure extension in two studies, Williams et al.[40] examined the intrarater reliability of three clinicians using the modified-modified Schober technique on 15 subjects with low back pain, reporting correlation coefficients ranging from .69 to .91 (Pearson's *r*

Table 10–2. TAPE MEASURE: INTERTESTER RELIABILITY FOR LUMBAR FLEXION					
STUDY	**TECHNIQUE**	***n***	**SAMPLE**	**CORRELATION**	
				ICC*	***r*†**
Fitzgerald et al.[11]	Schober	17	Healthy adults (20–82 yr)		1.0
Burdett et al.[7]	Modified Schober	23	Healthy adults (20–40 yr)	.72	.71
Hyytiainen et al.[18]	Modified Schober	30	Healthy adults (35–44 yr)		.87
Williams et al.[40]	Modified–Modified Schober	15	Low back pain adults (25–53 yr; $\bar{x} = 35.7$)	.72‡	

* Intraclass correlation
† Pearson's *r*
‡ Three testers performed measurements.

Table 10–3. TAPE MEASURE: VALIDITY FOR LUMBAR FLEXION				
STUDY	**TECHNIQUE**	**n**	**SAMPLE**	**CORRELATION (r*)**
Macrae & Wright[22]	Schober vs. Modified Schober		Not able to determine	Schober: .90 Modified: .97
Portek et al.[35]	Modified Schober	11	Healthy adults (25–36 yr; x̄ = 29.5)	.43

* Pearson's r

and ICC). Using a similar measurement technique in the examination of 100 patients with low back pain and 100 individuals without low back pain, Beattie et al.[2] reported slightly higher intrarater reliability than Williams et al.[40] Test-retest reliability for the individuals with low back pain was .93, and for those without low back pain reliability was .90 (ICC). Beattie et al.[2] also examined intertester reliability in 11 subjects without low back pain, reporting a correlation coefficient of .94 (ICC).

Using a slightly different technique than the Schober method, Frost et al.[13] used a tape measure to examine the changed distance between the spinous process of C7 and the posterior superior iliac spine during spinal extension. Examining 24 subjects, Frost et al.[13] reported an intrarater reliability of .78 and an inter-rater reliability of .79 (Pearson's r). An ANOVA performed to analyze the difference between the first and second measurements (intrarater) indicated no significant difference. However, the ANOVA performed to analyze the difference between examiners (inter-rater) indicated that a significant difference existed ($p < .05$).

Tables 10–4 and 10–5 provide a summary of reliability studies using the tape measure to examine extension of the spine. As indicated in the tables, intrarater reliability ranged from .69 to .93 (Table 10–4) and inter-rater reliability was reported as .79 and .94 (Table 10–5).

Lateral Flexion

Fingertip to Floor

The fingertip-to-floor method measures the distance from the third fingertip to the floor after the patient laterally flexes the spine (a detailed description is presented in Chapter 8). Frost et al.[13] examined right lateral flexion in 24

Table 10–4. TAPE MEASURE: INTRATESTER RELIABILITY FOR LUMBAR EXTENSION					
STUDY	**TECHNIQUE**	**n**	**SAMPLE**	**CORRELATION**	
				ICC*	**r†**
Frost et al.[13]	PSIS/C7	24	Healthy adults (20–55 yr; x̄ = 33.8)		.78
Williams et al.[40]	Modified– Modified Schober	15	Low back pain adults (25–53 yr; x̄ = 35.7)	.76*	.79, .91, .69‡
Beattie et al.[2]	Modified Schober	(A) 100	Healthy adults (20–76 yr; x̄ = 32.4)	.93	
		(B) 100	Low back pain adults (16–65 yr; x̄ = 37.6)	.90	

* Intraclass correlation
† Pearson's r
‡ Three testers performed measurements.

Table 10–5. TAPE MEASURE: INTERTESTER RELIABILITY FOR LUMBAR EXTENSION

STUDY	TECHNIQUE	*n*	SAMPLE	CORRELATION ICC*	*r*[†]
Frost et al.[13]	PSIS/C7	24	Healthy adults (20–55 yr; $\bar{x} = 33.8$)		.79
Beattie et al.[2]	Modified Schober	11	Healthy adults (20–76 yr; $\bar{x} = 32.4$)	.94	

* Intraclass correlation
† Pearson's *r*

individuals using the fingertip-to-floor method. Both intrarater reliability and inter-rater reliability were reported as .91. However, follow-up ANOVA revealed a significant difference ($p < .01$) between measurements for both intrarater and inter-rater reliability.

Marks at Lateral Thigh

A second technique for measuring lateral flexion is to place marks at the points on the lateral thigh that the third fingertip touches during erect standing and after lateral flexion (a detailed description is presented in Chapter 8). Measuring 18 subjects, Rose[38] reported intrarater reliability of .89 for right lateral flexion and .78 for left lateral flexion (Pearson's *r*). The least significant difference (defined as the extent to which repeated measures must differ for significant difference to occur) was reported as 3.0 cm and 4.0 cm for right and left lateral flexion, respectively.

Hyytiainen et al.[18] examined 30 subjects and reported intrarater reliability of .85 and inter-rater reliability of .86 (Pearson's *r*). Follow-up testing using an ANOVA for both intrarater and inter-rater reliability indicated no significant differences between the measurements taken. Slightly higher intertester reliability was reported by Alaranta et al.,[1] who reported a correlation of .91 (Pearson's *r*) in the measurement of 24 individuals. Follow-up testing using a paired *t* test revealed no significant difference between testers.

Marks at Lateral Trunk

A third method for measuring lateral flexion is to place two marks on the lateral trunk and to measure the change in the distance between these two marks before and after lateral flexion (a detailed description is presented in Chapter 8). Using marks on the lateral trunk to measure lateral flexion in six children between the ages of 5 and 9 years, Haley et al.[15] reported intratester reliability correlations of .89 and .77 for right and left lateral flexion, respectively (ICC).

Summary: Tape Measure for Measurement of Lateral Flexion

A summary of studies investigating reliability of examination of lateral flexion using a tape measure is presented in Tables 10–6 and 10–7. As indicated, intratester reliability across all methods ranged from .77 to .91 (Table 10–6) and intertester reliability ranged from .86 to .91 (Table 10–7).

Table 10–6. TAPE MEASURE: INTRATESTER RELIABILITY FOR LUMBAR LATERAL FLEXION

STUDY	TECHNIQUE	n	SAMPLE	CORRELATION ICC*	r†
Frost et al.[13]	Finger to floor	24	Healthy adults (20–55 yr; x̄ = 33.8)		.91
Hyytiainen et al.[18]	Marks at lateral thigh	30	Healthy adults (35–44 yr)		.85
Rose[38]	Marks at lateral thigh	18	Healthy adults (x̄ = 19.5 yr)		.89 (right) .78 (left)
Haley et al.[15]	Marks at lateral trunk	6	Healthy children (5–9 yr)	.89 (right) .77 (left)	

* Intraclass correlation
† Pearson's r

Rotation

A unique method for measuring rotation of the thoracolumbar spine using a tape measure was described by Frost et al.,[13] measuring the distance between ipsilateral acromion and the contralateral greater trochanter before and after the subject rotates the spine (a detailed description is presented in Chapter 8). Only one study has attempted to document the use of the tape measure to examine the amount of spinal rotation. Frost et al.[13] not only provided a description but also determined the reliability of the rotation technique using the tape measure. Intratester reliability on 24 subjects was reported as .71; intertester reliability was extremely low, with a reliability coefficient of .13. Follow-up testing using ANOVA indicated no significant difference between measurements related to intrarater reliability, but a significant difference ($p < .05$) between testers related to intertester reliability. The authors indicated that the inability of the two testers to accurately define the landmarks was a limiting factor in this measurement technique and the cause of the low correlation for inter-rater reliability.

GONIOMETER

Goniometry is a relatively quick and easy method for measuring spinal mobility. In addition, goniometers are readily accessible to the clinician and commonly used.[11]

Table 10–7. TAPE MEASURE: INTERTESTER RELIABILITY FOR LUMBAR LATERAL FLEXION

STUDY	TECHNIQUE	n	SAMPLE	CORRELATION (r*)
Frost et al.[13]	Finger to floor	24	Healthy adults (20–55 yr; x̄ = 33.8)	.91
Hyytiainen et al.[18]	Marks at lateral thigh	30	Healthy adults (35–44 yr)	.86
Alaranta et al.[1]	Marks at lateral thigh	24	Healthy adults	.91†

* Pearson's r
† Total = left and right lateral flexion combined.

Table 10–8. GONIOMETER: INTRATESTER RELIABILITY FOR FLEXION AND EXTENSION OF LUMBAR SPINE				
STUDY	*n*	**SAMPLE**	**CORRELATION**	
			ICC*	*r*[†]
Flexion				
Nitschke et al.[32]	34	LBP (20–65 yr)	.92	.92
Extension				
Nitschke et al.[32]	34	LBP (20–65 yr)	.81	.82

* Intraclass correlation
[†] Pearson's *r*
LBP, low back pain

Flexion and Extension

Burdett et al.[7] examined intertester reliability by using goniometry to measure flexion and extension in 23 subjects. These authors reported intertester reliability coefficients of .85 (ICC and Pearson's *r*) for flexion and .75 (ICC) and .77 (Pearson) for extension. Testing using ANOVA indicated no significant difference between testers for measurements of lumbar flexion or extension.

Although similar results for intertester correlation coefficients were reported by Nitschke et al.,[32] the authors' interpretation of the findings were quite different. Examining intertester reliability in measuring flexion and extension in 34 patients with low back pain, Nitschke et al.[32] reported correlations of .84 (ICC) and .90 (Pearson's *r*) for flexion. The 95% confidence interval (CI) for flexion was 30.37 degrees, and the *t* test showed no significant difference. For extension, the correlation reported was .63 (ICC) and .76 (Pearson's *r*) (95% CI = 18.34 degrees; *t* test not significant). In addition, this study examined these 34 patients for test-retest intrarater reliability, reporting correlations of .92 (ICC and Pearson's *r*) for flexion (95% CI = 29.12 degrees; *t* test not significant), and .81 (ICC) and .82 (Pearson's *r*) for extension (95% CI = 17.15 degrees; *t* test not significant). Nitschke et al.[32] suggested that although the *t* test performed did not indicate systematic error, the large 95% CI indicated the presence of random error, indicating that "the measurement with a long arm goniometer had poor reliability."

Tables 10–8 and 10–9 present a summary of the studies related to use of the goniometer to measure lumbar flexion and extension. As indicated in the tables, only one study reported intratester reliability (Table 10–8), and the range for intertester reliability was from .63 to .90 (Table 10–9).

Table 10–9. GONIOMETER: INTERTESTER RELIABILITY FOR FLEXION AND EXTENSION OF LUMBAR SPINE				
STUDY	*n*	**SAMPLE**	**CORRELATION**	
			ICC*	*r*[†]
Flexion				
Burdett et al.[7]	23	Healthy adults (20–40 yr)	.85	.85
Nitschke et al.[32]	34	LBP	.84	.90
Extension				
Burdett et al.[7]	23	Healthy adults (20–40 yr)	.75	.77
Nitschke et al.[32]	34	LBP (20–65 yr)	.63	.76

* Intraclass correlation
[†] Pearson's *r*
LBP, low back pain

Lateral Flexion

Fitzgerald et al.[11] examined intertester reliability for lateral flexion using two testers and 17 subjects. Intertester correlations reported were .76 for right lateral flexion and .91 for left lateral flexion (Pearson's *r*). Although the Pearson correlation was not followed up with an appropriate test to analyze random or systematic error (refer to Chapter 2), this study was included because only one other study exists related to the reliability of the goniometer to measure lateral flexion. The authors suggested that the goniometer was "an objective and reliable method for measuring spinal range of motion."

Nitschke et al.[32] also established intertester reliability for lateral flexion as part of their study previously described. Intertester reliability correlations were .62 (ICC and Pearson's *r*) for right lateral flexion (95% CI = 14.23 degrees; *t* test not significant) and .80 (ICC and Pearson's *r*) for left lateral flexion (95% CI = 10.33 degrees; *t* test not significant). In addition to examining intertester reliability, Nitschke et al.[32] examined these same 34 patients with low back pain to establish intratester reliability. The authors reported intratester reliabilities of .76 (ICC and Pearson's *r*) for right lateral flexion (95% CI = 10.91 degrees; *t* test not significant) and .84 (ICC and Pearson's *r*) for left lateral flexion (95% CI = 9.43 degrees; *t* test not significant). Based on these results, the authors suggested that the use of the goniometer for measurement of spinal range of motion "is inadequate."

A summary of intertester reliabilities for use of the goniometer for measurement of lateral flexion is presented in Table 10–10. As indicated in the table, the range of intertester reliability was from .62 to .91.

INCLINOMETER

Expressing the concern that "joint movements in the spine are still being assessed largely by clinical observation and subjective impression" and not objective measurement, in 1967 Loebl[21] described the use of the inclinometer, which he referred to as "a new, simple method for accurate clinical measure of spinal posture and movement." Although his study was descriptive in nature, with no reliability data to support any contention of accuracy, Loebl[21] was one of the first to describe the use of the inclinometer.

Since Loebl's article,[21] much needed research has been published on the reliability and validity of the inclinometer to measure spinal mobility. Unlike the reliability reported for the tape measure procedures, which is relatively consistent and high, the reliability of the accuracy of measurement using the inclinometer reported in the literature varies widely.

Table 10–10. GONIOMETER: INTERTESTER RELIABILITY FOR LATERAL FLEXION OF LUMBAR SPINE				
STUDY	***n***	**SAMPLE**	**CORRELATION**	
			ICC*	***r*[†]**
Fitzgerald et al.[11]	17	Healthy adults (20–82 yr)		.76 (right) .91 (left)
Nitschke et al.[32]	34	Low back pain (20–65 yr)	.62 (right) .80 (left)	.62 (right) .80 (left)

* Intraclass correlation
† Pearson's *r*

Flexion and Extension

Several studies used a test-retest design, with one tester performing the inclinometer technique to determine intrarater reliability for measurements of flexion and extension. Other studies used two testers to perform the inclinometer technique, comparing the results obtained by the two testers to determine inter-rater reliability. Because of the number of publications related to reliability of using inclinometers to measure flexion and extension, this section is divided into the following subsections for clarity: studies dealing with intrarater reliability, investigations related to intertester reliability, and research comparing results obtained with the inclinometer to data from radiographic (x-ray) examination (validity).

Techniques used for each study vary, with some authors placing the inclinometer at locations similar to those used with the Schober technique previously described in the tape measure section of Chapter 8. This inclinometer technique is designated measurement of lumbar flexion and extension. Other authors placed one inclinometer at the sacral base and a second inclinometer at the level of the C7/T1 spinous process. This measurement is designated thoracolumbar flexion and extension.

Finally, some studies reported not only reliability of flexion and extension, but also reliability of "total" movement. Total movement is the measurement of maximal flexion added to maximal extension, with a correlation performed on the sum.

Intrarater Reliability

Using an inclinometer, Mellin[27] reported intrarater reliability coefficients in the examination of 10 subjects as .86 for lumbar flexion, .93 for thoracolumbar flexion, .93 for extension, and .98 for thoracolumbar extension (Pearson's r). However, matched t tests comparing the first measure to the second measure for each motion indicated that a significant difference ($p < .05$) existed for each motion. A second study in which Mellin was involved provided somewhat different results. Mellin et al.[28] examined 27 subjects, resulting in an intratester reliability of .91 for lumbar flexion, .94 for thoracolumbar flexion, .79 for lumbar extension, and .87 for thoracolumbar extension (Pearson's r). In this study, a matched t test comparing the first measurement to the second measurement resulted in no significant difference. The authors concluded that "the accuracy of the methods described (inclinometer) make them useful for measurement of thoracolumbar mobility. "

Nitschke et al.[32] and Rondinelli et al.[37] reported reliability coefficients similar to those reported in the studies just presented, but came to different conclusions in the analysis of their data. Measuring lumbar flexion and extension in 34 individuals with low back pain, Nitschke et al.[32] reported correlations of .90 (Pearson's r and ICC) for flexion and .70 (ICC) and .71 (Pearson's r) for extension. Although no systematic error was found (as determined by t tests between measurements that were not significant), the authors suggested that the large random error (95% CI = 28.46 degrees for flexion, 16.52 degrees for extension) indicated "poor intrarater reliability." Establishing intrarater reliability of two testers using three different inclinometer techniques, Rondinelli et al.[37] measured flexion in eight subjects. The authors reported correlations ranging from .70 to .90 for intrarater reliability for flexion (ICC) and concluded that "these findings appear to undermine the expectations that clinicians can reliably apply surface inclinometry."[37]

Establishing intratester reliability, Williams et al.[40] examined lumbar flexion and extension in 15 patients with low back pain using three testers.

Results for intratester reliability for each examiner ranged from .13 to .87 for flexion and .28 to .66 for extension (ICC). The conclusion reached by the authors was that the "inclinometer technique needs improvement."

The back range of motion (BROM) device is a specialized measurement tool consisting of two separate plastic frames that are secured to the individual with elastic straps. Within the plastic frames, inclinometers are mounted and allow measurement of flexion, extension, lateral flexion, and rotation. A detailed description of the BROM device is presented in Chapter 8. Using the BROM device to analyze intrarater reliability in two testers measuring lumbar flexion in eight subjects, Rondinelli et al.[37] reported reliability correlations of .81 and .90 (ICC). Expanding the study by Rondinelli et al.[37] to include not only flexion but also measurement of intratester reliability for extension in 47 subjects, Breum et al.[6] reported correlation coefficients (ICC) of .91 for flexion and .63 for extension. Breum et al.[6] concluded that the "BROM was found to be a reliable instrument in the measurement of lumbar mobility." Using the same basic design as was employed in the study by Breum et al.,[6] Madson et al.[23] analyzed the reliability of the BROM device in measuring lumbar range of motion in 40 subjects. Intrarater reliability was .67 for flexion and .78 for extension. The 95% CI was 5.0 degrees for both flexion and extension measurements.

Tables 10–11 and 10–12 provide a summary of studies investigating intrarater reliability for the measurement of flexion and extension using the inclinometer. As indicated, reliability coefficients across all studies ranged from .13 to .94 for measurement of flexion (Table 10–11) and from .28 to .87 for measurement of extension (Table 10–12). If the Williams et al.[40] data are removed from the tables, the range of reported reliability for flexion is .67 to .94 and for extension is .71 to .98.

Table 10–11. INCLINOMETER: INTRATESTER RELIABILITY FOR LUMBAR FLEXION					
STUDY	**TECHNIQUE**	***n***	**SAMPLE**	**CORRELATION**	
				ICC*	***r*[†]**
Mellin[27]	Single	10	Healthy adults ($\bar{x}$ = 31.3)		.86 .93 (T–L[‡])
Mellin et al.[28]	Single	27	Healthy adults (24–50 yr; $\bar{x}$ = 30.6)		.91 .94 (T–L[‡])
Williams et al.[40]	Double	15	LBP adults (25–53 yr; $\bar{x}$ = 35.7)	.60	.87, .76, .13[§]
Nitschke et al.[32]	Double	34	LBP adults (20–65 yr)	.90	.90
Breum et al.[6]	BROM[‖]	47	Healthy adults (18–38 yr; $\bar{x}$ = 25.8)	.91	
Madson et al.[23]	BROM	40	Healthy adults (20–40 yr; $\bar{x}$ = 25.5)	.67	
Rondinelli et al.[37]	Single, double, BROM	8	Healthy adults (18–30 yr)	.85, .86 (single)[¶] .70, .81 (double)[¶] .81, .90 (BROM)[¶]	

* Intraclass correlation
† Pearson's *r*
‡ Thoracolumbar range of motion
§ Three testers performed measurement.
‖ Back range of motion device (Performance Attainment Associates, Roseville, Minn)
¶ Two testers performed measurement.
LBP, Low back pain

Table 10–12. INCLINOMETER: INTRATESTER RELIABILITY FOR LUMBAR EXTENSION

STUDY	TECHNIQUE	n	SAMPLE	CORRELATION ICC*	CORRELATION $r^†$
Mellin[27]	Single	10	Healthy adults ($\bar{x}$ = 31.3)		.93 .98 (T–L‡)
Mellin et al.[28]	Single	27	Healthy adults (24–50 yr; $\bar{x}$ = 30.6)		.79 .87 (T–L)
Williams et al.[40]	Double	15	LBP (25–53 yr; $\bar{x}$ = 35.7)	.48	.28, .66, .55§
Nitschke et al.[32]	Double	34	LBP (20–65 yr)	.70	.71
Breum et al.[6]	BROM‖	47	Healthy adults (18–38 yr; $\bar{x}$ = 25.8)	.63	
Madson et al.[23]	BROM	40	Healthy adults (20–40 yr; $\bar{x}$ = 25.5)	.78	

* Intraclass correlation
† Pearson's r
‡ Thoracolumbar range of motion
§ Three testers performed measurements.
‖ Back range of motion device (Performance Attainment Associates, Roseville, Minn)
LBP, Low back pain

Inter-rater Reliability

Four groups of investigators who examined intrarater reliability also studied inter-rater reliability of measuring spinal flexion and extension using the inclinometer. Mellin[27] examined intertester reliability in 15 subjects, reporting correlation coefficients of .97 for lumbar flexion, .95 for thoracolumbar flexion, and .89 for both lumbar and thoracolumbar extension (Pearson's r). Matched t tests comparing the first tester to the second tester for each motion indicated that a significant difference ($p < .001$) existed for each motion. Nitschke et al.[32] examined 34 patients with low back pain and reported intertester reliability using the inclinometer of .52 (ICC) and .67 (Pearson's r) for flexion (95% CI = 28.46 degrees; t test = significant difference at $p < .05$) and .35 (ICC and Pearson's r) for extension (95% CI = 16.52 degrees; t test not significant). Intertester reliability for measuring eight subjects was reported by Rondinelli et al.[37] as correlations (ICC) of .76 for lumbar flexion using a single inclinometer, .69 using a double inclinometer, and .77 when using the BROM device. Identical correlations (.77) were reported for intertester reliability of the BROM device for measuring lumbar flexion by Breum et al.[6] in a study of 40 subjects (ICC). Reliability correlations reported when measuring lumbar extension with the BROM device were .35 (ICC). The conclusions and opinions proposed by the authors of these three studies as to the use of the inclinometer for the measurement of flexion and extension based on their data collection is exactly the same as the information already presented in the previous section discussing intratester reliability.

Several other groups of investigators examined only intertester reliability of spinal measurements using the inclinometer. Burdett et al.[7] reported reliability coefficients of .91 (ICC) and .93 (Pearson's r) for lumbar flexion and .71 (ICC) and .72 (Pearson's r) for lumbar extension in their single inclinometer examination of 23 subjects. Follow-up testing using ANOVA indicated no significant difference between testers for inter-rater reliability for extension, but a significant difference between testers for flexion ($p < .05$).

Slightly lower results were reported in a study of 12 subjects without back pain and six patients with back pain performed by Chiarello and Savidge.[9] Correlations (ICC) were reported as .74 for lumbar flexion for subjects without back pain, .64 for lumbar flexion for patients with low back pain, .65 for lumbar extension for subjects without back pain, and .83 for lumbar extension for patients with low back pain. The authors concluded that these results indicated "acceptable reliability," and that using the inclinometer "in a clinical setting to document lumbar spine range of motion represents a vast improvement over observational methods."

Newton and Waddell[30] examined intertester reliability for lumbar flexion and extension in 20 patients with low back pain. Reported reliability correlations (ICC) were good (.98) for flexion but relatively poor (.48) for extension. Examining 24 normal individuals for intertester reliability of lumbar flexion, Alaranta et al.[1] reported a correlation of .61 (Pearson's r). A t test between measurements by the two testers indicated a significant difference ($p < .05$). Authors of both studies concluded that the measurements using the inclinometer "were found to be generally good."[1]

Tables 10–13 and 10–14 summarize studies performed on inter-rater reliability for the use of the inclinometer to measure flexion and extension. As indicated, the intertester reliability ranged from .52 to .98 (Table 10–13) for flexion and from .35 to .89 for extension (Table 10–14).

Validity

In an effort to establish the validity of the use of the inclinometer to measure lumbar flexion and extension, investigators have compared results of their examination with the inclinometer to examination by radiographic (x-ray) assessment. Mayer et al.[26] examined flexion in 12 patients with low back pain with both an inclinometer (both single and double) and by x-ray. Results indicated no significant difference (ANOVA) between the x-ray examination and either the single or the double inclinometer method. The authors

STUDY	TECHNIQUE	n	SAMPLE	CORRELATION	
				ICC*	r†
Burdett et al.[7]	Single	23	Healthy adults (20–40 yr)	.91	.93
Mellin[27]	Single	15	Healthy adults ($\bar{x}$ = 31.3)		.97 .95 (T–L‡)
Newton & Waddell[30]	Single	20	Healthy adults (20–55 yr)	.98	
Chiarello & Savidge[9]	Single	12	Healthy adults (23–55 yr; $\bar{x}$ = 25.5)	.74	
		6	LBP (24–37 yr; $\bar{x}$ = 32.7)	.64	
Alaranta et al.[1]	Double	24	Healthy adults (35–54 yr)		.61
Nitschke et al.[32]	Double	34	LBP (20–65 yr)	.52	.67
Rondinelli et al.[32]	Single, double, BROM§	8	Healthy adults (18–30 yr)	.76 (single) .69 (double) .77 (BROM)	
Breum et al.[6]	BROM	47	Healthy adults (18–38 yr; $\bar{x}$ = 25.8)	.77	

Table 10–13. INCLINOMETER: INTERTESTER RELIABILITY FOR LUMBAR FLEXION

* Intraclass correlation
† Pearson's r
‡ Thoracolumbar range of motion
§ Back range of motion device (Performance Attainment Associates, Roseville, Minn)
LBP, Low back pain

Table 10–14. INCLINOMETER: INTERTESTER RELIABILITY FOR LUMBAR EXTENSION					
STUDY	**TECHNIQUE**	***n***	**SAMPLE**	**CORRELATION**	
				ICC*	***r*†**
Burdett et al.[7]	Single	23	Healthy adults (20–40 yr)	.71	.72
Mellin[27]	Single	15	Healthy adults (x̄ = 31.3)		.89 .89 (T–L‡)
Newton & Waddell[30]	Single	20	Healthy adults (20–55 yr)	.48	
Chiarello & Savidge[9]	Single	12	Healthy adults (23–55 yr; x̄ = 25.5)	.65	
		6	LBP (24–37 yr; x̄ = 32.7)	.83	
Nitschke et al.[32]	Double	34	LBP (20–65 yr)	.35	.35
Breum et al.[6]	BROM§	47	Healthy adults (18–38 yr; x̄ = 25.8)	.35	

* Intraclass correlation
† Pearson's *r*
‡ Thoracolumbar range of motion
§ Back range of motion device (Performance Attainment Associates, Roseville, Minn)
LBP, Low back pain

concluded that "inclinometer measurement of range of motion is a simple, effective, quantitative technique for assessing disability and measuring progress in rehabilitation."[26]

Additional studies have examined validity of the inclinometer. Examining flexion in 27 subjects with the inclinometer and comparing these results to an examination by x-ray, Burdett et al.[7] reported a correlation coefficient of .73 for lumbar flexion and .15 for extension (Pearson's *r*). An ANOVA indicated no significant difference between inclinometer and x-ray measurement techniques for either flexion or extension. Newton and Waddell[30] examined flexion only in 20 patients with low back pain, reporting a correlation of .76 between the results obtained from the use of an inclinometer and from an x-ray (ICC).

Lower correlations between radiologic examination and the inclinometer were reported by Portek et al.[35] Measuring flexion and extension in 11 subjects, these authors reported correlations of .42 for flexion and .55 for extension (Pearson's *r*). No significant difference was found between inclinometer and radiographic examination (*t* test). Due to the poor correlations, the authors concluded that "comparison with the radiologic technique showed that the clinical measure only gave indices of back movement." The summary of the results of the validity studies comparing results obtained by the inclinometer and by x-ray examination are presented in Tables 10–15 and 10–16.

Lateral Flexion

Although research on the use of the inclinometer for measurement of flexion and extension of the spine is relatively common, investigations reporting the reliability of the inclinometer for the measurement of lateral flexion are few in number. Mellin et al.[28] used the inclinometer to examine the intratester reliability for measurement of lateral flexion in 27 subjects, measuring right and left lateral lumbar flexion (inclinometer placed both at and 20 cm superior to the posterior superior iliac spine) and right and left lateral thoracolumbar flexion (inclinometer placed at the posterior superior iliac spine and at the spinous process of T1). Reported correlations for intratester

Table 10-15. VALIDITY: X-RAY VS. INCLINOMETER FOR FLEXION OF LUMBAR SPINE

STUDY	TECHNIQUE	n	SAMPLE	CORRELATION ICC*	r†
Portek et al.[35]	Single	11	Healthy adults (25–36 yr; x̄ = 29.5)		.42
Burdett et al.[6]	Single	23	Healthy adults (20–40 yr)		.73
Newton & Waddell[30]	Single	20	Healthy adults (20–55 yr)	.76	
Mayer et al.[26]	Single, double	12	Low back pain (19–51 yr; x̄ = 31.0)	No significant difference between x-ray and single inclinometer, nor between x-ray and double inclinometer (total)‡	

* Intraclass correlation
† Pearson's r
‡ Total = extension and flexion range of motion combined; analysis of variance with repeated measures was statistical analysis performed.

reliability were as follows: right lateral lumbar flexion = .84, left lateral lumbar flexion = .86, right lateral thoracolumbar flexion = .81, and left lateral thoracolumbar flexion = .85 (Pearson's r). The matched t tests analyzing differences between measurements were not significant for any motion examined. Newton and Waddell[30] reported similar correlations for intertester reliability in the measurement of 20 patients with low back pain. The correlation for right lateral flexion was .78 and for left lateral flexion was .84 (ICC).

Nitschke et al.[32] examined both intrarater and inter-rater reliability of lateral flexion measurements in 34 subjects. Results for analysis of intrarater reliability were reported at .90 (95% CI = 10.26 degrees; t test not significant) for right lateral lumbar flexion and .89 (95% CI = 10.77 degrees; t test not significant) for left lateral lumbar flexion irrespective of the correlation

Table 10-16. VALIDITY: X-RAY VS. INCLINOMETER FOR EXTENSION OF LUMBAR SPINE

STUDY	TECHNIQUE	n	SAMPLE	CORRELATION (r*)
Portek et al.[35]	Single	11	Healthy adults (25–36 yr; x̄ = 29.5)	.55
Burdett et al.[7]	Single	27	Healthy adults (20–40 yr)	.15
Mayer et al.[26]	Single, double	12	Low back pain (20–59 yr; x̄ = 34.0)	No significant difference between x-ray and single inclinometer, nor between x-ray and double inclinometer (total)†

* Pearson's r
† Total = extension and flexion range of motion combined; analysis of variance with repeated measures was statistical analysis performed.

Table 10–17. INCLINOMETER: INTRATESTER RELIABILITY FOR LATERAL LUMBAR FLEXION

STUDY	TECHNIQUE	*n*	SAMPLE	CORRELATION ICC*	*r*†
Mellin et al.[28]	Single	27	Healthy adults (24–50 yr; x̄ = 30.6)		.84 (right) .86 (left) .81 (right T–L)‡ .85 (left T–L)
Nitschke et al.[32]	Double	34	Healthy adults (20–65 yr)	.90 (right) .89 (left)	.90 (right) .89 (left)
Breum et al.[6]	BROM§	47	Healthy adults (18–38 yr; x̄ = 25.8)	.89 (right) .92 (left)	
Madson et al.[23]	BROM	40	Healthy adults (20–40 yr; x̄ = 25.5)	.91 (right) .95 (left)	

* Intraclass correlation
† Pearson's *r*
‡ Thoracolumbar range of motion
§ Back range of motion device (Performance Attainment Associates, Roseville, Minn)

analysis used (ICC or Pearson's *r*). However, data for inter-rater reliability were far less than acceptable; right lateral lumbar flexion was .18 (ICC) and .62 (Pearson's *r*) (95% CI = 15.79 degrees; *t* test was significant at $p < .05$), and left lateral lumbar flexion was .13 (ICC) and .55 (Pearson's *r*) (95% CI = 16.76 degrees; *t* test was significant at $p < .05$). Nitschke et al.[32] suggested that owing to "systematic and random error" their findings indicate the use of the inclinometer for "spinal range of motion measurements is inadequate."

Both Madson et al.[23] and Breum et al.[6] used the BROM device to investigate reliability of measuring lateral flexion. Examining only intratester reliability, Madson et al.[23] reported correlations (Pearson's *r*) on 40 subjects of .91 for right lateral flexion and .95 for left lateral flexion (95% CI = 5 degrees). Results of intrarater reliability on 47 subjects for right lateral flexion and left lateral flexion were reported by Breum et al.[6] to be .89 and .92, respectively (ICC). Inter-rater reliability was reported as .89 for right lateral flexion and .81 for left lateral flexion (ICC). Tables 10–17 and 10–18 provide a summary of the studies reviewed related to reliability of measurement of lateral flexion using an inclinometer.

Table 10–18. INCLINOMETER: INTERTESTER RELIABILITY FOR LATERAL LUMBAR FLEXION

STUDY	TECHNIQUE	*n*	SAMPLE	CORRELATION ICC*	*r*†
Newton & Waddell[30]	Single	20	Healthy adults (20–55 yr)	.78 (right) .84 (left)	
Nitschke et al.[32]	Double	34	Healthy adults (20–65 yr)	.18 (right) .13 (left)	.62 (right) .55 (left)
Breum et al.[6]	BROM‡	47	Healthy adults (18–38 yr; x̄ = 25.8)	.89 (right) .81 (left)	

* Intraclass correlation
† Pearson's *r*
‡ Back range of motion device (Performance Attainment Associates, Roseville, Minn)

Rotation

Similar to the number of investigations on the reliability of the inclinometer in measuring lateral flexion, few studies have been performed on the reliability of the inclinometer in measuring rotation. In the most extensive study investigating the intertester reliability of the inclinometer for the measurement of lumbar rotation, Boline et al.[5] measured 25 subjects without back pain and 25 patients with low back pain using a technique in which the subject fully flexes the lumbar spine and then rotates maximally. Reliability correlations (ICC and Pearson's r) for right rotation, left rotation, and total range of motion (sum of left and right rotation combined) for subjects (n = 25), patients (n = 25), and all individuals combined (n = 50) ranged from .52 to .86.

Using a different inclinometer technique for measuring rotation, Alaranta et al.[1] measured rotation with the subjects seated. Using the mean of the total range of motion of right and left rotation, the authors reported an intertester reliability correlation of .79 (Pearson's r). Paired t test between testers indicated no significant difference.

Breum et al.[6] examined the reliability of the BROM device to measure rotation. Intrarater reliability for right rotation was .57 and for left rotation was .56 (ICC). Inter-rater reliability was quite low, with the authors reporting a correlation of .35 for right rotation and of .37 for left rotation (ICC). Madson et al.[23] reported a much higher intratester reliability using the BROM device than Breum et al.[6]: .88 for right rotation and .93 for left rotation (ICC). Tables 10–19 and 10–20 summarize the studies presented in this section.

CERVICAL SPINE

As was evident in the previous sections of this chapter, much research has been performed on the lumbar spine, using a variety of techniques, in an attempt to establish appropriate methods of measuring lumbar spine range of motion. Although the same measurement devices have been used to measure cervical range of motion, far less research has been performed on these techniques.

TAPE MEASURE

A study by Hsieh and Yeung[17] evaluated the intratester reliability of two different clinicians using a tape measure to examine six cervical motions in 34 subjects. As indicated in Table 10–21, intratester reliability ranged from .78

Table 10–19. INCLINOMETER: NTRATESTER RELIABILITY FOR LUMBAR ROTATION				
STUDY	**TECHNIQUE**	**n**	**SAMPLE**	**CORRELATION (ICC*)**
Breum et al.[6]	Sitting (BROM†)	47	Healthy adults (18–38 yr; $\bar{x}$ = 25.8)	.57 (right) .56 (left)
Madson et al.[23]	Sitting (BROM)	40	Healthy adults (20–40 yr; $\bar{x}$ = 25.5)	.88 (right) .93 (left)

* Intraclass correlation
† Back range of motion device (Performance Attainment Associates; Roseville, Minn)

Table 10–20. INCLINOMETER: INTERTESTER RELIABILITY FOR LUMBAR ROTATION

STUDY	TECHNIQUE	n	SAMPLE	CORRELATION		
				ICC*	r[†]	
Boline et al.[5]	Full flexion and rotate (single)	50	25 healthy adults (x̄ = 33.0 yr) 25 LBP (x̄ = 28.0 yr)	.67	.69	R rot (all[‡])
				.84	.86	R rot (LBP[§])
				.53	.54	R rot (norm[∥])
				.71	.72	L rot (all)
				.53	.52	L rot (LBP)
				.71	.73	L rot (norm)
				.75	.75	Total[¶] rot (all)
				.78	.79	Total rot (LBP)
				.70	.70	Total rot (norm)
Alaranta et al.[1]	Sitting (single)	24	Healthy adults (35–54 yr)		.79 (mean)**	
Breum et al.[6]	Sitting (BROM[††])	47	Healthy adults (18–38 yr; x̄ = 25.8)	.35 (right) .37 (left)		

* Intraclass correlation
[†] Pearson's r
[‡] All subjects
[§] Subgroup of subjects with low back pain
[∥] Subgroup of subjects with no low back pain
[¶] Left and right rotation range of motion combined
** Mean of the total range of right and left rotation
[††] Back range of motion device (Performance Attainment Associates, Roseville, Minn)
R rot, right rotation; L rot, left rotation

to .94. The 99% CI ranged from 1 cm to 3 cm. The authors concluded that the tape measure method "is a reliable means for clinicians to assess neck range of motion."

GONIOMETER

While studies on the reliability of the goniometer have been published in the literature related to the lumbar spine, studies also have been performed to test intratester and intertester reliability in the use of the goniometer in measurements on the cervical spine. This section presents information on reliability studies related to cervical flexion, extension, lateral flexion, and rotation.

Procedures for measuring cervical range of motion of flexion, extension, lateral flexion, and rotation using goniometry techniques similar to those

Table 10–21. TAPE MEASURE: INTRATESTER RELIABILITY FOR RANGE OF MOTION OF CERVICAL SPINE

STUDY	n	SAMPLE	CORRELATION (r*)
Flexion			
Hsieh & Yeung[17]	34	Healthy adults (14–31 yr; x̄ = 18.2)	.86, .95[†]
Extension			
Hsieh & Yeung[17]	34	Healthy adults (14–31 yr; x̄ = 18.2)	.79, .94[†]
Lateral Flexion			
Hsieh & Yeung[17]	34	Healthy adults (14–31 yr; x̄ = 18.2)	.91, .88 (right)[†] .86, .87 (left)
Rotation			
Hsieh & Yeung[17]	34	Healthy adults (14–31 yr; x̄ = 18.2)	.78, .88 (right)[†] .81, .81 (left)

* Pearson's r
[†] Two testers performed measurements.

Table 10–22. GONIOMETER: INTRATESTER RELIABILITY FOR FLEXION OF CERVICAL SPINE				
STUDY	**n**	**SAMPLE**	**CORRELATION**	
			ICC*	**r†**
Defibaugh[10]	15	Healthy adults (20–40 yr)		.77
Youdas et al.[41]	20	Cervical pain (21–84 yr; x̄ = 59.1)	.83	

* Intraclass correlation
† Pearson's r

described in Chapter 8 were examined by Youdas et al.[41] and Zachman et al.[43] Youdas et al.[41] reported on the examination of 20 patients with cervical spine pain. Intratester reliability correlations (ICC) ranged from .78 to .90 (Tables 10–22 to 10–25), and intertester reliability (ICC) ranged from .54 to .79 (Tables 10–26 to 10–29). Zachman et al.[43] examined intertester reliability in 24 subjects. Reliability correlations (Pearson's r) ranged from .43 to .85 (standard error of the estimates ranged from 5 to 12); details are presented in Tables 10–26 to 10–29. These authors suggested that range of motion measurements made by the same physical therapist have good to high reliability.

Using one of the more unique adaptations to a goniometer, Defibaugh[10] examined intratester and intertester reliability in 15 subjects. The device used was a "head goniometer" and consisted of a mouthpiece (made of $\frac{1}{8}$-inch plastic, 2 inches wide, and 1 $\frac{1}{2}$ inches long) attached to a pendulum goniometer (consisting of a 3-inch plastic protractor). Flexion, extension, lateral flexion, and rotation range of motion of the cervical spine were measured while the subject held the device in the mouth. Intratester reliability correlation (Pearson's r) ranged from .71 to .86, and intertester reliability ranged from .80 to .94 (see Tables 10–22 to 10–29). Using a Fisher t statistic, Defibaugh[10] reported no significant difference between measurements (intratester reliability) or testers (intertester reliability). Although unique and "moderately to highly reliable" (Defibaugh[10]), no other research has appeared in the literature on the use of this device.

Another adaptation for the measurement of lateral flexion was suggested by Pellecchia and Bohannon[34] and consisted of modifying the goniometer by adding a paper clip through the axis of rotation. The paper clip then acted as a free-swinging pendulum and served as a pointer. To measure lateral flexion, both arms of the goniometer were aligned with the base of the subject's nose at the end range of lateral flexion. The paper clip was used to read the measurement scale of the goniometer. Using this technique and measuring 100 subjects, the authors reported intratester reliability correlation (ICC) of .94 for right lateral flexion and .91 for left lateral flexion (see Table

Table 10–23. GONIOMETER: INTRATESTER RELIABILITY FOR EXTENSION OF CERVICAL SPINE				
STUDY	**n**	**SAMPLE**	**CORRELATION**	
			ICC*	**r†**
Defibaugh[10]	15	Healthy adults (20–40 yr)		.86
Youdas et al.[41]	20	Cervical pain (21–84 yr; x̄ = 59.1)	.86	

* Intraclass correlation
† Pearson's r

Table 10–24. GONIOMETER: INTRATESTER RELIABILITY FOR LATERAL FLEXION OF CERVICAL SPINE

STUDY	n	SAMPLE	CORRELATION	
			ICC*	r[†]
Defibaugh[10]	15	Healthy adults (20–40 yr)		.83 (right) .81 (left)
Youdas et al.[41]	20	Cervical pain (21–84 yr; x̄ = 59.1)	.85 (right) .84 (left)	
Pellecchia & Bohannon[34]	100	Healthy adults (14–95 yr)	.94 (right) .91 (left)	

* Intraclass correlation
† Pearson's r

Table 10–25. GONIOMETER: INTRATESTER RELIABILITY FOR ROTATION OF CERVICAL SPINE

STUDY	n	SAMPLE	CORRELATION	
			ICC*	r[†]
Defibaugh[10]	15	Healthy adults (20–40 yr)		.81 (right) .71 (left)
Youdas et al.[41]	20	Cervical pain (21–84 yr; x̄ = 59.1)	.90 (right) .78 (left)	

* Intraclass correlation
† Pearson's r

Table 10–26. GONIOMETER: INTERTESTER RELIABILITY FOR FLEXION OF CERVICAL SPINE

STUDY	n	SAMPLE	CORRELATION	
			ICC*	r[†]
Defibaugh[10]	15	Healthy adults (20–40 yr)		.80
Zachman et al.[43]	24	Healthy adults (6–51 yr)		.54
Youdas et al.[41]	20	Cervical pain (21–84 yr; x̄ = 59.1)	.57	

* Intraclass correlation
† Pearson's r

Table 10–27. GONIOMETER: INTERTESTER RELIABILITY FOR EXTENSION OF CERVICAL SPINE

STUDY	n	SAMPLE	CORRELATION	
			ICC*	r[†]
Defibaugh[10]	15	Healthy adults (20–40 yr)		.90
Zachman et al.[43]	24	Healthy adults (6–51 yr)		.85
Youdas et al.[41]	20	Cervical pain (21–84 yr; x̄ = 59.1)	.79	

* Intraclass correlation
† Pearson's r

STUDY	n	SAMPLE	CORRELATION	
			ICC*	r†
Defibaugh[10]	15	Healthy adults (20–40 yr)		.85 (right) .86 (left)
Zachman et al.[43]	24	Healthy adults (6–51 yr)		.43 (right) .61 (left)
Youdas et al.[41]	20	Cervical pain (21–84 yr; x̄ = 59.1)	.72 (right) .79 (left)	
Pellecchia & Bohannon[34]	35	Healthy adults (14–95 yr)	.86 (right) .65 (left)	

Table 10–28. GONIOMETER: INTERTESTER RELIABILITY FOR LATERAL FLEXION OF CERVICAL SPINE

* Intraclass correlation
† Pearson's r

10–24). Further analysis of 35 subjects to examine intertester reliability indicated correlations (ICC) of .86 for right lateral flexion and .65 for left lateral flexion (see Table 10–28).

INCLINOMETER

The use of a double inclinometer (hand-held) to measure cervical flexion, extension, lateral flexion, and rotation was investigated by Mayer et al.[25] In the first part of this study, intratester reliability was examined using a test-retest design on 58 subjects. Excellent reliability (Pearson's r) was reported, with all correlations being greater than .97 (Tables 10–30 to 10–33). Although after performing a Pearson correlation, follow-up testing for random and systematic error is appropriate (refer to Chapter 2), Mayer et al.[25] did not perform any such tests. However, this study is included in this chapter because it is the only published investigation on the reliability of dual inclinometers for measuring cervical range of motion.

Attachment of Inclinometer to the Head

One of the first studies in which an inclinometer-type device was attached to the head was a study by Bennett et al.,[4] which used a "bubble goniometer" held in place by rubber straps in order to measure flexion and extension of the cervical spine. Two testers measured the same subject, and "the variation was ±5 degrees." No other statistical analysis of the reliability of this first attempt to attach an inclinometer to the head was provided.

STUDY	n	SAMPLE	CORRELATION	
			ICC*	r†
Defibaugh[10]	15	Healthy adults (20–40 yr)		.87 (right) .94 (left)
Zachman et al.[43]	24	Healthy adults (6–51 yr)		.52 (right) .47 (left)
Youdas et al.[41]	20	Cervical pain (21–84 yr; x̄ = 59.1)	.62 (right) .54 (left)	

Table 10–29. GONIOMETER: INTERTESTER RELIABILITY FOR ROTATION OF CERVICAL SPINE

* Intraclass correlation
† Pearson's r

Table 10–30. INCLINOMETER: INTRATESTER RELIABILITY FOR FLEXION OF CERVICAL SPINE

STUDY	TECHNIQUE	n	SAMPLE	CORRELATION ICC*	r[†]
Mayer et al.[25]	Double inclinometer	58	Healthy adults (17–62 yr)		.99
Youdas et al.[41]	CROM[‡]	20	Healthy adults (21–84 yr; $\bar{x}$ = 59.1)	.95	
Capuano-Pucci et al.[8]	CROM	20	Healthy adults ($\bar{x}$ = 23.5 yr)		.63, .91[§]
Youdas et al.[42]	CROM	6	Healthy adults (22–56 yr; $\bar{x}$ = 27.2)	.64, .76, .23 .88, .84[‖]	
Nilsson[31]	CROM	14	Healthy adults (23–45 yr)		.76

* Intraclass correlation
[†] Pearson's r
[‡] Cervical range of motion device (Performance Attainment Associates, Roseville, Minn)
[§] Two testers performed measurements.
[‖] Five testers performed measurements; ICC was performed for this study.

Other researchers took Bennett et al.'s[4] proposed method of attaching the inclinometer to the head with elastic straps one step further by applying more sophisticated research designs. In a study comparing cervical rotation range of motion of swimmers with that of healthy nonswimmers, Guth[14] used an inclinometer attached to the top of the head with an elastic band. The author reported correlations of .90 to .96 for intratester reliability (see Table 10–33) and .88 to .96 for intertester reliability (see Table 10–37); however, why a range of correlations was reported was not clear. The author reported no significant difference between measurements (intratester) or testers (intertester) using a t test.

Differing slightly from the previous studies, Alaranta et al.[1] used an inclinometer attached to a "cloth helmet." Instead of reporting reliability of each motion, the authors used the sum of flexion and extension, the mean of right

Table 10–31. INCLINOMETER: INTRATESTER RELIABILITY FOR EXTENSION OF CERVICAL SPINE

STUDY	TECHNIQUE	n	SAMPLE	CORRELATION ICC*	r[†]
Mayer et al.[25]	Double inclinometer	58	Healthy adults (17–62 yr)		.99
Youdas et al.[41]	CROM[‡]	20	Healthy adults (21–84 yr; $\bar{x}$ = 59.1)	.90	
Capuano-Pucci et al.[8]	CROM	20	Healthy adults ($\bar{x}$ = 23.5)		.90, .82[§]
Youdas et al.[42]	CROM	6	Healthy adults (22–56 yr; $\bar{x}$ = 27.2)	.96, .89, .96, .94, .93[‖]	
Nilsson[31]	CROM	14	Healthy adults (23–45 yr)		.85

* Intraclass correlation
[†] Pearson's r
[‡] Cervical range of motion device (Performance Attainment Associates, Roseville, Minn)
[§] Two testers performed measurements.
[‖] Five testers performed measurements; ICC was performed for this study.

Table 10–32. INCLINOMETER: INTRATESTER RELIABILITY FOR LATERAL FLEXION OF CERVICAL SPINE

STUDY	TECHNIQUE	n	SAMPLE	CORRELATION ICC*	CORRELATION r[†]
Mayer et al.[25]	Double inclinometer	58	Healthy adults (17–62 yr)		.97 (right) .98 (left)
Youdas et al.[41]	CROM[‡]	20	Healthy adults (21–84 yr; $\bar{x}$ = 59.1)	.92 (right) .84 (left)	
Capuano-Pucci et al.[8]	CROM	20	Healthy adults ($\bar{x}$ = 23.5 yr)		.79, .89 (right)[§] .84, .90 (left)
Youdas et al.[42]	CROM	6	Healthy adults (22–56 yr; $\bar{x}$ = 27.2)		.75, .60, .94, .88, .85[‖] (right) .77, .87, .90, .86, .67 (left)
Nilsson[31]	CROM	14	Healthy adults (23–45 yr)		.61 (right) .68 (left)

* Intraclass correlation
[†] Pearson's r
[‡] Cervical range of motion device (Performance Attainment Associates, Roseville, Minn)
[§] Two testers performed measurements.
[‖] Five testers performed measurements; ICC was performed for this study.

and left lateral flexion, and the mean of right and left rotation. Intertester reliability correlations ranged from .69 to .86 (Tables 10–34 to 10–37).

Instead of using elastic straps to secure the inclinometer to the head as previously described, Tucci et al.[39] placed an inclinometer on head gear constructed from a wood block with an arc cut into it, which was then padded and placed on the head of the subject and held in place with elastic straps. Using this device, inter-rater reliability performed on 10 subjects resulted in reliability correlations (ICC) ranging from .82 to .91 (see Tables 10–34 to 10–37), leading the authors to conclude that the device is "simple, inexpensive, and highly accurate."

Table 10–33. INCLINOMETER: INTRATESTER RELIABILITY FOR ROTATION OF CERVICAL SPINE

STUDY	TECHNIQUE	n	SAMPLE	CORRELATION ICC*	CORRELATION r[†]
Mayer et al.[25]	Double inclinometer	58	Healthy adults (17–62 yr)		.98 (right) .99 (left)
Youdas et al.[31]	CROM[‡]	20	Healthy adults (21–84 yr; $\bar{x}$ = 59.1)	.93 (right) .90 (left)	
Capuano-Pucci et al.[8]	CROM	20	Healthy adults ($\bar{x}$ = 23.5 yr)		.85, .62 (right)[§] .85, .89 (left)
Youdas et al.[42]	CROM	6	Healthy adults (22–56 yr; $\bar{x}$ = 27.2)		.80, .58, .99, .82, .71[‖] (right) .83, .84, .92, .95, .81 (left)
Guth[14]	Inclinometer "attached by an elastic band to top of head"	8	Healthy adolescents (14–17 yr)		.90–.96[¶]
Nilsson[31]	CROM	14	Healthy adults (23–45 yr)		.75 (right) .68 (left)

* Intraclass correlation
[†] Pearson's r
[‡] Cervical range of motion device (Performance Attainment Associates, Roseville, Minn)
[§] Two testers performed measurements.
[‖] Five testers performed measurements; ICC was performed for this study.
[¶] Refer to text for explanation.

Table 10-34. INCLINOMETER: INTERTESTER RELIABILITY FOR FLEXION OF CERVICAL SPINE					
STUDY	**TECHNIQUE**	***n***	**SAMPLE**	**CORRELATION**	
				ICC*	***r*[†]**
Tucci et al.[39]	Gravity goniometer (with "wooden head" adapter)	10	Healthy adults	.84	
Zachman et al.[43]	Pendulum goniometer fastened to headpiece (called "rangiometer")	24	Healthy adults (6–51 yr)		.64
Youdas et al.[41]	CROM[‡]	20	Healthy adults (21–84 yr; x̄ = 59.1)	.86	
Capuano-Pucci et al.[8]	CROM	20	Healthy adults (x̄ = 23.5 yr)		.80, .77[§]
Rheault et al.[36]	CROM	22	Healthy adults (x̄ = 37.4 yr)	.76	
Youdas et al.[42]	CROM	6	Healthy adults (22–56 yr; x̄ = 27.2)	.83[‖]	
Alaranta et al.[1]	Inclinometer attached to "cloth helmet"	24	Healthy adults		.69
Nilsson[31]	CROM	14	Healthy adults (23–45 yr)		.71

* Intraclass correlation
† Pearson's *r*
‡ Cervical range of motion device (Performance Attainment Associates, Roseville, Minn)
§ Intertester reliability was examined across two sessions.
‖ Intertester reliability analyzed using one ICC performed across five testers.

Table 10-35. INCLINOMETER: INTERTESTER RELIABILITY FOR EXTENSION OF CERVICAL SPINE					
STUDY	**TECHNIQUE**	***n***	**SAMPLE**	**CORRELATION**	
				ICC*	***r*[†]**
Tucci et al.[39]	Gravity goniometer (with "wooden head" adapter)	10	Healthy adults	.86	
Zachman et al.[43]	Pendulum goniometer fastened to headpiece (called "rangiometer")	24	Healthy adults (6–51 yr)		.89
Youdas et al.[41]	CROM[‡]	20	Healthy adults (21–84 yr; x̄ = 59.1)	.86	
Capuano-Pucci et al.[8]	CROM	20	Healthy adults (x̄ = 23.5 yr)		.83, .76[§]
Rheault et al.[36]	CROM	22	Healthy adults (x̄ = 37.4 yr)	.98	
Youdas et al.[42]	CROM	6	Healthy adults (22–56 yr; x̄ = 27.2)	.90[‖]	
Alaranta et al.[1]	Inclinometer attached to "cloth helmet"	24	Healthy adults		.69
Nilsson[31]	CROM	14	Healthy adults (23–45 yr)		.71 .85

* Intraclass correlation
† Pearson's *r*
‡ Cervical range of motion device (Performance Attainment Associates, Roseville, Minn)
§ Intertester reliability was examined across two sessions.
‖ Intertester reliability analyzed using one ICC performed across five testers.

				CORRELATION	
STUDY	**TECHNIQUE**	**_n_**	**SAMPLE**	**ICC***	**_r_[†]**
Tucci et al.[39]	Gravity goniometer (with "wooden head" adapter)	10	Healthy adults	.87 (right) .82 (left)	
Zachman et al.[43]	Pendulum goniometer fastened to headpiece (called "rangiometer")	24	Healthy adults (6–51 yr)		.84 (right) .79 (left)
Youdas et al.[41]	CROM[‡]	20	Healthy adults (21–84 yr; $\bar{x} = 59.1$)	.88 (right) .73 (left)	
Capuano-Pucci et al.[8]	CROM	20	Healthy adults ($\bar{x} = 23.5$ yr)		.84, .85 (right)[§] .87, .74 (left)
Rheault et al.[36]	CROM	22	Healthy adults ($\bar{x} = 37.4$ yr)	.87 (right) .86 (left)	
Youdas et al.[42]	CROM	6	Healthy adults (22–56 yr; $\bar{x} = 27.2$)	.87 (right)[∥] .89 (left)	
Alaranta et al.[1]	Inclinometer attached to "cloth helmet"	24	Healthy adults		.79 (mean)[¶]
Nilsson[31]	CROM	14	Healthy adults (23–45 yr)		.58 (right) .58 (left)

Table 10–36. INCLINOMETER: INTERTESTER RELIABILITY FOR LATERAL FLEXION OF CERVICAL SPINE

* Intraclass correlation
† Pearson's _r_
‡ Cervical range of motion device (Performance Attainment Associates, Roseville, Minn)
§ Intertester reliability was examined across two sessions.
∥ Intertester reliability analyzed using one ICC performed across five testers.
¶ Mean of the total range of right and left lateral flexion

In what appears to be a headpiece similar to instruments proposed by Tucci et al.,[39] Zachman et al.[43] introduced the "rangiometer," rigid head gear with an inclinometer mounted on top. Using the device to examine cervical range of motion in 24 subjects, Zachman et al.[43] reported intertester reliability coefficients (Pearson's _r_) ranging from .62 to .89 (standard errors of the estimate ranged from 5 degrees to 11 degrees), which were considered "moderately reliable" by the authors (see Tables 10–34 to 10–37).

Cervical Range of Motion (CROM)

The cervical range of motion (CROM) device consists of inclinometers mounted on a plastic frame that is placed over the subject's head and aligned on the bridge of the nose and ears. A detailed description is provided in Chapter 9.

Several studies have examined the intertester and intratester reliability of the CROM device using essentially the same procedures for measurement of cervical flexion, extension, right and left lateral flexion, and right and left rotation. Results are summarized in Tables 10–30 to 10–37. Youdas et al.[41] examined 20 patients with cervical pain, reporting correlation coefficients (ICC) ranging from .84 to .95 for intratester reliability and .73 to .90 for intertester reliability. Similar results were found by Capuano-Pucci et al.,[8] who examined 20 subjects without cervical pain using two testers. Intrarater reliability for each tester ranged from .62 to .91 (Pearson's r) (see Tables 10–30 to 10–33). Two separate testing sessions were performed to measure inter-rater reliability between the two testers. Reliability correlations ranged for the first session from .80 to .87 and for the second session from .74 to .85 (Pearson's r) (see Tables 10–34 to 10–37). Paired t tests analyzing the differences between measurements (intratester) and testers (intertester) revealed no significant difference across all measurements. Rheault et al.[36] reported equally high correlations, but they only examined intertester reliability. Examining 22 subjects, the authors reported intertester reliability correlations ranging from .76 to .98 (ICC) (see Tables 10–34 to 10–37). Each of these authors agreed with the conclusion that the CROM was "a reliable and useful tool for assessing cervical range of motion" (Capuano-Pucci et al.[8]).

In a study designed to provide normative data for cervical range of motion across nine decades of age, Youdas et al.[42] established reliability in two

Table 10–37. INCLINOMETER: INTERTESTER RELIABILITY FOR ROTATION OF CERVICAL SPINE

STUDY	TECHNIQUE	n	SAMPLE	CORRELATION ICC*	r[†]
Tucci et al.[39]	Gravity goniometer (with "wooden head" adapter)	10	Healthy adults	.91 (right) .87 (left)	
Zachman et al.[43]	Pendulum goniometer fastened to headpiece (called "rangiometer")	24	Healthy adults (6–51 yr)		.62 (right) .69 (left)
Youdas et al.[41]	CROM[‡]	20	Healthy adults (21–84 yr; $\bar{x} = 59.1$)	.90 (right) .82 (left)	
Capuano-Pucci et al.[8]	CROM	20	Healthy adults ($\bar{x} = 23.5$ yr)		.84, .82 (right)[§] .84, .79 (left)
Rheault et al.[36]	CROM	22	Healthy adults ($\bar{x} = 37.4$ yr)	.81 (right) .82 (left)	
Youdas et al.[42]	CROM	6	Healthy adults (22–56 yr; $\bar{x} = 27.2$)	.82 (right)[‖] .66 (left)	
Alaranta et al.[1]	Inclinometer attached to "cloth helmet"	24	Healthy adults		.86 (mean)[¶]
Guth[14]	Inclinometer "attached by an elastic band to top of head"	8	Healthy adolescents (14–17 yr)		.88–.96**
Nilsson[31]	CROM	14	Healthy adults (23–45 yr)		.66 (right) .29 (left)

* Intraclass correlation
† Pearson's r
‡ Cervical range of motion device (Performance Attainment Associates, Roseville, Minn)
§ Intertester reliability was examined across two sessions.
‖ Intertester reliability analyzed using one ICC performed across five testers.
¶ Mean of the total range of right and left rotation
** Refer to text for explanation.

pilot studies prior to collecting data on 337 subjects. For intrarater reliability, five testers measured six subjects twice. The reliability correlations for each tester are presented in Tables 10–30 to 10–33. The authors also reported the median ICCs for intratester reliability as "fair" for cervical flexion (ICC = .76), "high" for cervical extension (ICC = .94), and "good" for left lateral cervical flexion (ICC = .86), right lateral cervical flexion (ICC = .85), left cervical rotation (ICC = .84), and right cervical rotation (ICC = .80). For intertester reliability, a "random, unique triplet of testers" was used for a sample of 20 subjects. Intertester reliability (ICC) ranged from .66 to .90 (see Tables 10–34 to 10–37). The authors concluded that "measurement of the cervical spine with the CROM instrument demonstrates good intra-tester and inter-tester reliability" (Youdas et al.[42]).

In the only study to use the CROM to measure *passive* flexion, extension, lateral flexion, and rotation range of motion of the cervical spine, Nilsson[31] examined 14 subjects. The author reported intrarater reliability (Pearson's *r*) of *passive* motion of the cervical spine ranging from .61 to .85 (see Tables 10–30 to 10–33) and for inter-rater reliability (Pearson's *r*) ranging from .29 to .85 (see Tables 10–34 to 10–37). Follow-up testing using a paired *t* test indicated no significant differences between measurements (intratester) for all measurements of cervical range of motion. However, the paired *t* test indicated significant differences between testers (intertester) for the cervical motion of flexion ($p < .05$), extension ($p < .05$), and lateral flexion ($p < .05$). (Note: No significant difference between testers was found for cervical rotation.) Given the lower correlations with intertester reliability as related to intratester reliability, as well as the significant *t* tests with inter-rater reliability, the author concluded that the CROM "has an acceptable reliability as long as all measurements are carried out by the same examiner."

Validity

Herrmann[16] examined the total range of motion (flexion and extension combined) in 11 subjects using an inclinometer attached to a headband and compared these measurements to a radiographic examination. The correlation between the inclinometer and the x-ray was .98 (ICC and Pearson's *r*), and no significant difference was found between measurements taken by the two devices (Fisher *t* test). Based on the statistics, the authors concluded that the method was a "valid tool for measuring neck flexion and extension range of motion."

For the second part of their study, Mayer et al.[25] examined consistency of measurement of cervical flexion between the double inclinometer and radiographic examination in three subjects, reporting a correlation of .99 (Pearson's *r*). As indicated previously, no follow-up statistical analysis to the Pearson correlation was performed, and this study is included only because no other study on the reliability and validity of the double inclinometer measurement of cervical range of motion has been published.

Investigating validity, Ordway et al.[33] measured cervical flexion and extension using the CROM device and examination by x-ray on 20 subjects. Statistical analysis using ANOVA indicated no significant differences between measurements using the CROM device and x-ray. These results support the contention that the CROM device is a valid instrument for measuring cervical flexion and extension range of motion. Table 10–38 provides information on studies investigating the validity of measurement of cervical range of motion using inclinometers.

Table 10–38. INCLINOMETER: VALIDITY FOR FLEXION AND EXTENSION OF CERVICAL SPINE					
STUDY	TECHNIQUE	*n*	SAMPLE	CORRELATION	
				ICC*	*r*†
Hermann[16]	Pendulum goniometer attached to "head band"	11	Healthy adults (21–68 yr)	.98 (total)	.98‡
Mayer et al.[25]	Double inclinometer	3	Healthy adults (17–62 yr)		.99§
Ordway et al.[33]	CROM‖	20	Healthy adults (20–49 yr; $\bar{x} = 31.0$)		No significant difference in range of motion between CROM and x-ray (flexion, extension)¶

* Intraclass correlation
† Pearson's *r*
‡ Total = flexion and extension combined
§ Flexion only
‖ Cervical range of motion device (Performance Attainment Associates, Roseville, Minn)
¶ Analysis of variance with repeated measures

TEMPOROMANDIBULAR JOINT

Iglarsh and Snyder-Mackler[19] have suggested that mandibular depression (opening), protrusion, and lateral deviation are important range of motion parameters of the temporomandibular joint (TMJ) that should be measured at the initial examination, and, if impairment exists, measured before and after each intervention. Although several references support Iglarsh and Snyder-Mackler's suggestion of the importance of examining the range of motion of the TMJ and provide descriptions of the measurement procedure (Magee,[24] Freidman and Weisberg,[12] Bell,[3] Kaplan[20]), no studies could be found in which reliability of any of these measurements was investigated.

References

1. Alaranta H, Hurri H, Heliovaara M, et al.: Flexibility of the spine: Normative values of goniometric and tape measurements. Scand J Rehab Med 1994;26:147–154.
2. Beattie P, Rothstein JM, Lamb RL: Reliability of the attraction method for measuring lumbar spine backward bending. Phys Ther 1987;67:364–369.
3. Bell WE: Temporomandibular Disorders, 3rd ed. Chicago: Yearbook Medical Publishers, 1986.
4. Bennett JG, Bergmanis LE, Carpenter JK, Skowlund HV: Range of motion of the neck. Phys Ther 1963;43:45–47.
5. Boline PD, Keating JC, Haas M, Anderson AV: Inter examiner reliability and discriminant validity of inclinometric measurement of lumbar rotation in chronic low-back pain patients and subjects without low-back pain. Spine 1992;17:335–338.
6. Breum J, Wiberg J, Bolton JE: Reliability and concurrent validity of the BROM II for measuring lumbar mobility. J Manipulative Physiol Ther 1995;18:497–502.
7. Burdett RG, Brown KE, Fall MP: Reliability and validity of four instruments for measuring lumbar spine and pelvic positions. Phys Ther 1986;66:677–684.
8. Capuano-Pucci D, Rheault W, Aukai J, et al.: Intratester and intertester reliability of the cervical range of motion device. Arch Phys Med Rehabil 1991;72:338–340.

9. Chiarello CM, Savidge R: Interrater reliability of the Cybex EDI-320 and fluid goniometer in normals and patients with low back pain. Arch Phys Med Rehabil 1993;74:32–37.

10. Defibaugh JJ: Part II: An experimental study of head motion in adult males. Phys Ther 1964;44:163–168.

11. Fitzgerald GK, Wynveen KJ, Rheault W, Rothschild B: Objective assessment with establishment of normal values for lumbar spinal range of motion. Phys Ther 1983;63:1776–1781.

12. Freidman MH, Weisberg J: The temporomandibular joint. In Gould JA: Orthopaedic and Sports Physical Therapy, 2nd ed. St. Louis: Mosby, 1990, pp 575–598.

13. Frost M, Stuckey S, Smalley LA, Dorman G: Reliability of measuring trunk motions in centimeters. Phys Ther 1982;62:1431–1437.

14. Guth EH: A comparison of cervical rotation in age-matched adolescent competitive swimmers and healthy males. J Orthop Sports Phys Ther 1995;21:21–27.

15. Haley SM, Tada WL, Carmichael EM: Spinal mobility in young children. Phys Ther 1986;66:1697–1703.

16. Herrmann DB: Validity study of head and neck flexion-extension motion comparing measurements of a pendulum goniometer and roentgenograms. J Orthop Sports Phys Ther 1990;11:414–418.

17. Hsieh C, Yeung B: Active neck motion measurements with a tape measure. J Orthop Sports Phys Ther 1986;8:88–92.

18. Hyytiainen K, Salminen JJ, Suvitie T, et al.: Reproducibility of nine tests to measure spinal mobility and trunk muscle strength. Scand J Rehab Med 1991;23:3–10.

19. Iglarsh A, Snyder-Mackler L: Temporomandibular joint and the cervical spine. In Richardson JK, Iglarsh ZA: Clinical Orthopaedic Physical Therapy. Philadelphia: WB Saunders, 1994, pp 1–72.

20. Kaplan AS: Examination and diagnosis—Chapter 4. In Kaplan AS, Assael LA: Temporomandibular Disorders. Philadelphia: WB Saunders, 1991.

21. Loebl WY: Measurement of spinal posture and range of spinal motion. Ann Phys Med 1967;9:103–110.

22. Macrae IF, Wright V: Measurement of back movement. Ann Rheum Dis 1969;28:584–589.

23. Madson TJ, Youdas JW, Suman VJ: Reproducibility of lumbar spine range of motion measurements using the back range of motion device. J Orthop Sports Phys Ther 1999;29:470–477.

24. Magee DJ: Orthopedic Physical Assessment, 3rd ed. Philadelphia: WB Saunders, 1997.

25. Mayer T, Brady S, Bovasso E, et al.: Noninvasive measurement of cervical tri-planar motion in normal subjects. Spine 1993;18:2191–2195.

26. Mayer TG, Tencer AF, Kristoferson S, Mooney V: Use of noninvasive techniques for quantification of spinal range-of-motion in normal subjects and chronic low-back dysfunction patients. Spine 1984;9:588–595.

27. Mellin GP: Measurement of thoracolumbar posture and mobility with a Myrin inclinometer. Spine 1986;11:759–762.

28. Mellin GP, Kiiski R, Weckstrom A: Effects of subject position on measurements of flexion, extension, and lateral flexion of the spine. Spine 1991;16:1108–1110.

29. Moll JMV, Wright V: Normal range of motion: An objective clinical study. Ann Rheum Dis 1971;30:381–386.

30. Newton M, Waddell G: Reliability and validity of clinical measurement of the lumbar spine in patients with chronic low back pain. Physiotherapy 1991;77:796–800.

31. Nilsson N: Measuring passive cervical motion: A study of reliability. J Manipulative Physiol Ther 1995;18:293–297.

32. Nitschke J, Nattrass C, Disler P, et al.: Reliability of the American Medical Association Guides' model for measuring spinal range of motion. Spine 1999;24:262–268.

33. Ordway NR, Seymour R, Donelson RG, et al.: Cervical sagittal range-of-motion analysis using three methods. Spine 1997;22:501–508.

34. Pellecchia GL, Bohannon RW: Active lateral neck flexion range of motion measurements obtained with a modified goniometer: Reliability and estimates of normal. J Manipulative Physiol Ther 1998;21:443–447.

35. Portek I, Pearcy MJ, Reader GP, Mowat AG: Correlation between radiographic and clinical measurement of lumbar spine movement. Br J Rheumatol 1983;22:197–205.

36. Rheault W, Albright B, Byers C, et al.: Intertester reliability of the cervical range of motion device. J Orthop Sports Phys Ther 1992;15:147–150.

37. Rondinelli R, Murphy J, Esler A, et al.: Estimation of normal lumbar flexion with surface inclinometry. Am J Phys Med Rehabil 1992;71:219–224.

38. Rose MJ: The statistical analysis of the intra-observer repeatability of four clinical measurement techniques. Physiotherapy 1991;77:89–91.

39. Tucci SM, Hicks JE, Gross EG, et al.: Cervical motion assessment: A new, simple and accurate method. Arch Phys Med Rehabil 1986;67:225–230.

40. Williams R, Binkley J, Bloch R, et al.: Reliability of the modified-modified Schober and double inclinometer methods for measuring lumbar flexion and extension. Phys Ther 1993;73:26–37.

41. Youdas JW, Carey TR, Garrett TR: Reliability of measurement of cervical spine range of motion—Comparison of three methods. Phys Ther 1991;71:98–104.

42. Youdas JW, Garrett TR, Suman VJ, et al.: Normal range of motion of the cervical spine: An initial goniometric study. Phys Ther 1992;72:770–780.

43. Zachman ZJ, Traina AD, Keating JC, et al.: Interexaminer reliability and concurrent validity of two instruments for the measurement of cervical ranges of motion. J Manipulative Physiol Ther 1989;12:205–210.

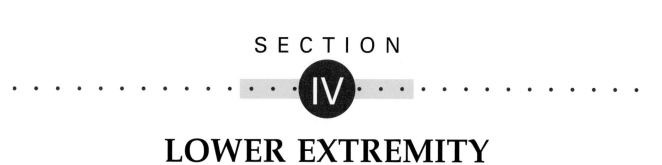

SECTION

IV

LOWER EXTREMITY

11

MEASUREMENT of RANGE of MOTION of the HIP

ANATOMY AND OSTEOKINEMATICS

The hip is a ball-and-socket joint that consists of an articulation between the convex head of the femur and the concave acetabulum of the pelvis, or hip bone. Movement at the hip, which occurs in all three of the cardinal planes, consists of flexion, extension, abduction, adduction, medial rotation, and lateral rotation. These motions may be achieved by movement of the femur on the pelvis or by movement of the pelvis on the femur. An additional motion, circumduction, has been described as occurring at the hip joint. This motion is a sequence of flexion, abduction, extension, and adduction and is not normally measured with a goniometer.[4, 10]

LIMITATIONS OF MOTION: HIP JOINT

The majority of the motions at the hip are limited by the ligaments (iliofemoral, ischiofemoral, and pubofemoral) that surround the joint, as well as by the hip joint capsule. The primary exception to this rule is hip flexion, which is limited by approximation of the soft tissue between the anterior thigh and the abdomen when the knee is flexed, and by tension in the hamstring muscles when the hip is flexed with the knee extended. Thus, normal end-feels for hip extension, abduction, adduction, medial rotation, and lateral rotation are firm, as a result of capsular and ligamentous limitations of motion. The normal end-feel for hip flexion with the knee flexed is soft (soft tissue approximation), whereas the normal end-feel for hip flexion with the knee extended is firm, owing to muscular tension in the hamstring group.[4, 10] Information on normal ranges of motion for all motions of the hip is found in Appendix C.

TECHNIQUES OF MEASUREMENT: HIP FLEXION/EXTENSION

A variety of techniques have been employed to measure hip flexion. Measurements have been taken with the patient in the supine position with the contralateral hip either flexed or extended (Figs. 11–1 and 11–2),[1, 3, 7, 15] and with the patient in a sidelying position using either the Mundale[14] (Fig. 11–3) or the pelvifemoral angle technique[11] (Fig. 11–4). These techniques vary in patient positioning, in specific landmarks used for goniometric alignment, and in the degree to which each method controls for pelvic motion. Values for the normal maximum amount of hip flexion that are provided in the literature vary widely (see www.wbsaunders.com/SIMON/Reese/joint/). Such discrepancies in standards for the normal hip appear to be caused by

Fig. 11–1. Hip flexion measured with contralateral hip flexed; recommended by AAOS and AMA; allows little control of pelvic motion.

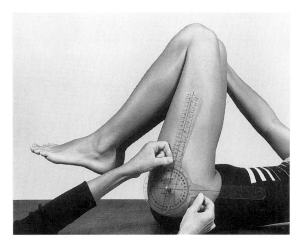

the technique used and the degree to which each of the different techniques controls for pelvic motion. Of the techniques in the preceding list, the one recommended by both the American Academy of Orthopaedic Surgeons (AAOS) and the American Medical Association (AMA) places the least emphasis on controlling pelvic motion.[1, 7]

Motions of the pelvis on the lumbar spine during the measurement of hip flexion or extension can artificially inflate the range of motion measurement obtained. To control for this phenomenon, one should either use landmarks on the pelvis to eliminate the possibility of including lumbar spine motion in the measurement, or manually ensure that the pelvis remains in a neutral position at the beginning and end of the range of motion measurement. The neutral position of the pelvis has been described as the position in which a line drawn through the anterior superior iliac spines (ASIS) and the symphysis pubis is vertical and lies in the frontal plane.[9, 17] With the pelvis in this position, a line connecting the anterior and posterior superior iliac spines of the pelvis is horizontal and lies in the transverse plane.[10]

According to the Mundale technique,[14] the line through the iliac spines is used as the pelvic reference for hip flexion and extension goniometry, and the stationary arm of the goniometer is positioned perpendicular to this line (see Fig. 11–3). Using the pelvis for alignment of the stationary arm of the

Fig. 11–2. Hip flexion measured with contralateral hip extended, providing more pelvic stability.

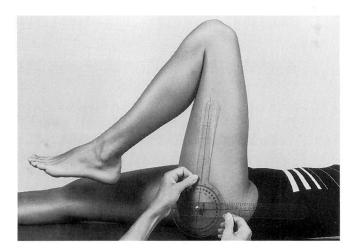

Fig. 11–3. Mundale technique for measuring hip motion. Goniometer is aligned as follows: Stationary arm perpendicular to a line through the iliac spines; axis over greater trochanter; moving arm along lateral midline of femur toward lateral femoral epicondyle. (Modified from Reese NB: Muscle and Sensory Testing. Philadelphia, WB Saunders, 1999, with permission.)

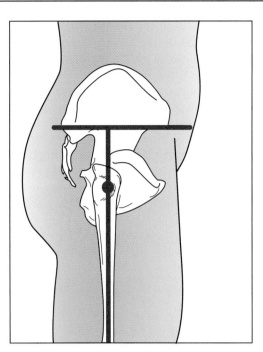

goniometer eliminates the possibility of including motion of the lumbar spine in goniometric measurements of hip flexion and extension. A second technique, which uses landmarks on the pelvis for alignment of the stationary arm of the goniometer, is the pelvifemoral angle technique.[12] When using this technique, the examiner aligns the stationary arm of the goniometer parallel to a line extending from the ASIS through the ischial tuberosity of the pelvis (see Fig. 11–4). When using either the Mundale or the pelvifemoral angle technique, alignment of the moving arm of the goniometer is

Fig. 11–4. Pelvifemoral angle technique for measuring hip motion. Goniometer is aligned as follows: Stationary arm parallel to a line extending from the ASIS through the ischial tuberosity; axis over the greater trochanter; moving arm along lateral midline of femur toward lateral femoral epicondyle. (Modified from Reese NB: Muscle and Sensory Testing. Philadelphia, WB Saunders, 1999, with permission.)

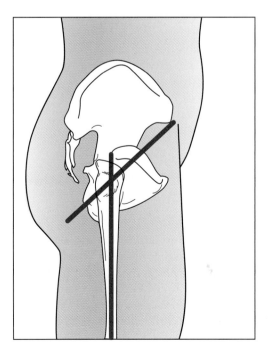

along the midline of the femur toward the lateral femoral epicondyle, while the axis is placed on the greater trochanter.[12, 14] With either technique, the patient is placed in a sidelying position to allow the examiner access to the indicated bony landmarks.

Other techniques recommended for measuring hip flexion and extension use landmarks on the trunk or the examining table for alignment of the stationary arm of the goniometer.[1, 3, 7, 13] The danger in using these landmarks is the possibility that lumbar motion may be included in measurements of hip motion, thus creating unreliable goniometric measurements. However, if the pelvis is maintained in a neutral position (see the previous description), then a line through the midline of the trunk will parallel a line connecting the ASIS and the pubic symphysis, thus providing a reliable reference for the stationary arm of the goniometer. The use of such a reference is advantageous because it allows the patient to be placed in a supine (flexion) or a prone (extension) position during the measurement, thus providing greater stability of the pelvis. Additionally, the need for marking lines on, or taping, the patient is avoided. Whenever landmarks on the trunk are used for alignment of the goniometer's stationary arm, extreme care must be taken, as indicated previously, to maintain the pelvis in a neutral position through manual monitoring of pelvic motion and patient positioning. While both the AAOS and the AMA direct that the patient's contralateral hip be flexed during measurements of ipsilateral hip flexion,[1, 7] maintaining the contralateral thigh against the examining table is necessary in order to minimize pelvic motion during the measurement.[9] Therefore, the technique of measuring hip flexion described in this text recommends extension of the contralateral hip during the measurement.

Measurement of hip extension range of motion also can be accomplished using the Mundale and pelvifemoral angle techniques. Additionally, the AAOS describes two methods of measuring hip extension, both of which use a proximal goniometer alignment that is parallel to the table top and to a line through the lateral midline of the trunk.[7] The patient is placed in the prone position for both AAOS techniques, the only difference in the two techniques being that the patient's contralateral hip is extended in one technique and flexed over the end of the examining table in the other. Some examiners also use the Thomas technique (used for measuring hip flexion contracture; see Chapter 14) to measure hip extension.[2] In a comparison of four of these techniques, Bartlett et al.[2] reported the highest intrarater and inter-rater reliabilities for the AAOS (contralateral hip flexed) and Thomas techniques in children with myelomeningocele and spastic diplegia (see Chapter 15). While the contralateral hip may be extended or flexed during measurements of hip extension range of motion (ROM), fewer patients may have difficulty extending the hip while lying prone than while standing and leaning over an examining table.

TECHNIQUES OF MEASUREMENT: HIP ABDUCTION/ADDUCTION

Measurement of hip abduction and adduction is most commonly done with the patient positioned supine and the ipsilateral hip positioned in 0 degrees of extension. The hip is maintained in 0 degrees of extension throughout the measurement.[1, 7, 13] However, hip abduction occasionally is measured with the ipsilateral hip maintained in 90 degrees of flexion throughout the measurement.[7] This technique appears to be used primarily in the pediatric population and may be less reliable than measurement of hip abduction with the hip extended.[5]

TECHNIQUES OF MEASUREMENT: HIP MEDIAL/LATERAL ROTATION

Rotation of the hip is generally measured either with the patient's hip in 90 degrees of flexion (patient seated) or with the hip in the anatomical position of 0 degrees of extension (patient prone or supine). In the literature a disagreement exists over which position, if either, allows the greater amount of hip rotation. Haley[8] reported a decrease in both medial and lateral active hip rotation in the supine, as compared with the seated, position, whereas Simoneau et al.[16] reported increased active hip lateral, but not medial, rotation when measured in the prone, as compared with the seated, position. Ellison et al.[6] found no difference in the amount of medial and lateral rotation of the hip in the prone compared with the seated position, although this group measured passive, but not active, hip rotation. Unfortunately, most sources reporting standards for hip rotation range of motion (e.g., AAOS, AMA) do not include descriptions of the position in which rotation of the hip was measured. Available data for normal ranges of hip rotation are reported in Appendix C.

As there appears to be no difference in the reliability of measurements of hip rotation taken with the hip flexed or extended,[16] the examiner may choose either method for performing measurements of this motion. However, care should be taken, as always, to use identical techniques whenever repeated measures are taken, since the amount of motion may vary depending on patient position.[8, 16] In the technique described in this text for measuring hip rotation, the patient's hip is flexed.

Hip Flexion

Fig. 11–5. Starting position for measurement of hip flexion. Bony landmarks for goniometer alignment (lateral midline of pelvis/trunk, greater trochanter, lateral femoral epicondyle) indicated by orange line and dots.

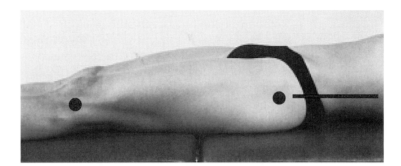

Patient position:	Supine, with lower extremities in anatomical position (Fig. 11–5).
Stabilization:	Over anterior aspect of ipsilateral pelvis (Fig. 11–6).
Examiner action:	After instructing patient in motion desired, stabilize ipsilateral pelvis with one hand and flex patient's hip through available ROM with other hand. Ipsilateral knee should be allowed to flex as well. Hip should not be flexed past the point at which pelvic motion begins to occur (as detected by superior movement of ipsilateral ASIS under examiner's stabilizing hand). Return limb to starting position. Performing passive movement provides an estimate of the ROM and demonstrates to patient exact motion desired (see Fig. 11–6).
Goniometer alignment:	Palpate following bony landmarks (shown in Fig. 11–5) and align goniometer accordingly (Fig. 11–7).
Stationary arm:	Lateral midline of pelvis and trunk.*

---

* Lateral midline of pelvis should parallel midline of trunk as long as pelvic motion is prevented and neutral pelvis is maintained (see description of neutral pelvis in Techniques of Measurement: Hip Flexion/Extension).

Fig. 11–6. End of hip flexion ROM, showing proper hand placement for stabilizing pelvis and detecting pelvic motion. Bony landmarks for goniometer alignment (lateral midline of pelvis/trunk, greater trochanter, lateral femoral epicondyle) indicated by orange line and dots.

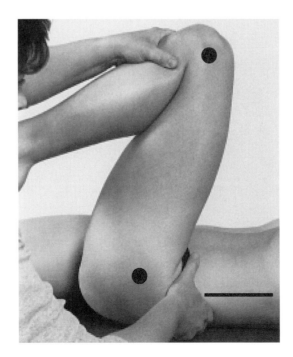

Fig. 11–7. Starting posi-tion for measurement of hip flexion, demonstrating proper initial alignment of goniometer.

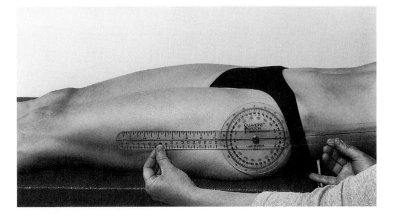

Axis:	Greater trochanter of femur.
Moving arm:	Lateral midline of femur toward lateral femoral epicondyle.

Read scale of goniometer.

Patient/Examiner action: Perform passive, or have patient perform active, hip flexion (Fig. 11–8). In either case, hip flexion should not be allowed to continue past point at which pelvic motion is detected (see Examiner action).

Confirmation of alignment: Repalpate landmarks and confirm proper goniometric alignment at end of ROM, correcting alignment as necessary (see Fig. 11–8). Read scale of goniometer.

Documentation: Record patient's ROM.

Precaution: Should hip be allowed to flex past point at which pelvic motion begins to occur, motion measured will include both hip and lumbar flexion. In order to isolate hip flexion, pelvic motion must not be permitted.

Alternative patient position: Sidelying. Stabilization of pelvis more difficult with patient in this position. Goniometer alignment remains the same.

Fig. 11–8. End of hip flex-ion ROM, demonstrating proper alignment of go-niometer at end of range.

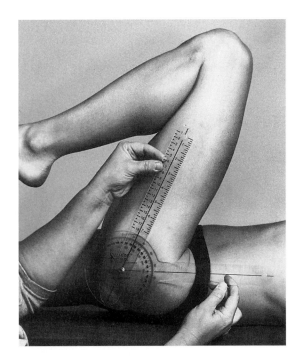

Hip Extension

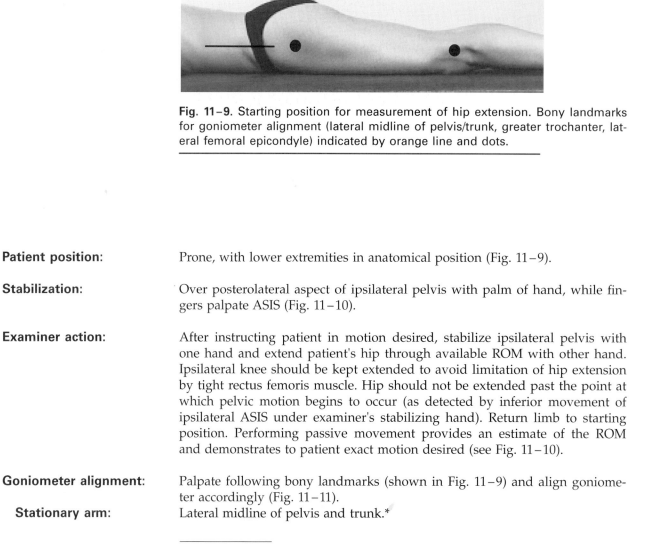

Fig. 11-9. Starting position for measurement of hip extension. Bony landmarks for goniometer alignment (lateral midline of pelvis/trunk, greater trochanter, lateral femoral epicondyle) indicated by orange line and dots.

Patient position:	Prone, with lower extremities in anatomical position (Fig. 11-9).
Stabilization:	Over posterolateral aspect of ipsilateral pelvis with palm of hand, while fingers palpate ASIS (Fig. 11-10).
Examiner action:	After instructing patient in motion desired, stabilize ipsilateral pelvis with one hand and extend patient's hip through available ROM with other hand. Ipsilateral knee should be kept extended to avoid limitation of hip extension by tight rectus femoris muscle. Hip should not be extended past the point at which pelvic motion begins to occur (as detected by inferior movement of ipsilateral ASIS under examiner's stabilizing hand). Return limb to starting position. Performing passive movement provides an estimate of the ROM and demonstrates to patient exact motion desired (see Fig. 11-10).
Goniometer alignment:	Palpate following bony landmarks (shown in Fig. 11-9) and align goniometer accordingly (Fig. 11-11).
Stationary arm:	Lateral midline of pelvis and trunk.*

---

* Lateral midline of pelvis should parallel midline of trunk as long as pelvic motion is prevented and neutral pelvis is maintained (see description of neutral pelvis in Techniques of Measurement: Hip Flexion/Extension).

Fig. 11-10. End of hip extension ROM, showing proper hand placement for stabilizing pelvis and detecting pelvic motion. Bony landmarks for goniometer alignment (lateral midline of pelvis/trunk, greater trochanter, lateral femoral epicondyle) indicated by orange line and dots.

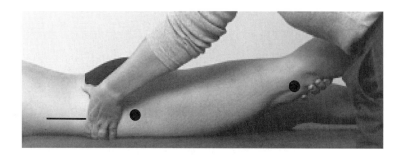

Fig. 11–11. Starting position for measurement of hip extension, demonstrating proper initial alignment of goniometer.

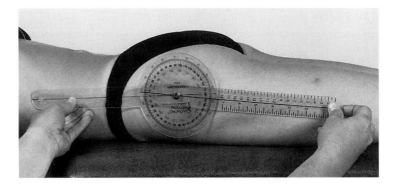

Axis:	Greater trochanter of femur.
Moving arm:	Lateral midline of femur toward lateral femoral epicondyle.
	Read scale of goniometer.
Patient/Examiner action:	Perform passive, or have patient perform active, hip extension (Fig. 11–12). In either case, hip extension should not be allowed to continue past point at which pelvic motion is detected (see Examiner action).
Confirmation of alignment:	Repalpate landmarks and confirm proper goniometric alignment at end of ROM, correcting alignment as necessary (see Fig. 11–12). Read scale of goniometer.
Documentation:	Record patient's ROM.
Precaution:	Should hip be allowed to extend past point at which pelvic motion begins to occur, motion measured will include both hip and lumbar extension. In order to isolate hip extension, pelvic motion must not be permitted.
Alternative patient position:	Sidelying. Stabilization of pelvis more difficult with patient in this position. Goniometer alignment remains the same.

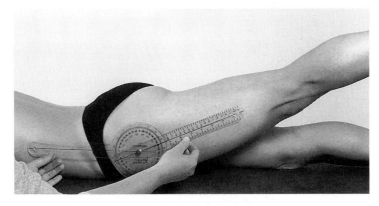

Fig. 11–12. End of hip extension ROM, demonstrating proper alignment of goniometer at end of range.

Hip Abduction

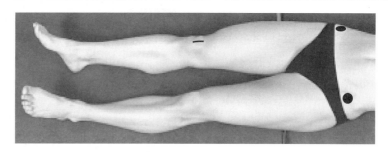

Fig. 11–13. Starting position for measurement of hip abduction. Bony landmarks for goniometer alignment (ipsilateral ASIS, contralateral ASIS, midline of patella) indicated by orange dots and line.

Patient position:	Supine, with lower extremities in anatomical position (Fig. 11–13).
Stabilization:	Over anterior aspect of ipsilateral pelvis (Fig. 11–14).
Examiner action:	After instructing patient in motion desired, abduct patient's hip through available ROM, avoiding hip rotation. Return limb to starting position. Performing passive movement provides an estimate of the ROM and demonstrates to patient exact motion desired (see Fig. 11–14).
Goniometer alignment:	Palpate following bony landmarks (shown in Fig. 11–13) and align goniometer accordingly (Fig. 11–15).
Stationary arm:	Toward contralateral ASIS.
Axis:	Ipsilateral ASIS.

Fig. 11–14. End of hip abduction ROM, showing proper hand placement for stabilizing pelvis. Bony landmarks for goniometer alignment (ipsilateral ASIS, contralateral ASIS, midline of patella) indicated by orange dots and line.

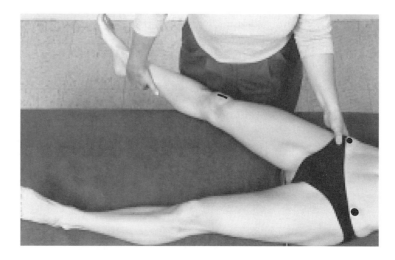

Fig. 11–15. Starting position for measurement of hip abduction, demonstrating proper initial alignment of goniometer.

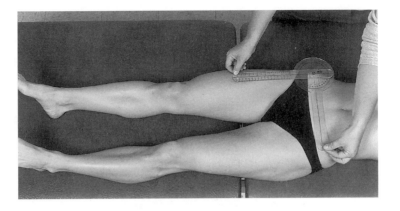

Moving arm:	Anterior midline of ipsilateral femur, using midline of patella as reference.
	Read scale of goniometer.
Patient/Examiner action:	Perform passive, or have patient perform active, hip abduction (Fig. 11–16).
Confirmation of alignment:	Repalpate landmarks and confirm proper goniometric alignment at end of ROM, correcting alignment as necessary (see Fig. 11–16) (see Note). Read scale of goniometer.
Documentation:	Record patient's ROM.
Note:	Confirmation of alignment of stationary arm is critical to avoid including lateral pelvic tilting in hip abduction ROM.

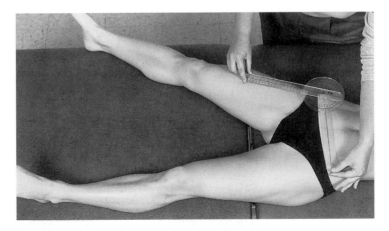

Fig. 11–16. End of hip abduction ROM, demonstrating proper alignment of goniometer at end of range.

Hip Adduction

Fig. 11–17. Starting position for measurement of hip adduction. Contralateral hip is abducted to allow room for adduction of ipsilateral hip. Bony landmarks for goniometer alignment (ipsilateral ASIS, contralateral ASIS, midline of patella) indicated by orange dots and line.

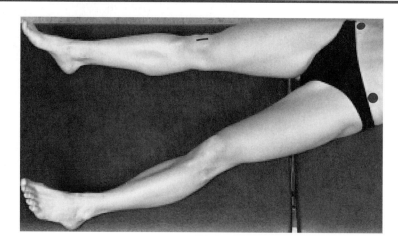

Patient position:	Supine with ipsilateral lower extremity in anatomical position; contralateral hip abducted (Fig. 11–17).
Stabilization:	Over anterior aspect of ipsilateral pelvis (Fig. 11–18).
Examiner action:	After instructing patient in motion desired, adduct patient's hip through available ROM, avoiding hip rotation. Return limb to starting position. Performing passive movement provides an estimate of the ROM and demonstrates to patient exact motion desired (see Fig. 11–18).
Goniometer alignment:	Palpate following bony landmarks (shown in Fig. 11–17) and align goniometer accordingly (Fig. 11–19).
Stationary arm:	Toward contralateral ASIS.
Axis:	Ipsilateral ASIS.

Fig. 11–18. End of hip adduction ROM, showing proper hand placement for stabilizing pelvis. Bony landmarks for goniometer alignment (ipsilateral ASIS, contralateral ASIS, midline of patella) indicated by orange dots and line.

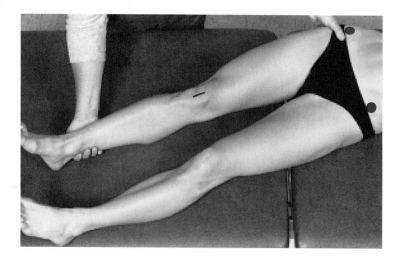

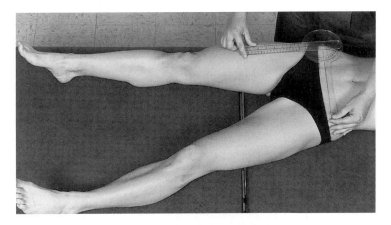

Fig. 11–19. Starting position for measurement of hip adduction, demonstrating proper initial alignment of goniometer.

Moving arm:	Anterior midline of femur, using midline of patella as reference.
	Read scale of goniometer.
Patient/Examiner action:	Perform passive, or have patient perform active, hip adduction (Fig. 11–20).
Confirmation of alignment:	Repalpate landmarks and confirm proper goniometric alignment at end of ROM, correcting alignment as necessary (see Fig. 11–20) (see Note). Read scale of goniometer.
Documentation:	Record patient's ROM.
Note:	Confirmation of alignment of stationary arm is critical to avoid including lateral pelvic tilting in hip adduction ROM.

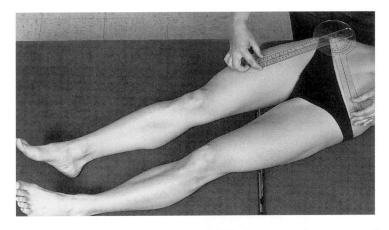

Fig. 11–20. End of hip adduction ROM, demonstrating proper alignment of goniometer at end of range.

Hip Lateral Rotation

Fig. 11–21. Starting position for measurement of hip lateral rotation. Weight is distributed evenly over both ischial tuberosities. Towel roll is placed under ipsilateral thigh to position femur in horizontal plane. Bony landmarks for goniometer alignment (midpoint of patella, tibial crest) indicated by orange dot and line.

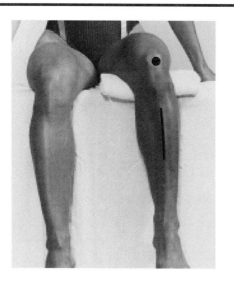

Patient position:	Seated, with hip and knee flexed to 90 degrees, folded towel under thigh; weight equally distributed over both ischial tuberosities (Fig. 11–21).
Stabilization:	None needed; pelvis is stabilized by patient's weight.
Examiner action:	After instructing patient in motion desired, laterally rotate patient's hip through available ROM by keeping the thigh stationary and moving the leg, foot, and ankle medially. Return limb to starting position. Performing passive movement provides an estimate of the ROM and demonstrates to patient exact motion desired (Fig. 11–22).
Goniometer alignment:	Palpate following bony landmarks (shown in Fig. 11–21) and align the goniometer accordingly (Fig. 11–23).
Stationary arm:	Perpendicular to floor.
Axis:	Midpoint of patella.
Moving arm:	Anterior midline of tibia, along tibial crest.
	Read scale of goniometer.

Fig. 11–22. End of hip lateral rotation ROM. Examiner's hand stabilizes thigh against table. Bony landmarks for goniometer alignment (midpoint of patella, tibial crest) indicated by orange dot and line.

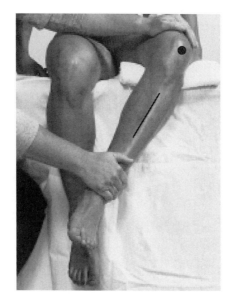

Fig. 11–23. Starting position for measurement of hip lateral rotation, demonstrating proper initial alignment of goniometer.

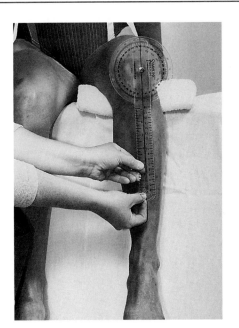

Patient/Examiner action:	Perform passive, or have patient perform active, hip lateral rotation. Patient should be instructed to maintain equal weight on both ischial tuberosities (Fig. 11–24).
Confirmation of alignment:	Repalpate landmarks and confirm proper goniometric alignment at end of ROM, correcting alignment as necessary (see Fig. 11–24). Read scale of goniometer.
Documentation:	Record patient's ROM.
Precaution:	Do not allow patient to laterally flex trunk to ipsilateral side or lift ipsilateral thigh from table during measurement, as doing so will result in a falsely increased ROM.
Alternative position:	Supine with hip and knee flexed 90 degrees. Stationary arm of goniometer is aligned parallel to anterior midline of trunk. Alignment of rest of goniometer remains the same.

Fig. 11–24. End of hip lateral rotation ROM, demonstrating proper alignment of goniometer at end of range.

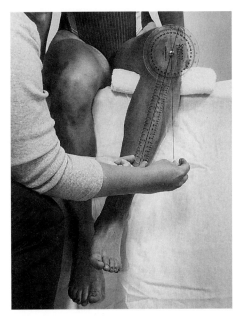

Hip Medial Rotation

Fig. 11–25. Starting position for measurement of hip medial rotation. Weight is distributed evenly over both ischial tuberosities. Towel roll is placed under ipsilateral thigh to position femur in horizontal plane. Bony landmarks for goniometer alignment (midpoint of patella, tibial crest) indicated by orange dot and line.

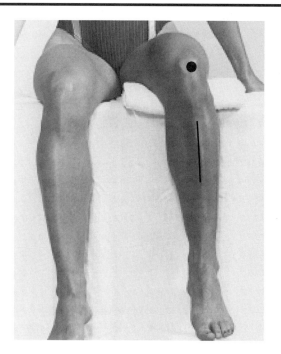

Patient position:	Seated, with hip and knee flexed to 90 degrees, folded towel under thigh; weight equally distributed over both ischial tuberosities (Fig. 11–25).
Stabilization:	None needed; pelvis is stabilized by patient's weight.
Examiner action:	After instructing patient in motion desired, medially rotate patient's hip through available ROM by keeping the thigh stationary and moving the leg, foot, and ankle laterally. Return limb to starting position. Performing passive movement provides an estimate of the ROM and demonstrates to patient exact motion desired (Fig. 11–26).
Goniometer alignment:	Palpate following bony landmarks (shown in Fig. 11–25) and align goniometer accordingly (Fig. 11–27).
Stationary arm:	Perpendicular to floor.
Axis:	Midpoint of patella.

Fig. 11–26. End of hip medial rotation ROM. Examiner's hand stabilizes thigh against table. Bony landmarks for goniometer alignment (midpoint of patella, tibial crest) indicated by orange dot and line.

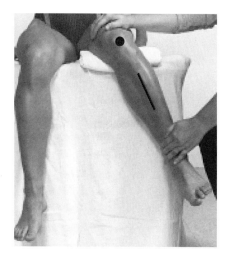

Fig. 11–27. Starting position for measurement of hip medial rotation, demonstrating proper initial alignment of goniometer.

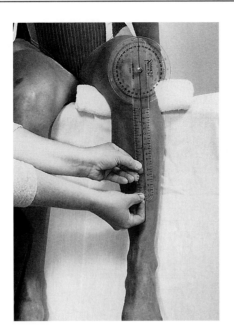

Moving arm:	Anterior midline of tibia, along tibial crest.
	Read scale of goniometer.
Patient/Examiner action:	Perform passive, or have patient perform active, hip medial rotation. Patient should be instructed to maintain equal weight on both ischial tuberosities (Fig. 11–28).
Confirmation of alignment:	Repalpate landmarks and confirm proper goniometric alignment at end of ROM, correcting alignment as necessary (see Fig. 11–28). Read scale of goniometer.
Documentation:	Record patient's ROM.
Precaution:	Do not allow patient to laterally flex trunk to contralateral side or lift ipsilateral thigh from table during measurement, as doing so will result in a falsely increased ROM.
Alternative patient position:	Supine with hip and knee flexed to 90 degrees. Stationary arm of goniometer is aligned parallel to anterior midline of trunk. Alignment of rest of goniometer remains the same.

Fig. 11–28. End of hip medial rotation ROM, demonstrating proper alignment of goniometer at end of range.

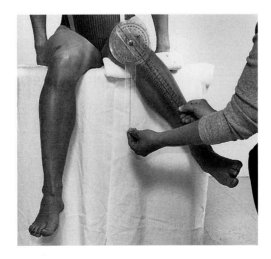

References

1. American Medical Association: Guides to the Evaluation of Permanent Impairment, 4th ed. Chicago, 1993.
2. Bartlett MD, Wolf LS, Shurtleff DB, et al.: Hip flexion contractures: A comparison of measurement methods. Arch Phys Med Rehabil 1985;66:620–625.
3. Clarkson HM: Musculoskeletal Assessment: Joint Range of Motion and Manual Muscle Strength, 2nd ed. Baltimore, Williams & Wilkins, 2000.
4. Clemente CD (ed.). Gray's Anatomy of the Human Body. Philadelphia, Lea & Febiger, 1985.
5. Drews JE, Vraciu JK, Pellino G: Range of motion of the joints of the lower extremities of newborns. Phys Occup Ther Pediatr 1984;4:49–62.
6. Ellison JB, Rose SJ, Sahrmann SA: Patterns of hip rotation range of motion: A comparison between healthy subjects and patients with low back pain. Phys Ther 1990;70:537–541.
7. Greene WB, Heckman JD: The Clinical Measurement of Joint Motion. Rosemont, Ill, American Academy of Orthopaedic Surgeons, 1994.
8. Haley ET: Range of hip rotation and torque of hip rotator muscle groups. Am J Phys Med 1953;32:261–270.
9. Kendall FP, McCreary EK, Provance PG: Muscles: Testing and Function, 4th ed. Baltimore, Williams & Wilkins, 1993.
10. Levangie PK, Norkin CC: Joint Structure and Function, 3rd ed. Philadelphia, F.A. Davis, 2001.
11. Milch H: The pelvifemoral angle. J Bone Joint Surg 1942;24:148–153.
12. Milch H: The measurement of hip motion in the sagittal and coronal planes. J Bone Joint Surg 1959;41A:731–736.
13. Moore ML: Clinical assessment of joint motion. In Basmajian JV (ed.): Therapeutic Exercise, 3rd ed. Philadelphia, Williams & Wilkins, 1978. pp 151–190.
14. Mundale MO, Hislop HJ, Babideau RJ, et al.: Evaluation of extension of the hip. Arch Phys Med Rehabil 1956;37:75–80.
15. Norkin CC, White DJ: Measurement of Joint Motion: A Guide to Goniometry, 2nd edition. Philadelphia, F.A. Davis, 1995.
16. Simoneau CC, Hoenig KJ, Lepley JE, et al.: Influence of hip position and gender on active hip internal and external rotation. J Orthop Sports Phys Ther 1998;28:158–164.
17. Steindler A: Mechanics of Normal and Pathological Motion in Man. Springfield, Ill, Charles C Thomas, 1935.

12

MEASUREMENT of RANGE of MOTION of the KNEE

ANATOMY AND OSTEOKINEMATICS

The knee joint consists of three separate articulations within a single joint capsule, one articulation between each convex femoral condyle and the corresponding tibial condyle and intervening meniscus, and a third articulation between the patella and the anterior aspect of the distal femur.[2, 4, 11] Each of the two articulations between the femoral and the tibial condyles and the menisci can be described as separate joints[2, 6] but are treated as a single joint, the tibiofemoral joint, during range of motion (ROM) measurements. Motion at the articulation between the patella and the anterior femur, the patellofemoral joint, typically is not measured clinically using a goniometer. Therefore, only tibiofemoral motion is considered in the following discussion of the knee joint.

Classic explanations of motion occurring at the knee joint describe active motion as including flexion and extension, which occur around a medial-lateral axis passing through the femoral condyles,[3] and rotation of the tibia, which occurs around a longitudinal axis passing through the medial intercondylar tubercle.[8] According to this description of knee motion, the axis for flexion and extension of the knee is not fixed but moves as the knee flexes.[3, 10] Other investigators have challenged this classic description, asserting that flexion and extension of the knee occur around a fixed, oblique axis that extends from the lateral, posterior, inferior aspect of the knee to its medial, anterior, superior aspect.[7] This axis is described as passing through the lateral and medial femoral epicondyles (at the point of attachment of the collateral ligaments) and superior to the decussation of the cruciate ligaments. As such, the axis for knee flexion and extension lies not in the transverse plane but at an angle to all three cardinal planes, producing combined motions of flexion, adduction, medial rotation or extension, abduction, and lateral rotation.

Rotation at the knee, which occurs passively during flexion and extension motions and is associated with the locking mechanism of the knee, also may be produced actively, but only when the knee is flexed.[8, 13] Active rotation is impossible when the knee is extended fully, owing to the tightness of the collateral and cruciate ligaments.[2, 8] Typically, only flexion and extension of the knee, and not rotation, are measured clinically.

LIMITATIONS OF MOTION: KNEE JOINT

Knee flexion is limited by soft tissue approximation between the structures of the posterior thigh and calf, provided that the hip also is in some degree of flexion.[8, 12] Flexion of the knee may be limited prematurely if the hip is

(Text continues on page 306.)

Knee Flexion

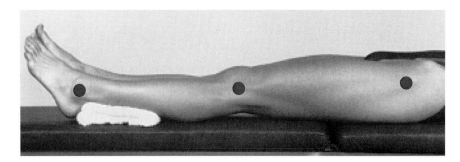

Fig. 12-1. Starting position for measurement of knee flexion. Towel roll under ipsilateral ankle to promote full knee extension. Bony landmarks for goniometer alignment (greater trochanter, lateral femoral epicondyle, lateral malleolus) indicated by orange dots.

Patient position:	Supine, with lower extremities in anatomical position; towel roll under ipsilateral ankle (Fig. 12–1).
Stabilization:	Over anterior aspect of thigh (Fig. 12–2).
Examiner action:	After instructing patient in motion desired, flex patient's knee through available ROM by sliding patient's foot along table toward pelvis. Return to starting position. Performing passive movement provides an estimate of the ROM and demonstrates to patient the exact motion desired (see Fig. 12–2).

Fig. 12-2. End of knee flexion ROM, showing proper hand placement for stabilization of ipsilateral thigh. Bony landmarks for goniometer alignment (greater trochanter, lateral femoral epicondyle, lateral malleolus) indicated by orange dots.

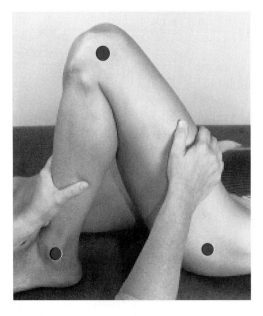

Fig. 12–3. Starting position for measurement of knee flexion demonstrating proper initial alignment of goniometer.

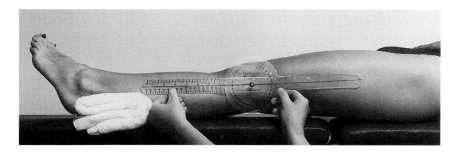

Goniometer alignment:	Palpate following bony landmarks (shown in Fig. 12–1) and align goniometer accordingly (Fig. 12–3).
Stationary arm:	Lateral midline of femur toward greater trochanter.
Axis:	Lateral epicondyle of femur.
Moving arm:	Lateral midline of fibula, in line with fibular head and lateral malleolus.
	Read scale of goniometer.
Patient/Examiner action:	Perform passive, or have patient perform active, knee flexion by sliding foot toward pelvis (Fig. 12–4).
Confirmation of alignment:	Repalpate landmarks and confirm proper goniometric alignment at end of ROM, correcting alignment as necessary (see Fig. 12–4). Read scale of goniometer.
Documentation:	Record patient's ROM.
Note:	Knee flexion may be measured with patient in prone position, but knee flexion ROM in prone may be limited owing to tightness of rectus femoris muscle.
Alternative patient position:	Prone (see preceding Note) or sidelying. In either case, goniometer alignment remains the same.

Fig. 12–4. End of knee flexion ROM, demonstrating proper alignment of goniometer at end of range.

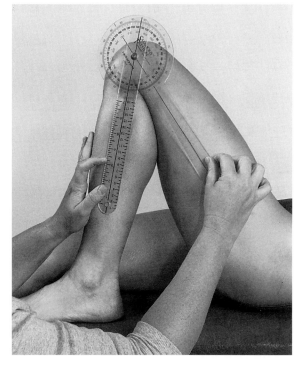

Knee Extension

Fig. 12–5. Starting position for measurement of knee extension. Towel roll under ipsilateral ankle to promote full knee extension. Bony landmarks for goniometer alignment (greater trochanter, lateral femoral epicondyle, lateral malleolus) indicated by orange dots.

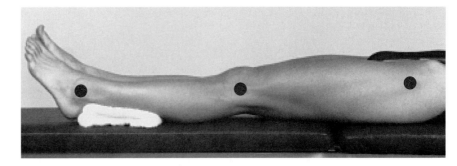

Patient position:	Supine, with knee extended as far as possible; towel roll under ipsilateral ankle (Fig. 12–5).
Stabilization:	None needed.
Examiner action:	Determine whether knee is extended as far as possible by either: a) asking patient to straighten knee as far as possible (if measuring active ROM), or b) providing passive pressure on the knee in the direction of extension (if measuring passive ROM) (Fig. 12–6).

Fig. 12–6. End of knee extension ROM. Examiner is ensuring complete knee extension through posteriorly directed pressure on the distal thigh. Bony landmarks for goniometer alignment (greater trochanter, lateral femoral epicondyle, lateral malleolus) indicated by orange dots.

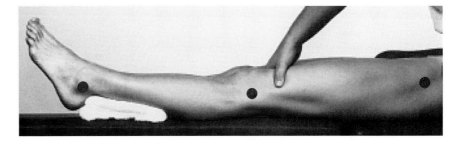

Fig. 12–7. Measurement of knee extension demonstrating proper alignment of goniometer.

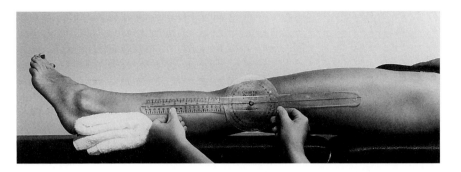

Goniometer alignment:	Palpate the following bony landmarks (shown in Fig. 12–5) and align goniometer accordingly (Fig. 12–7).
Stationary arm:	Lateral midline of femur toward greater trochanter.
Axis:	Lateral epicondyle of femur.
Moving arm:	Lateral midline of fibula, in line with fibular head and lateral malleolus.
	Read scale of goniometer.
Documentation:	Record patient's ROM.
Alternative patient position:	Prone or sidelying. If prone position is used, it may be necessary to place a towel roll under the anterior aspect of the patient's thigh, and the patient's foot must be off the table in order to obtain full knee extension. With either position, goniometer alignment remains the same.

extended, owing to tension in the rectus femoris muscle, which crosses the anterior aspect of both the hip and the knee joints.[9] The preferred position for measurement of knee flexion is with the patient supine and the hip flexed in order to avoid such premature stoppage of the motion. Capsular and ligamentous structures provide the primary limitation of knee extension, provided the hip is extended as well.[8, 10] When the hip is flexed, extension of the knee may be limited by tension in the hamstring muscle group.[9, 13] Thus, normal end-feels for knee flexion are soft (soft tissue approximation) with the hip flexed and firm (muscular) with the hip extended. Normal end-feels for knee extension are firm (capsular/ligamentous) with the hip extended and firm (muscular) with the hip flexed. Information regarding normal ranges of motion for the knee is found in Appendix C.

TECHNIQUES OF MEASUREMENT: KNEE FLEXION/EXTENSION

Motion of the knee may be measured with the subject in either the supine or the prone position. The American Academy of Orthopaedic Surgeons[5] lists both supine and prone as optional starting positions for the measurement of knee motion. However, tightness in the rectus femoris muscle may limit knee flexion when the subject is positioned in prone. Therefore, the supine position for measuring knee flexion, which is recommended by the American Medical Association,[1] is preferred.

References

1. American Medical Association: Guides to the Evaluation of Permanent Impairment, 4th ed. Chicago, 1993.
2. Clemente CD (ed): Gray's Anatomy of the Human Body, 13th ed. Philadelphia, Lea & Febiger, 1985.
3. Frankel VH, Burstein AH: Orthopedic Biomechanics. Philadelphia, Lea & Febiger, 1970.
4. Gill DG, Corbacio EJ, Lauchle LE: Anatomy of the knee. In Engle RP (ed): Knee Ligament Rehabilitation. New York, Churchill Livingstone, 1991.
5. Greene WB, Heckman JD: The Clinical Measurement of Joint Motion. Rosemont, Ill, American Academy of Orthopaedic Surgeons, 1994.
6. Greenfield BH: Functional anatomy of the knee. In Greenfield, BH: Rehabilitation of the Knee. Philadelphia, FA Davis, 1993.
7. Hollister AM, Jatana S, Singh AK, et al.: The axes of rotation of the knee. Clin Orthop 1993;290:259–268.
8. Kapandji IA: The Physiology of Joints, vol 1, 5th ed. New York, Churchill Livingstone, 1987.
9. Kendall FP, McCreary EK, Provance PG: Muscles: Testing and Function, 4th ed. Baltimore, Williams & Wilkins, 1993.
10. Levangie PK, Norkin CC: Joint Structure and Function: A Comprehensive Analysis, 3rd ed. Philadelphia, FA Davis, 2001.
11. Mangine R, Heckman T: The Knee. In Sanders B (ed): Sports Physical Therapy. Norwalk, Conn, Appleton & Lange, 1990.
12. Smith LK, Weiss EL, Lehmkuhl LD: Brunnstrom's Clinical Kinesiology, 5th ed. Philadelphia, FA Davis, 1996.
13. Soderberg GL: Kinesiology: Application to Pathological Motion, 2nd ed. Baltimore, Williams & Wilkins, 1997.

MEASUREMENT of RANGE of MOTION of the ANKLE and FOOT

ANATOMY AND OSTEOKINEMATICS: ANKLE, SUBTALAR, AND MIDTARSAL JOINTS

Traditional anatomical descriptions of motion at the ankle (talocrural), subtalar, and midtarsal joints depict motions occurring at these joints as dorsiflexion, plantarflexion, inversion, and eversion in their classical definitions (see Chapter 1).[5] However, more contemporary explanations describe motion at these joints as occurring around oblique axes that lie at angles to all three cardinal planes.[7, 15, 23] These so-called triplanar axes allow motion in all three planes simultaneously. The motions thus produced have been termed pronation (a combination of dorsiflexion, abduction, and eversion) and supination (a combination of plantarflexion, adduction, and inversion).[7, 23] However, much confusion surrounds these terms in the literature, with some authors using supination and pronation instead of, or interchangeably with, inversion and eversion.[13, 16, 19, 24] For purposes of this text, motion occurring at the ankle, subtalar, and midtarsal joints is termed pronation and supination, with emphasis placed on the component motion(s) of pronation or supination that is greatest at each joint (e.g., the dorsiflexion component of pronation at the ankle).

The ankle, or talocrural, joint consists of the articulation of the concave distal tibia, along with the fibular malleolus, with the convex proximal surface of the talus. Motion at this joint consists of pronation and supination around an oblique axis that angles, from lateral to medial, anteriorly and dorsally and falls slightly distal to the malleoli.[7] Movement around such an axis causes the major components of pronation and supination at the talocrural joint to be dorsiflexion and plantarflexion, respectively, which are the motions measured clinically to examine pronation and supination at this joint.

The subtalar, or talocalcaneal, joint is formed by two articulations, a posterior and an anterior, between the talus and the calcaneus. The posterior articulation occurs between the convex posterior talar facet of the calcaneus and the concave posterior calcaneal facet of the talus. The anterior articulation, formed by contact between the convex head of the talus and the concave middle and anterior talar facets of the calcaneus, is also part of the talocalcaneonavicular joint (an articulation between the anterior aspects of the talus and the calcaneus and the posterior aspect of the navicular).[5] Motion at the subtalar joint consists of pronation and supination around an oblique axis that extends, from lateral to medial, in an anterior and dorsal direction, falling through the head of the talus.[17] Because of the location and angulation of the subtalar joint axis, the principle components of pronation and supination at this joint are eversion and inversion and abduction and adduction.[15] Inversion and eversion are the motions measured clinically to examine supination and pronation of this joint.[7]

The midtarsal (or transverse tarsal) joint is a collective term used for the combined calcaneocuboid joint and the talonavicular portion of the talocalcaneonavicular joint. Although these articulations do not share a joint capsule, their joint lines traverse the foot from medial to lateral in a roughly **S** shape, allowing motion to occur across the combined joints.[5] The primary components of pronation and supination that occur at this joint add to the component motions of dorsiflexion/plantarflexion at the ankle and eversion/inversion at the subtalar joint. Because no adequate means of measuring isolated midtarsal motion exists, motion at this joint is measured in this text in conjunction with subtalar motion as foot inversion and eversion.

Limitations of Motion: Ankle, Subtalar, and Midtarsal Joints

The dorsiflexion and plantarflexion components of ankle pronation and supination are limited by the joint capsule, as well as by ligaments and muscles crossing the joint. Ankle plantarflexion is limited initially by tension in the muscles that dorsiflex the ankle and then by anterior capsular and ligamentous structures. Thus, the normal end-feel for ankle plantarflexion is firm (muscular, then capsular/ligamentous). Ankle dorsiflexion is limited by tension in the soleus and gastrocnemius muscles, causing a firm (muscular) end-feel, particularly if the knee is extended when the movement occurs. Posterior capsular and ligamentous structures also limit ankle dorsiflexion, particularly with the knee flexed. Inversion and eversion of the subtalar and midtarsal joints are limited by tension in the collateral ligaments of the ankle, producing a firm (ligamentous) end-feel with either motion.[13] Information on normal ranges of motion for the dorsiflexion, plantarflexion, inversion, and eversion components of pronation and supination is found in Appendix C.

Techniques of Goniometry: Ankle Dorsiflexion/Plantarflexion Components of Pronation/Supination

The dorsiflexion and plantarflexion components of ankle pronation and supination may be measured using a variety of techniques and landmarks. The most common proximal landmark used for these measurements is the fibular shaft,[22] with the axis of the goniometer generally placed over, or distal to but aligned with, the lateral malleolus.[19] Several distal landmarks have been used to measure ankle dorsiflexion and plantarflexion, including the shaft of the fifth metatarsal,[2, 19, 20] the heel,[2, 19] and the plantar surface of the foot.[2, 8] While each of these distal landmarks appears to be reliable in the measurement of ankle dorsiflexion, techniques employing the heel as a distal landmark are less reliable than those in which the fifth metatarsal or plantar surface of the foot are used.[2] Values obtained during the measurement of ankle dorsiflexion range of motion (ROM) have been shown to vary significantly according to the landmarks used during the measurement and according to the type of motion (active or passive) measured,[2] reinforcing the need for standardized positioning and technique during the measurement of range of motion. Position of the patient's knee during the measurement may also influence the values obtained during dorsiflexion measurement, as tension in the calcaneal tendon may limit dorsiflexion with the knee extended.[12]

Many examiners recommend measuring the components of ankle motion, and in particular dorsiflexion, while maintaining the subtalar joint in a neutral position.[1, 2, 6, 26, 27] The rationale behind such positioning is an attempt to minimize motion of the midtarsal joint while isolating talocrural motion.[26] Although the use of neutral positioning of the subtalar joint during ankle dorsiflexion does not completely eliminate forefoot motion,[1] a significant difference has been demonstrated in the amount of ankle dorsiflexion obtained when performing the measurement with the subtalar joint in the neutral compared with the pronated position.[26] However, measurements of ankle dorsiflexion taken while maintaining the subtalar joint in neutral may require extensive examiner training in order to be reliable[6] because of problems in the reliability of determining the neutral position of the subtalar joint.[9, 21]

Techniques of Goniometry: Subtalar Inversion/Eversion Components of Pronation/Supination

The literature describes a variety of methods of measuring range of motion of inversion and eversion that occur as the principle components of supination and pronation at the subtalar joint. If one attempts to isolate and measure the amount of inversion and eversion occurring only at the subtalar joint, one must make the decision whether or not to reference the motion from the neutral position of the subtalar joint (STJN). This position of the subtalar joint, STJN, is the position of the joint in which it is neither pronated nor supinated.[23] Many individuals advocate measuring subtalar joint motion from a reference point of STJN,[14, 25] while others use anatomical zero as a reference.[10, 18] Unless the examiner is highly trained in determining the neutral position of the subtalar joint, measurements of subtalar motion referenced from subtalar neutral may be less reliable than those referenced from anatomical zero.[6, 9]

Should one choose to reference measurements of subtalar motion from STJN, two basic methods may be used to establish the neutral position of the subtalar joint. One method uses a mathematical calculation based on measurements of calcaneal inversion and eversion to determine subtalar neutral,[28] whereas the other method establishes subtalar neutral by palpating for talonavicular congruency.[18] Since there is no general agreement as to which of these two techniques for establishing STJN is preferred, and since the latter technique requires fewer steps, palpating for talonavicular congruency is used in this text for determining STJN. To establish STJN by palpation, grasp the medial and lateral sides of the talar head with the thumb and index finger of one hand while passively pronating and supinating the foot with the other hand until the talar head is felt equally against both the thumb and the index finger. This position of the talus is STJN. Once the neutral position of the subtalar joint has been located, measurement of inversion and eversion is then performed by placing the axis of the goniometer on the posterior aspect of the subtalar joint at the level of the malleoli, aligning the proximal arm with a line bisecting the lower leg, and aligning the distal arm with a line bisecting the calcaneus. These measurements may be taken with the subject standing in a weight-bearing position or prone in a non–weight-bearing position, with the amount of motion obtained varying significantly depending on the patient's position.[14]

The inversion and eversion components of supination and pronation also can be measured across the joints of the entire foot, resulting in the measurement of motion that occurs at several joints, including the talocrural, subtalar, and transverse tarsal joints.[4, 19] Although measurement of foot inversion and eversion does not measure isolated motion at a single joint, such measurements are commonly used, easily performed, and are useful as screening techniques.

ANATOMY AND OSTEOKINEMATICS: METATARSOPHALANGEAL AND INTERPHALANGEAL JOINTS

The metatarsophalangeal (MTP) joints of the foot are similar in structure to the metacarpophalangeal joints of the hand in that they are condyloid joints, allowing motion in two cardinal body planes.[7, 13] The articulations at the MTP joints take place between the convex metatarsal heads, which are interconnected on their plantar surfaces by the deep transverse metatarsal ligaments, and the concave bases of the proximal phalanges.[5] Active motions at these joints, as at the metacarpophalangeal joints, consist of flexion, extension, abduction, and adduction, although the range of abduction and adduction available in the toes is much less than that seen in the fingers, with active abduction and adduction of the 1st MTP joint being impossible for some individuals.[5, 13]

The interphalangeal (IP) joints of the toes are classified as hinge joints, and, as such, are capable of the motions of flexion and extension. Each interphalangeal joint is composed of an articulation between the convex head of the more proximal phalanx and the concave base of the more distal phalanx. Nine such interphalangeal joints are found in the toes, two (one proximal and one distal) in each of the lateral four toes, and one interphalangeal joint in the great (1st) toe.[5, 13]

Limitations of Motion: Metatarsophalangeal and Interphalangeal Joints

Both MTP and IP joint flexion is limited by tension in the toe extensor muscles and tendons, whereas extension is limited by tension in the toe flexors and tendons and the plantar ligaments. Thus, the normal end-feel for both flexion and extension at all these joints is firm, owing to limitation by muscular, or muscular and ligamentous, structures. Abduction and adduction at the MTP joints are limited by the collateral ligaments of the joints or by approximation with adjacent toes.[5] Information regarding the normal ranges of motion for the MTP joints is found in Appendix C.

Techniques of Goniometry: Metatarsophalangeal and Interphalangeal Flexion/Extension

Clinically, extension of the 1st MTP joint is the motion of the toes of most common concern, as limitation of that motion can cause significant impairment of foot function during gait. In fact, only articles examining MTP extension,[3, 11] and none examining MTP flexion or IP flexion or extension, were found in the literature. The focus in the literature on measuring MTP extension is probably due to the need for sufficient MTP extension, more than other motions of the toes, in normal functioning of the foot.

No fewer than four different methods for measuring extension of the 1st MTP joint have been described in the literature. The methods vary according to the technique used by the examiner and according to the position in which the patient is placed during the measurement. Two basic measuring techniques and a variety of patient positions are described in the four methods. One measuring technique uses an approach in which the motion is measured from the medial aspect of the joint, with the goniometer aligned so that the axis is at the medial joint line, the moving arm is positioned along the medial midline of the proximal phalanx of the great toe, and the stationary arm is positioned along the medial midline of the first metatarsal.[3] A second technique involves measuring extension with the goniometer aligned on the dorsum of the great toe, with the axis on the dorsal joint space, the moving arm on the dorsal midline of the proximal phalanx, and the stationary arm on the dorsal midline of the first metatarsal.[19] Subjects may be placed in a variety of positions when these measuring techniques are used, including non–weight-bearing with the talocrural joint in neutral, partial weight-bearing with the subject seated, and weight-bearing with the subject standing.[11]

Ankle Supination: Plantarflexion Component

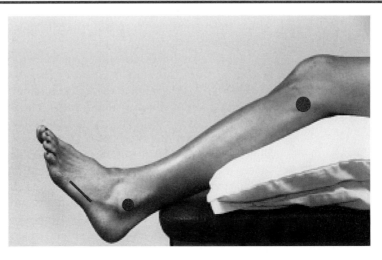

Fig. 13–1. Starting position for measurement of ankle supination: Plantarflexion component. Bony landmarks for goniometer alignment (fibular head, lateral malleolus, lateral midline of 5th metatarsal) indicated by orange line and dots.

Patient position:	Supine or sitting (see Note), with knee flexed (as shown) or extended, ankle in anatomical position (Fig. 13–1).
Stabilization:	Over posterior aspect of distal leg (Fig. 13–2).
Examiner action:	After instructing patient in motion desired, plantarflex patient's ankle through available ROM. Return to starting position. Performing passive movement provides an estimate of the ROM and demonstrates to patient exact motion desired (see Fig. 13–2).
Goniometer alignment:	Palpate following bony landmarks (shown in Fig. 13–1) and align goniometer accordingly (Fig. 13–3).

Fig. 13–2. End of ankle supination: plantarflexion component ROM, showing proper hand placement for stabilizing leg. Bony landmarks for goniometer alignment (fibular head, lateral malleolus, lateral midline of 5th metatarsal) indicated by orange line and dots.

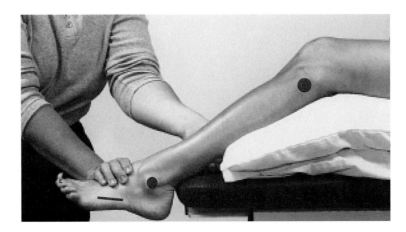

Fig. 13–3. Starting position for measurement of ankle supination: Plantarflexion component, demonstrating proper initial alignment of goniometer. Note that axis of goniometer is positioned at the intersection point of lines through the lateral midline of the fibula and the 5th metatarsal.

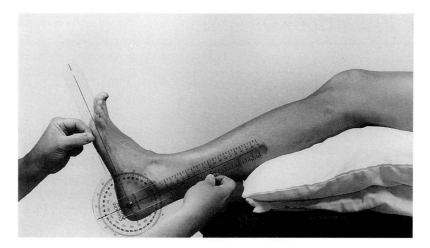

Stationary arm:	Lateral midline of fibula, in line with fibular head.
Axis:	Distal to, but in line with lateral malleolus, at intersection of lines through lateral midline of fibula and lateral midline of 5th metatarsal.
Moving arm:	Lateral midline of 5th metatarsal.
	Read scale of goniometer.
Patient/Examiner action:	Perform passive, or have patient perform active, ankle plantarflexion (Fig. 13–4).
Confirmation of alignment:	Repalpate landmarks and confirm proper goniometric alignment at end of ROM, correcting alignment as necessary. Read scale of goniometer (Fig. 13–4).
Documentation:	Record patient's ROM.
Note:	Supine position is preferred over sitting position for measurements of ankle motion, as bony landmarks are placed more easily at the examiner's eye level when the patient is supine.
Alternative patient position:	Prone or sidelying. In either case, goniometer alignment remains the same.

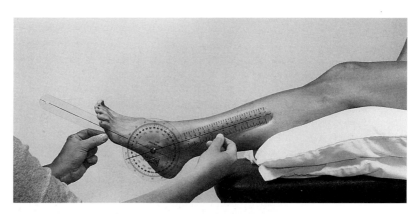

Fig. 13–4. End of ankle supination: plantarflexion component ROM, demonstrating proper alignment of goniometer at end of range.

Ankle Pronation: Dorsiflexion Component

Fig. 13–5. Starting position for measurement of ankle pronation: dorsiflexion component. Bony landmarks for goniometer alignment (fibular head, lateral malleolus, lateral midline of 5th metatarsal) indicated by orange line and dots.

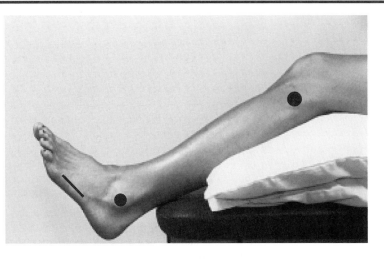

Patient position:	Supine or sitting (see Note), with knee flexed at least 30 degrees, ankle in anatomical position (Fig. 13–5).
Stabilization:	Over anterior aspect of distal leg (Fig. 13–6).
Examiner action:	After instructing patient in motion desired, dorsiflex patient's ankle through available ROM. Return to starting position. Performing passive movement provides an estimate of the ROM and demonstrates to patient exact motion desired (see Fig. 13–6).
Goniometer alignment:	Palpate following bony landmarks (shown in Fig. 13–5) and align goniometer accordingly (Fig. 13–7).

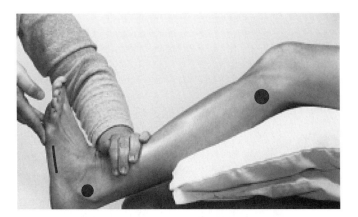

Fig. 13–6. End of ankle pronation: dorsiflexion component ROM, showing proper hand placement for stabilizing leg and dorsiflexing joint. Note that motion is achieved through upward pressure on the plantar surfaces of metatarsals 4 and 5. Bony landmarks for goniometer alignment (fibular head, lateral malleolus, lateral midline of 5th metatarsal) indicated by orange line and dots.

Fig. 13–7. Starting position for measurement of ankle pronation: dorsiflexion component, demonstrating proper initial alignment of goniometer. Note that axis of goniometer is positioned at the intersection point of lines through the lateral midline of the fibula and the 5th metatarsal.

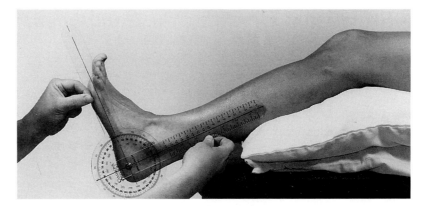

Stationary arm:	Lateral midline of fibula, in line with fibular head.
Axis:	Distal to, but in line with lateral malleolus, at intersection of lines through lateral midline of fibula and lateral midline of 5th metatarsal.
Moving arm:	Lateral midline of 5th metatarsal.
	Read scale of goniometer.
Patient/Examiner action:	Perform passive, or have patient perform active, ankle dorsiflexion (Fig. 13–8).
Confirmation of alignment:	Repalpate landmarks and confirm proper goniometric alignment at end of ROM, correcting alignment as necessary. Read scale of goniometer (Fig. 13–8).
Documentation:	Record patient's ROM.
Note:	Supine position is preferred over sitting position for measurements of ankle motion, as bony landmarks are placed more easily at the examiner's eye level when the patient is supine.
Alternative patient position:	Prone or sidelying. In either case, goniometer alignment remains the same. Motion also can be measured with knee extended, providing an estimation of gastrocnemius tightness (see Figs. 14–32 through 14–34).

Fig. 13–8. End of ankle pronation: dorsiflexion component ROM, demonstrating proper alignment of goniometer at end of range.

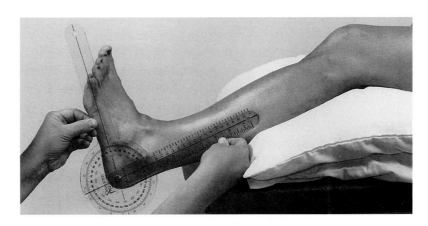

Ankle Pronation: Dorsiflexion Component in Subtalar Neutral Position

Fig. 13–9. Starting position for measurement of ankle pronation: dorsiflexion component, with subtalar joint in neutral position. Bony landmarks for goniometer alignment (fibular head, lateral malleolus, lateral midline of 5th metatarsal) indicated by orange line and dots.

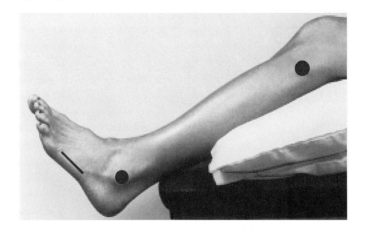

An assistant is needed to perform this measurement correctly.

Patient position:	Supine or sitting, with knee flexed at least 30 degrees, ankle in anatomical position (Fig. 13–9).
Stabilization:	Over head of talus (see Examiner action).

Examiner action (Examiner #1):	1. Place patient's subtalar joint in neutral position as follows:
	   a. Grasp medial and lateral sides of talar head with thumb and index finger of one hand.
	   b. With other hand, passively pronate and supinate foot until talar head is felt equally against both thumb and index finger. This position is subtalar neutral.

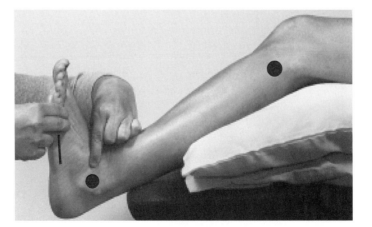

Fig. 13–10. End of ankle pronation: dorsiflexion component ROM, with subtalar joint maintained in neutral position. The examiner's left hand is grasping the talar head to ensure the maintenance of a neutral subtalar joint position, while the right hand is dorsiflexing the ankle through upward pressure on the plantar surfaces of metatarsals 4 and 5. Bony landmarks for goniometer alignment (fibular head, lateral malleolus, lateral midline of 5th metatarsal) indicated by orange line and dots.

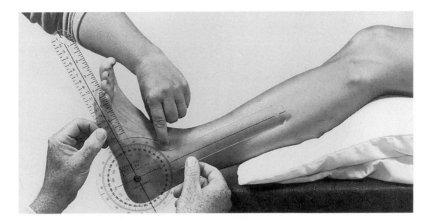

Fig. 13–11. Starting position for measurement of ankle pronation: dorsiflexion component, with subtalar joint maintained in neutral position, demonstrating proper initial alignment of goniometer. Examiner #1 maintains the subtalar joint in a neutral position by grasping the talar head, while examiner #2 aligns the goniometer. Note that axis of goniometer is positioned at the intersection point of lines through the lateral midline of the fibula and the 5th metatarsal.

2. Passively dorsiflex patient's ankle through available ROM with one hand, while maintaining grasp on talus with opposite hand, assuring that subtalar neutral position is maintained during entire range of dorsiflexion (Fig. 13–10). Return to starting position.

Goniometer alignment (Examiner #2):	Examiner #2 aligns goniometer as described for ankle dorsiflexion test (landmarks shown in Fig. 13–9) and reads scale of goniometer (Fig. 13–11).
Patient/Examiner action:	Examiner #1 performs passive, or has patient perform active, ankle dorsiflexion while maintaining subtalar joint in neutral position (Fig. 13–12).
Confirmation of alignment:	Examiner #2 repalpates landmarks and confirms proper alignment at end of ROM, correcting alignment as necessary. Examiner #2 reads scale of goniometer (Fig. 13–12).
Documentation:	Record patient's ROM.
Precaution:	Reliability of this measurement technique may be poor owing to questionable reliability of establishing neutral position of subtalar joint.

Fig. 13–12. End of ankle pronation: dorsiflexion component ROM, with subtalar joint maintained in neutral position, demonstrating proper alignment of goniometer at end of range. Examiner #1 maintains subtalar joint in neutral position while passively dorsiflexing the ankle. Examiner #2 performs goniometric measurement of motion.

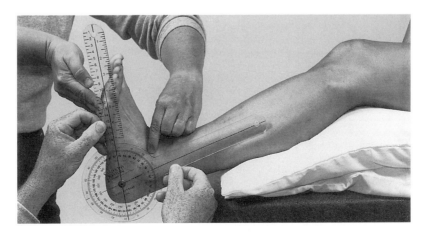

Ankle/Foot Supination: Inversion Component

Fig. 13–13. Starting position for measurement of combined ankle/foot supination: inversion component. Bony landmarks for goniometer alignment (tibial crest, anterior midline of talocrural joint, anterior midline of 2nd metatarsal) indicated by orange lines and dot.

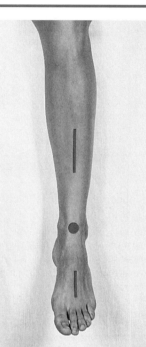

Patient position:	Seated, with ankle in anatomical position (Fig. 13–13).
Stabilization:	Over posterior aspect of distal leg (Fig. 13–14).
Examiner action:	After instructing patient in motion desired, invert patient's foot/ankle through available ROM. Return to starting position. Performing passive movement provides an estimate of the ROM and demonstrates to patient exact motion desired (see Fig. 13–14).
Goniometer alignment:	Palpate following bony landmarks (shown in Fig. 13–13) and align goniometer accordingly (Fig. 13–15).
Stationary arm:	Anterior midline of tibia, in line with tibial crest.

Fig. 13–14. End of combined ankle/foot supination: inversion component ROM, showing proper hand placement for stabilizing tibia and inverting ankle/foot. Bony landmarks for goniometer alignment (tibial crest, anterior midline of talocrural joint, anterior midline of 2nd metatarsal) indicated by orange lines and dot.

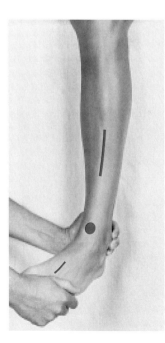

Fig. 13–15. Starting position for measurement of ankle/foot supination: inversion component, demonstrating proper initial alignment of goniometer.

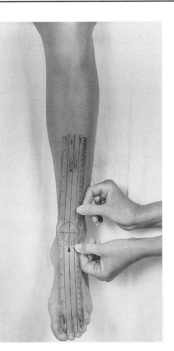

Axis:	Anterior aspect of talocrural joint, midway between medial and lateral malleoli.
Moving arm:	Anterior midline of 2nd metatarsal.
	Read scale of goniometer.
Patient/Examiner action:	Perform passive, or have patient perform active, ankle/foot inversion (Fig. 13–16).
Confirmation of alignment:	Repalpate landmarks and confirm proper goniometric alignment at end of ROM, correcting alignment as necessary. Read scale of goniometer (Fig. 13–16).
Documentation:	Record patient's ROM.
Alternative patient position:	Supine, with ankle in anatomical position; goniometer alignment remains the same.

Fig. 13–16. End of ankle/foot supination: inversion component ROM, demonstrating proper alignment of goniometer at end of range.

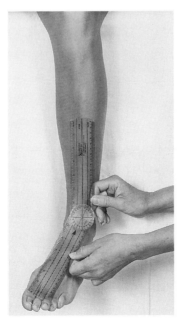

Ankle/Foot Pronation: Eversion Component

Fig. 13–17. Starting position for measurement of combined ankle/foot pronation: eversion component. Bony landmarks for goniometer alignment (tibial crest, anterior midline of talocrural joint, anterior midline of 2nd metatarsal) indicated by orange lines and dot.

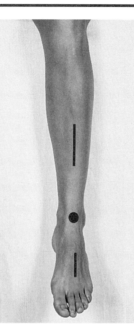

Patient position:	Seated, with ankle in anatomical position (Fig. 13–17).
Stabilization:	Over posterior aspect of distal leg (Fig. 13–18).
Examiner action:	After instructing patient in motion desired, evert patient's foot/ankle through available ROM. Return to starting position. Performing passive movement provides an estimate of the ROM and demonstrates to patient exact motion desired (see Fig. 13–18).
Goniometer alignment:	Palpate following bony landmarks (shown in Fig. 13–17) and align goniometer accordingly (Fig. 13–19).
Stationary arm:	Anterior midline of tibia, in line with tibial crest.
Axis:	Anterior aspect of talocrural joint, midway between medial and lateral malleoli.

Fig. 13–18. End of combined ankle/foot pronation: eversion component ROM, showing proper hand placement for stabilizing tibia and inverting ankle/foot. Bony landmarks for goniometer alignment (tibial crest, anterior midline of talocrural joint, anterior midline of 2nd metatarsal) indicated by orange lines and dot.

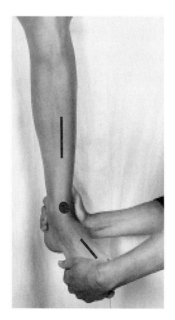

Fig. 13–19. Starting position for measurement of ankle/foot pronation: eversion component, demonstrating proper initial alignment of goniometer.

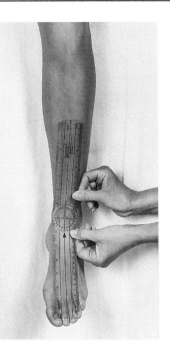

Moving arm:	Anterior midline of 2nd metatarsal.
	Read scale of goniometer.
Patient/Examiner action:	Perform passive, or have patient perform active, ankle/foot eversion (Fig. 13–20).
Confirmation of alignment:	Repalpate landmarks and confirm proper goniometric alignment at end of ROM, correcting alignment as necessary. Read scale of goniometer (Fig. 13–20).
Documentation:	Record patient's ROM.
Alternative patient position:	Supine, with ankle in anatomical position; goniometer alignment remains the same.

Fig. 13–20. End of ankle/foot pronation: eversion component ROM, demonstrating proper alignment of goniometer at end of range.

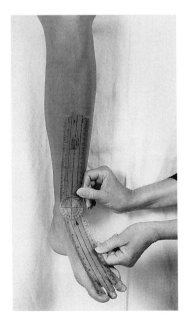

Subtalar Supination: Inversion Component (Referenced from Anatomical Zero)

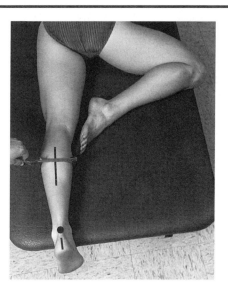

Fig. 13-21. Starting position for measurement of subtalar supination: inversion component, referenced from anatomical zero. Position of contralateral lower extremity places ipsilateral calcaneus in the frontal plane. Calipers are used to determine posterior midline of leg and calcaneus (see text for instructions). Landmarks for goniometer alignment (posterior midline of leg, calcaneal tendon in line with malleoli, posterior midline of calcaneus) indicated by orange lines and dot.

Patient position:	Prone, with lower extremity to be measured in anatomical position; foot off end of table. Opposite lower extremity positioned in hip flexion, abduction, and external rotation with knee flexed (Fig. 13–21).
Stabilization:	Over distal aspect of ipsilateral leg (Fig. 13–22).
Examiner action:	After instructing patient in procedure to be performed, invert patient's calcaneus by moving it medially. Performing passive movement provides an estimate of the ROM and demonstrates procedure to patient (see Fig. 13–22).
Goniometer alignment:	Palpate following landmarks (shown in Fig. 13–21) and align goniometer accordingly (Fig. 13–23).

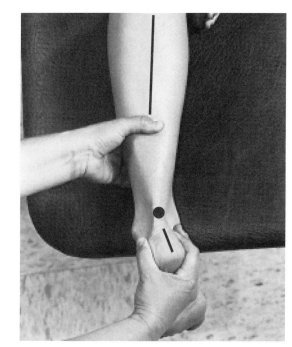

Fig. 13-22. End of subtalar supination: inversion component ROM, showing proper hand placement for stabilizing tibia and inverting subtalar joint. Landmarks for goniometer alignment (posterior midline of leg, calcaneal tendon in line with malleoli, posterior midline of calcaneus) indicated by orange lines and dot.

Fig. 13–23. Starting position for measurement of subtalar supination: inversion component, demonstrating proper alignment of goniometer. Calcaneus is positioned so that goniometer reads 0 degrees at beginning of ROM.

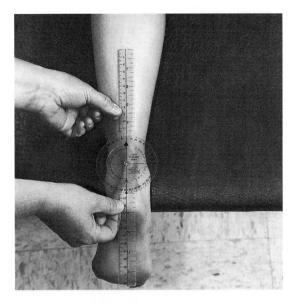

Stationary arm:	Posterior midline of leg (use of calipers* is recommended for determining this line; see Fig. 13–21).
Axis:	Over calcaneal tendon in line with malleoli.
Moving arm:	Posterior midline of calcaneus (use of calipers* is recommended for determining this line).
	Move patient's calcaneus until scale of goniometer reads 0 degrees. This is the 0-degree starting position.
Examiner action:	Perform passive, or have patient perform active, calcaneal inversion (Fig. 13–24).
Confirmation of alignment:	Repalpate landmarks and confirm proper goniometric alignment at end of ROM, correcting alignment as necessary. Read scale of goniometer (Fig. 13–24).
Documentation:	Record patient's ROM.

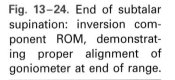

* Caliper use: Calipers are placed near proximal end of structure (leg or calcaneus) with vertical arms contacting medial and lateral aspects of structure (without compressing tissue). Dot is made on structure at midpoint between vertical arms. Calipers are then moved to distal aspect of structure and above procedure repeated. Line connecting proximal and distal dots, which will accurately represent midline of structure, is drawn.

Fig. 13–24. End of subtalar supination: inversion component ROM, demonstrating proper alignment of goniometer at end of range.

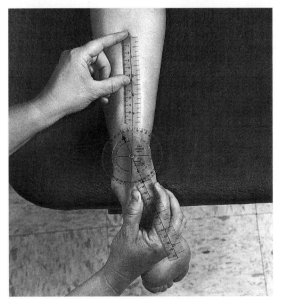

Subtalar Pronation: Eversion Component (Referenced from Anatomical Zero)

Fig. 13-25. Starting position for measurement of subtalar pronation: eversion component, referenced from anatomical zero. Position of contralateral lower extremity places ipsilateral calcaneus in the frontal plane. Calipers are used to determine posterior midline of leg and calcaneus (see text for instructions). Landmarks for goniometer alignment (posterior midline of leg, calcaneal tendon in line with malleoli, posterior midline of calcaneus) indicated by orange lines and dot.

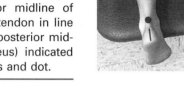

Patient position:	Prone, with lower extremity to be measured in anatomical position; foot off end of table. Opposite lower extremity position in hip flexion, abduction, and external rotation with knee flexed (Fig. 13-25).
Stabilization:	Over distal aspect of ipsilateral leg (Fig. 13-26).
Examiner action:	After instructing patient in procedure to be performed, evert patient's calcaneus by moving it laterally. Performing passive movement provides an estimate of the ROM and demonstrates procedure to patient (see Fig. 13-26).
Goniometer alignment:	Palpate following landmarks (shown in Fig. 13-25) and align goniometer accordingly (Fig. 13-27).

Fig. 13-26. End of subtalar pronation: eversion component ROM, showing proper hand placement for stabilizing tibia and everting subtalar joint. Landmarks for goniometer alignment (posterior midline of leg, calcaneal tendon in line with malleoli, posterior midline of calcaneus) indicated by orange lines and dot.

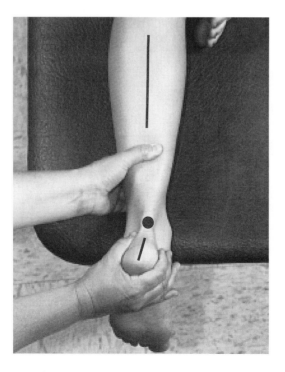

Fig. 13–27. Starting position for measurement of subtalar pronation: eversion component, demonstrating proper alignment of goniometer. Calcaneus is positioned so that goniometer reads 0 degrees at beginning of ROM.

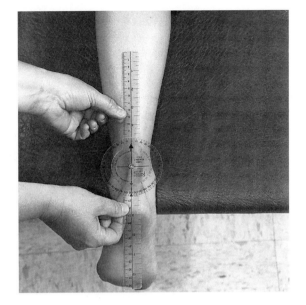

Stationary arm:	Posterior midline of leg (use of calipers* is recommended for determining this line; see Fig. 13–25).
Axis:	Over calcaneal tendon in line with malleoli.
Moving arm:	Posterior midline of calcaneus (use of calipers* is recommended for determining this line).

Move patient's calcaneus until scale of goniometer reads 0 degrees. This is the 0-degree starting position.

Examiner action:	Perform passive, or have patient perform active, calcaneal eversion (Fig. 13–28).
Confirmation of alignment:	Repalpate landmarks and confirm proper goniometric alignment at end of ROM, correcting alignment as necessary. Read scale of goniometer (Fig. 13–28).
Documentation:	Record patient's ROM.

---

* Caliper use: See the footnote under Subtalar Supination: Inversion Component.

Fig. 13–28. End of subtalar pronation: eversion component ROM, demonstrating proper alignment of goniometer at end of range.

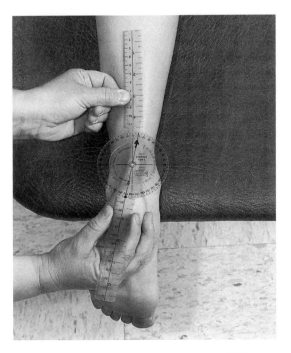

First Metatarsophalangeal (MTP) Joint Flexion (Plantarflexion)

Fig. 13–29. Starting position for measurement of 1st MTP joint flexion. Bony landmarks for goniometer alignment (medial midline of 1st metatarsal, medial aspect of 1st MTP joint, medial midline of proximal phalanx) indicated by orange lines and dot.

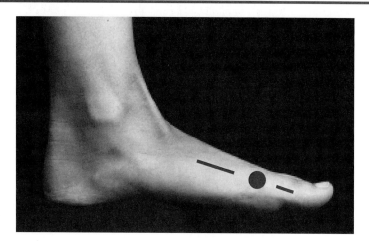

Patient position:	Supine or seated with ankle in neutral position (Fig. 13–29).
Stabilization:	Over 1st metatarsal (Fig. 13–30).
Examiner action:	After instructing patient in motion desired, flex patient's 1st MTP joint through available ROM. Return limb to starting position. Performing passive movement provides an estimate of the ROM and demonstrates to patient exact motion desired (see Fig. 13–30).

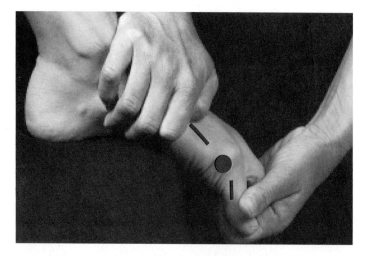

Fig. 13–30. End of 1st MTP joint flexion ROM, showing proper hand placement for stabilizing 1st metatarsal and flexing MTP joint. Bony landmarks for goniometer alignment (medial midline of 1st metatarsal, medial aspect of 1st MTP joint, medial midline of proximal phalanx) indicated by orange lines and dot.

Fig. 13–31. Starting position for measurement of 1st MTP joint flexion, demonstrating proper initial alignment of goniometer.

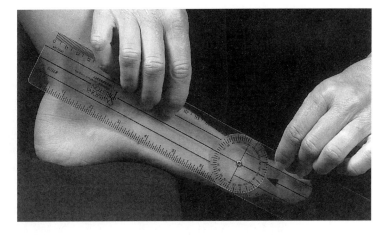

Goniometer alignment:	Palpate following bony landmarks (shown in Fig. 13–29) and align goniometer accordingly (Fig. 13–31).
Stationary arm:	Medial midline of 1st metatarsal.
Axis:	Medial aspect of 1st MTP joint.
Moving arm:	Medial midline of proximal phalanx of great toe.

Read scale of goniometer.

Patient/Examiner action: Perform passive, or have patient perform active, MTP flexion (Fig. 13–32).

Confirmation of alignment: Repalpate landmarks and confirm proper goniometric alignment at end of ROM, correcting alignment as necessary. Read scale of goniometer (Fig. 13–32).

Documentation: Record patient's ROM.

Note: Alternative alignment is with goniometer positioned over dorsum of the joint, similar to MTP flexion of lateral four toes (see Metatarsophalangeal [MTP] or Interphalangeal [PIP, DIP, IP] Flexion).

Fig. 13–32. End of 1st MTP joint flexion ROM, demonstrating proper alignment of goniometer at end of range.

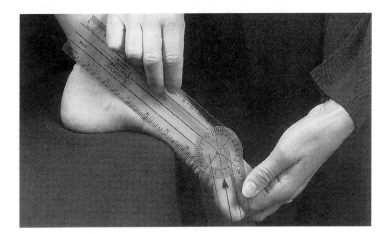

First Metatarsophalangeal (MTP) Joint Extension (Dorsiflexion)

Fig. 13–33. Starting position for measurement of 1st MTP joint extension. Bony landmarks for goniometer alignment (medial midline of 1st metatarsal, medial aspect of 1st MTP joint, medial midline of proximal phalanx) indicated by orange lines and dot.

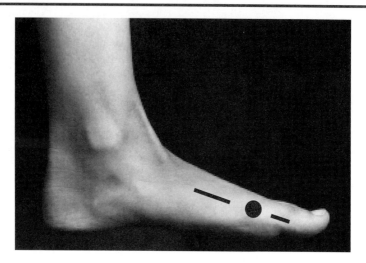

Patient position: Supine or seated, with ankle in neutral position (Fig. 13–33).

Stabilization: Over 1st metatarsal (Fig. 13–34).

Examiner action: After instructing patient in motion desired, extend patient's 1st MTP joint through available ROM. Return limb to starting position. Performing passive movement provides an estimate of the ROM and demonstrates to patient exact motion desired (see Fig. 13–34).

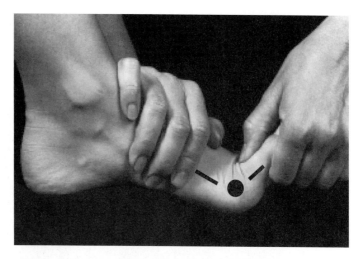

Fig. 13–34. End of 1st MTP joint extension ROM, showing proper hand placement for stabilizing 1st metatarsal and extending MTP joint. Bony landmarks for goniometer alignment (medial midline of 1st metatarsal, medial aspect of 1st MTP joint, medial midline of proximal phalanx) indicated by orange lines and dot.

Fig. 13–35. Starting position for measurement of 1st MTP joint extension, demonstrating proper initial alignment of goniometer.

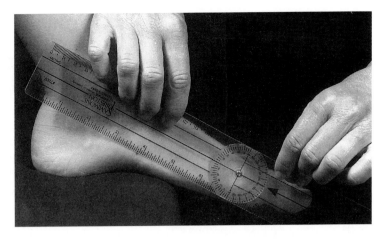

Goniometer alignment:	Palpate following bony landmarks (shown in Fig. 13–33) and align goniometer accordingly (Fig. 13–35).
Stationary arm:	Medial midline of 1st metatarsal.
Axis:	Medial aspect of 1st MTP joint.
Moving arm:	Medial midline of proximal phalanx of great toe.
	Read scale of goniometer.
Patient/Examiner action:	Perform passive, or have patient perform active, MTP extension (Fig. 13–36).
Confirmation of alignment:	Repalpate landmarks and confirm proper goniometric alignment at end of ROM, correcting alignment as necessary. Read scale of goniometer (Fig. 13–36).
Documentation:	Record patient's ROM.
Note:	Alternative alignment is with goniometer positioned over dorsum of the joint, similar to MTP flexion of lateral four toes (see Metatarsophalangeal [MTP] or Interphalangeal [PIP, DIP, IP] Flexion).

Fig. 13–36. End of 1st MTP joint extension ROM, demonstrating proper alignment of goniometer at end of range.

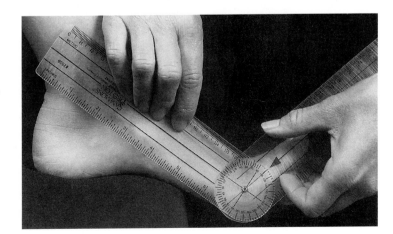

First Metatarsophalangeal (MTP) Joint Abduction

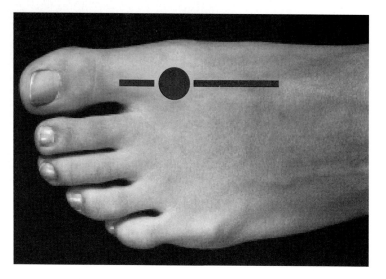

Fig. 13-37. Starting position for measurement of 1st MTP joint abduction. Bony landmarks for goniometer alignment (dorsal midline of 1st metatarsal, dorsal aspect of 1st MTP joint, dorsal midline of proximal phalanx) indicated by orange lines and dot.

Patient position:	Supine or seated, with ankle in neutral position (Fig. 13–37).
Stabilization:	Over 1st metatarsal (Fig. 13–38).
Examiner action:	After instructing patient in motion desired, abduct patient's 1st MTP joint through available ROM. Return limb to starting position. Performing passive movement provides an estimate of the ROM and demonstrates to patient exact motion desired (see Fig. 13–38).

Fig. 13-38. End of 1st MTP joint abduction ROM, showing proper hand placement for stabilizing 1st metatarsal and abducting MTP joint. Bony landmarks for goniometer alignment (dorsal midline of 1st metatarsal, dorsal aspect of 1st MTP joint, dorsal midline of proximal phalanx) indicated by orange lines and dot.

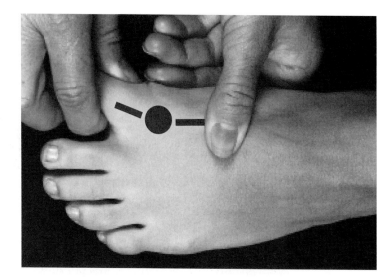

Fig. 13–39. Starting position for measurement of 1st MTP joint abduction, demonstrating proper initial alignment of goniometer.

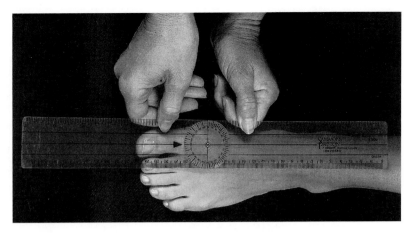

Goniometer alignment:	Palpate following bony landmarks (shown in Fig. 13–37) and align goniometer accordingly (Fig. 13–39).
Stationary arm:	Dorsal midline of 1st metatarsal.
Axis:	Dorsal midline of 1st MTP joint.
Moving arm:	Dorsal midline of proximal phalanx of great toe.
	Read scale of goniometer.
Patient/Examiner action:	Perform passive MTP abduction (Fig. 13–40; see Note).
Confirmation of alignment:	Repalpate landmarks and confirm proper goniometric alignment at end of ROM, correcting alignment as necessary. Read scale of goniometer (Fig. 13–40).
Documentation:	Record patient's ROM.
Note:	Active abduction of the 1st MTP joint may be difficult or impossible for many individuals.

Fig. 13–40. End of 1st MTP joint abduction ROM, demonstrating proper alignment of goniometer at end of range.

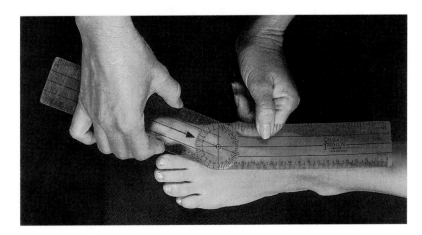

First Metatarsophalangeal (MTP) Joint Adduction

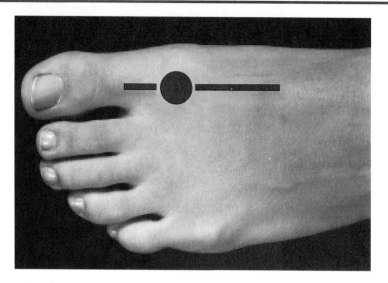

Fig. 13–41. Starting position for measurement of 1st MTP joint adduction. Bony landmarks for goniometer alignment (dorsal midline of 1st metatarsal, dorsal aspect of 1st MTP joint, dorsal midline of proximal phalanx) indicated by orange lines and dot.

Patient position: Supine or seated, with ankle in neutral position (Fig. 13–41).

Stabilization: Over 1st metatarsal (Fig. 13–42).

Examiner action: After instructing patient in motion desired, adduct patient's 1st MTP joint through available ROM. Return limb to starting position. Performing passive movement provides an estimate of the ROM and demonstrates to patient exact motion desired (see Fig. 13–42).

Fig. 13–42. End of 1st MTP joint adduction ROM, showing proper hand placement for stabilizing 1st metatarsal and adducting MTP joint. Bony landmarks for goniometer alignment (dorsal midline of 1st metatarsal, dorsal aspect of 1st MTP joint, dorsal midline of proximal phalanx) indicated by orange lines and dot.

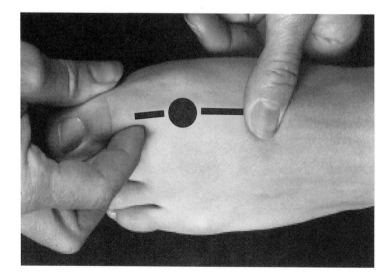

Fig. 13–43. Starting position for measurement of 1st MTP joint adduction, demonstrating proper initial alignment of goniometer.

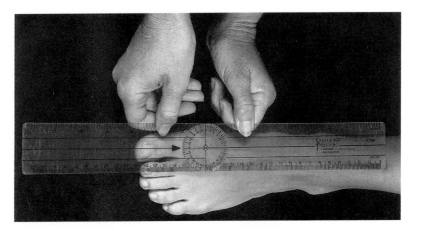

Goniometer alignment:	Palpate following bony landmarks (shown in Fig. 13–41) and align goniometer accordingly (Fig. 13–43).
Stationary arm:	Dorsal midline of 1st metatarsal.
Axis:	Dorsal midline of 1st MTP joint.
Moving arm:	Dorsal midline of proximal phalanx of great toe.
	Read scale of goniometer.
Patient/Examiner action:	Perform passive MTP adduction (Fig. 13–44; see Note).
Confirmation of alignment:	Repalpate landmarks and confirm proper goniometric alignment at end of ROM, correcting alignment as necessary. Read scale of goniometer (Fig. 13–44).
Documentation:	Record patient's ROM.
Note:	Active adduction of the 1st MTP joint may be difficult or impossible for many individuals.

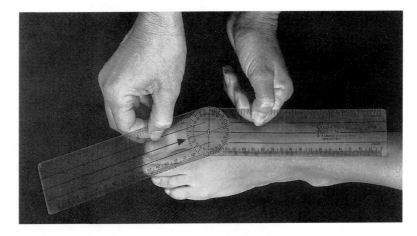

Fig. 13–44. End of 1st MTP joint adduction ROM, demonstrating proper alignment of goniometer at end of range.

Metatarsophalangeal (MTP) or Interphalangeal (PIP, DIP, IP) Flexion

Fig. 13–45. Starting position for measurement of MTP joint flexion. Bony landmarks for goniometer alignment (dorsal midline of metatarsal, dorsal aspect of MTP joint, dorsal midline of proximal phalanx) indicated by orange lines and dot.

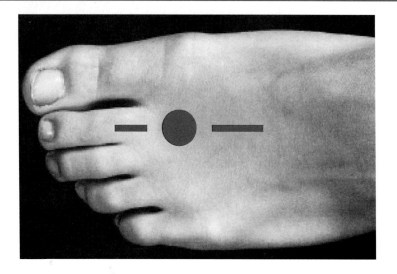

Measurement of 2nd MTP Joint Shown

Patient position:	Supine or seated, with ankle in neutral position (Fig. 13–45).
Stabilization:	Over more proximal bone of joint to be measured (in this case, stabilization of metatarsals is shown) (Fig. 13–46).
Examiner action:	After instructing patient in motion desired, flex joint to be measured through available ROM. Return toe to starting position. Performing passive movement provides an estimate of the ROM and demonstrates to patient exact motion desired (see Fig. 13–46).

Fig. 13–46. End of MTP joint flexion ROM, showing proper hand placement for stabilizing metatarsal and flexing MTP joint. Bony landmarks for goniometer alignment (dorsal midline of metatarsal, dorsal aspect of MTP joint) indicated by orange line and dot.

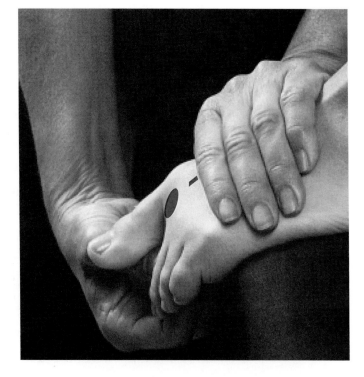

Fig. 13–47. Starting position for measurement of MTP joint flexion, demonstrating proper initial alignment of goniometer.

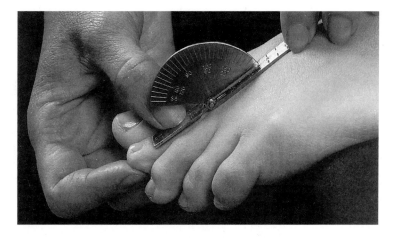

Goniometer alignment:	Palpate following bony landmarks (shown in Fig. 13–45) and align go-niometer accordingly (Fig. 13–47).
Stationary arm:	Dorsal midline of more proximal bone of joint to be measured (in this case, the metatarsal).
Axis:	Dorsal midline of joint to be measured (in this case, the MTP joint).
Moving arm:	Dorsal midline of more distal bone of joint to be measured (in this case, the proximal phalanx).
	Read scale of goniometer.
Patient/Examiner action:	Perform passive, or have patient perform active, flexion of joint to be measured (Fig. 13–48).
Confirmation of alignment:	Repalpate landmarks and confirm proper goniometric alignment at end of ROM, correcting alignment as necessary. Read scale of goniometer (Fig. 13–48).
Documentation:	Record patient's ROM.
Alternative patient position:	Sidelying; goniometer alignment remains same.
Note:	This technique may be used to measure flexion of the MTP, DIP, or PIP joints of the lateral four toes, or flexion of the MTP or IP joint of the great toe. The figures shown here depict the measurement of MTP flexion of the 2nd toe.

Fig. 13–48. End of MTP joint flexion ROM, demonstrating proper alignment of goniometer at end of range.

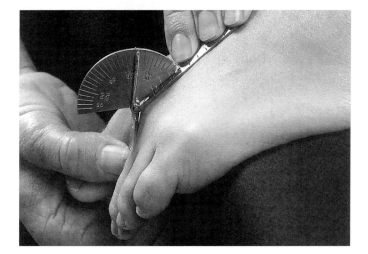

Metatarsophalangeal (MTP) or Interphalangeal (PIP, DIP, IP) Extension

Fig. 13–49. Starting position for measurement of MTP joint extension. Bony landmarks for goniometer alignment (dorsal midline of metatarsal, dorsal aspect of MTP joint, dorsal midline of proximal phalanx) indicated by orange lines and dot.

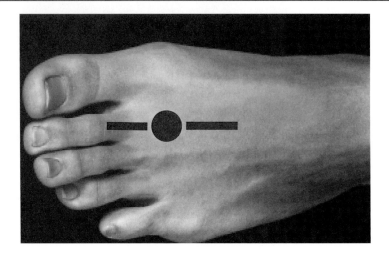

Measurement of 2nd MTP Joint Shown

Patient position:	Supine or seated, with ankle in neutral position (Fig. 13–49).
Stabilization:	Over more proximal bone of joint to be measured (in this case, stabilization of metatarsals is shown) (Fig. 13–50).
Examiner action:	After instructing patient in motion desired, extend joint to be measured through available ROM. Return limb to starting position. Performing passive movement provides an estimate of the ROM and demonstrates to patient exact motion desired (see Fig. 13–50).

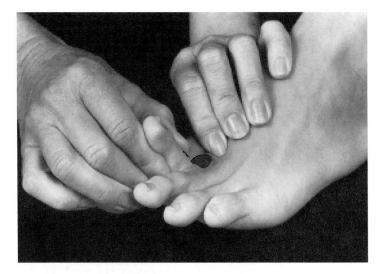

Fig. 13–50. End of MTP joint extension ROM, showing proper hand placement for stabilizing metatarsal and extending MTP joint. Bony landmarks for goniometer alignment (dorsal aspect of MTP joint, dorsal midline of proximal phalanx) indicated by orange line and dot.

Fig. 13–51. Starting position for measurement of MTP joint extension, demonstrating proper initial alignment of goniometer.

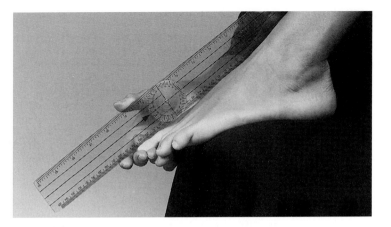

Goniometer alignment:	Palpate following bony landmarks (shown in Fig. 13–49) and align goniometer accordingly (Fig. 13–51).
Stationary arm:	Dorsal midline of more proximal bone of joint to be measured (in this case, the metatarsal).
Axis:	Dorsal midline of joint to be measured (in this case, MTP joint).
Moving arm:	Dorsal midline of more distal bone of joint to be measured (in this case, the proximal phalanx).
	Read scale of goniometer.
Patient/Examiner action:	Perform passive, or have patient perform active, extension of joint to be measured (Fig. 13–52).
Confirmation of alignment:	Repalpate landmarks and confirm proper goniometric alignment at end of ROM, correcting alignment as necessary. Read scale of goniometer (Fig. 13–52).
Documentation:	Record patient's ROM.
Alternative patient position:	Sidelying; goniometer alignment remains same.
Note:	This technique may be used to measure extension of the MTP, DIP, or PIP joints of the lateral four toes, or extension of the MTP or IP joint of the great toe. The figures shown here depict the measurement of MTP extension of the 2nd toe.

Fig. 13–52. End of MTP joint extension ROM, demonstrating proper alignment of goniometer at end of range.

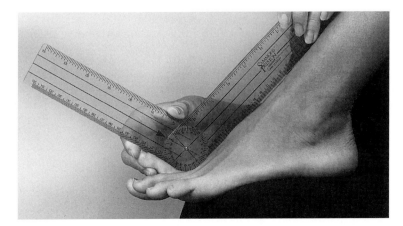

References

1. Bohannon RW, Tiberio D, Waters G: Motion measured from forefoot and hindfoot landmarks during passive ankle dorsiflexion range of motion. J Orthop Sports Phys Ther 1991;13:20–22.

2. Bohannon RW, Tiberio D, Zito M: Selected measures of ankle dorsiflexion range of motion: Differences and intercorrelations. Foot Ankle Int 1989;10:99–103.

3. Buell T, Green DR, Risser J: Measurement of the first metatarsophalangeal joint range of motion. J Am Podiatr Med Assoc 1988;78:439–448.

4. Clarkson HM: Musculoskeletal Assessment: Joint Range of Motion and Manual Muscle Strength, 2nd ed. Baltimore, Williams & Wilkins, 2000.

5. Clemente CD: Gray's Anatomy, 30th American edition. Philadelphia, Lea & Febiger, 1985.

6. Diamond JE, Mueller MJ, Delitto A, et al.: Reliability of a diabetic foot evaluation. Phys Ther 1989;69:797–802.

7. Donatelli R: The Biomechanics of the Foot and Ankle, 2nd ed. Philadelphia, F.A. Davis, 1996.

8. Ekstrand J, Wiktorsson M, Oberg B, et al.: Lower extremity goniometric measurements: A study to determine their reliability. Arch Phys Med Rehabil 1982;63:171–175.

9. Elveru RA, Rothstein JM, Lamb RL: Goniometric reliability in a clinical setting: Subtalar and ankle joint measurements. Phys Ther 1988;68:672–677.

10. Greene WB, Heckman JD: Joint motion: Method of measuring and recording. Rosemont, Ill, American Academy of Orthopaedic Surgeons, 1994.

11. Hopson MM, McPoil TG, Cornwall MW: Motion of the first metatarsophalangeal joint: Reliability and validity of four measurement techniques. J Am Podiatr Med Assoc 1995;85: 198–204.

12. Hornsby TM, Nicholson GG, Gossman MR, et al.: Effect of inherent muscle length on isometric plantar flexion torque in healthy women. Phys Ther 1987;67:1119–1197.

13. Kapandji IA: The Physiology of the Joints, vol 2, 5th ed. New York, Churchill Livingston, 1987.

14. Lattanza L, Gray GW, Kantner RM: Closed versus open kinematic chain measurements of subtalar joint eversion: Implications for clinical practice. J Orthop Sports Phys Ther 1988;9:310–314.

15. Levangie PK, Norkin CC: Joint Structure and Function: A Comprehensive Analysis, 3rd ed. Philadelphia, F.A. Davis, 2001.

16. Lundberg A, Kalin B, Selvik G: Kinematics of the ankle/foot complex: Plantarflexion and dorsiflexion. Foot Ankle Int 1989;9:194–200.

17. Manter JT: Movements of the subtalar and transverse tarsal joints. Anat Rec 1941;80: 397–410.

18. McPoil TG, Brocato RS: The foot and ankle: Biomechanical evaluation and treatment. In Gould JA, Davies GJ (eds): Orthopaedic and Sports Physical Therapy. St. Louis, Mosby, 1985, pp 313–325.

19. Norkin CC, White DJ: Measurement of Joint Motion: A Guide to Goniometry. Philadelphia, F.A. Davis, 1995.

20. Pandya S, Florence JM, King WM, et al.: Reliability of goniometric measurements in patients with Duchenne muscular dystrophy. Phys Ther 1985;65:1339–1342.

21. Picciano AM, Rowlands MS, Worrell T: Reliability of open and closed kinetic chain subtalar joint neutral positions and navicular drop test. J Orthop Sports Phys Ther 1993;18:553–558.

22. Rome, K: Ankle joint dorsiflexion measurement studies: A review of the literature. J Am Podiatr Med Assoc 1996;86:205–211.

23. Root ML, Orien WP, Weed JH: Clinical biomechanics: Normal and abnormal function of the foot, vol 2. Los Angeles, Clinical Biomechanics Corp., 1977.

24. Smith LK, Weiss EL, Lehmkuhl LD: Brunnstrom's Clinical Kinesiology, 5th ed. Philadelphia, F.A. Davis, 1996.

25. Smith-Oricchio K, Harris BA: Interrater reliability of subtalar neutral, calcaneal inversion and eversion. J Orthop Sports Phys Ther 1990;12:10–15.

26. Tiberio D, Bohannon RW, Zito MA: Effect of subtalar joint position on the measurement of maximum ankle dorsiflexion. Clin Biomech (Bristol, Avon) 1989;4:189–191.

27. Tiberio D: Evaluation of functional ankle dorsiflexion using subtalar neutral position: A clinical report. Phys Ther 1987;67:955–957.

28. Wooden MJ: Podiatric Physical Therapy. Albany, NY, Clinical Education Associates, Inc., 1987.

14

MUSCLE LENGTH TESTING of the LOWER EXTREMITY

TESTS FOR MUSCLE LENGTH: ILIOPSOAS

Developed in 1876 as a method of measuring hip flexion contractures in children with tuberculosis, the Thomas test for determining iliopsoas muscle length has become "probably the most widely known and performed test for detecting decreased hip extension."[15] The original Thomas test was defined by Kendall et al.[13] as follows:

> The Thomas flexion test is founded upon our inability to extend a diseased hip without producing a lordosis. If there is flexion deformity, the patient is unable to extend the thigh on the diseased side, and it remains at an angle.

The original Thomas test has undergone modifications over the years, and today the most frequent variation in the original technique is to use a goniometer to measure the amount of hip flexion while the subject holds the contralateral knee toward the chest.

A second technique that can be used to measure iliopsoas muscle length is a modification of the technique used by the American Academy of Orthopaedic Surgeons (AAOS) to measure hip extension.[7] This technique is performed with the patient in the prone position with the knee flexed to 90 degrees.

TESTS FOR MUSCLE LENGTH: RECTUS FEMORIS

The Thomas test position also can be used to measure the length of the rectus femoris muscle. Kendall et al.[13] suggested that the Thomas test technique could be used not only to examine the iliopsoas muscle by taking measurements at the hip, but also to examine the length of the rectus femoris muscle (a two-joint muscle) by taking measurements at the knee.

The length of the rectus femoris muscle also can be examined in the prone position. The knee is fully flexed through the full available range of motion (ROM), ensuring that the ipsilateral hip is not allowed to flex.

TESTS FOR MUSCLE LENGTH: HAMSTRINGS

According to Gajdosik et al.,[4] the straight leg raise is the most common clinical test for measurement of hamstring muscle length. A second type of test used for the measurement of hamstring muscle length is the knee extension test, which is described in the literature as being performed in two ways: active and passive. Magee[16] refers to these tests as the "90/90 test." Measurements similar to the 90/90 knee extension test have been described in the pediatric medical literature for examination of infants and referred to as measurement of the "popliteal angle."[12, 20]

Sit and Reach Test

The sit and reach test, a field test used to measure hamstring flexibility, is a part of most health-related physical fitness test batteries.[11] The test is performed by having the subject assume the long sitting posture and reach forward with both hands as far as possible, not allowing the knees to flex. A score is given based on the most distant point on a standardized box reached by both hands (Fig. 14–1).[1]

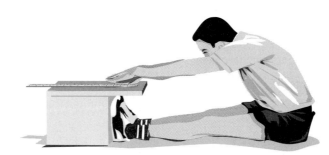

Fig. 14–1. Illustration of the sit and reach test, a composite test measuring multiple motions and muscles that is not included in this chapter.

Although the sit and reach test has been shown to be reliable,[11, 22] some authors suggest that the ability to reach is influenced by hamstring flexibility, range of motion of the lumbar and thoracic spine, anthropometric factors such as legs short or arms long relative to the length of the trunk, and the amount of scapular abduction allowing a greater reach with the arms.[1, 11] Jackson and Langford[11] suggest that "the sit and reach test does not possess criterion-related validity as a field test for hamstring and low back flexibility."

Included in Chapter 1 is information defining composite tests (tests that measure more than one motion or muscle) and a rationale for avoiding these types of tests when examining muscle length. Given that the sit and reach test is influenced by so many factors, including muscle length of the upper and lower extremities and range of motion of the spine, a detailed description of this technique is not included in this chapter.

TESTS FOR MUSCLE LENGTH: ILIOTIBIAL BAND AND TENSOR FASCIAE LATAE

Description of Tests

In 1935, Ober[18] described a test to examine the relationship between tightness in the tensor fasciae latae and iliotibial band and low back pain and sciatica. The test, known today as the Ober test, originally was used to examine the length of the iliotibial band and of the tensor fasciae latae in individuals with low back pain, but it now is used to examine muscle length in all individuals. In addition, use of the Ober test on patients with anterior knee pain and iliotibial band friction syndrome also has been documented.[2, 3, 9]

In 1952, Kendall et al.[14] presented a modification of the original Ober test, suggesting that the examiner should keep the knee extended in the extremity to be tested (as opposed to flexing the knee to 90 degrees as originally described by Ober) while performing the examination. Referred to as the Modified Ober, the following reasons have been offered for modifying the original Ober test: less stress to the medial knee joint, less tension on the patella, less potential interference by a tight rectus femoris muscle,[13] and a more functional test position.[17] Based on a review of the literature, the Ober test and the Modified Ober test appear to be used with equal frequency; neither test has been shown to be more popular, more accurate, or easier to perform than the other.

Expressing concern that the Ober test was too difficult to be used "satisfactorily," Gautam and Anand[8] suggested the use of an alternative test for examining iliotibial band and tensor fasciae latae muscle length. These authors suggested that the problem with the Ober test arose from the difficulty in maintaining the hip in 0 degrees extension while at the same time attempting to examine the amount of hip adduction. They suggested that the Ober test is, therefore, a "two-plane" test (extension, abduction). Gautam and Anand[8] proposed a "new" test for estimating iliotibial band contracture to be performed with the patient prone, thus eliminating the need to control hip extension. In this way, the two-plane Ober test is converted into a one-plane test of abduction. This "new test" for iliotibial band and tensor fasciae latae length is referred to in this text as the prone technique.

Quantification

The methods of quantifying the results of the Ober test and of the modifications of the Ober test range from observation[5, 10, 18] to use of the goniometer,[19, 21] the tape measure,[2] and the inclinometer.[17]

Ober[18] relied on observation to quantify the results, stating that "if there is no contracture present, the thigh will adduct beyond the median line." Hoppenfeld[10] suggested that when the Ober test is performed, if the iliotibial tract is "normal," the thigh should drop to the adducted position, and if "contracture" is present in the tensor fasciae latae or the iliotibial band, the thigh remains abducted. Gose and Schweizer[5] presented a slightly more sophisticated classification system, describing the position of the lower extremity relative to the horizontal body plane.

> If the leg can be passively stretched to a position horizontal but not completely adducted to the table, it constitutes "minimal" tightness, especially in the proximal fascia. If the leg can be passively adducted to horizontal at best, it constitutes "moderate" tightness of the iliotibial band and proximal fascia. . . . If the leg cannot passively be adducted to horizontal, this constitutes a maximal contracture of the iliotibial band throughout its expanse.

Reid et al.[21] suggested the use of a goniometer to quantify length of the iliotibial band and tensor fasciae latae muscles during performance of the Ober test. The axis of the goniometer was placed at the anterior superior iliac spine, the stationary arm of the goniometer was placed parallel to the support surface (horizontal), and the moving arm was aligned along the long axis of the adducting thigh, pointed toward the mid-patella. A value of 0 degrees was documented when the thigh was horizontal, positive values were recorded if the thigh was adducted past horizontal, and negative values were recorded if the thigh did not adduct to horizontal.

The use of a tape measure to quantify muscle length was described by Doucette and Goble.[2] Subjects were placed in the Ober test position, and the distance between the medial border of the patella and the support surface was measured. Melchione and Sullivan[17] described using an inclinometer placed at the distal lateral thigh of the extremity on which the Modified Ober test was performed.

TESTS FOR MUSCLE LENGTH: GASTROCNEMIUS AND SOLEUS

The key to differentiating between muscle length testing of the gastrocnemius and of the soleus muscles is to realize that because of its origin on the femur and insertion on the calcaneus, the gastrocnemius crosses two joints (the knee and the ankle joints). The soleus originates from the posterior surface of the fibula and tibia and crosses only the ankle joint as it inserts into the posterior surface of the calcaneus.

Therefore, flexing the knee during muscle length testing causes the gastrocnemius to become slack across the knee, and the amount of dorsiflexion is limited only by the soleus muscle. In testing muscle length of the gastrocnemius, the knee is extended, which elongates the muscle across the knee and the ankle.[6, 13, 23]

Iliopsoas Muscle Length: Thomas Test

Fig. 14–2. Starting position for measurement of iliopsoas muscle length using Thomas test. Bony landmarks for goniometer alignment (lateral midline of trunk, greater trochanter, lateral femoral epicondyle) indicated by orange line and dots.

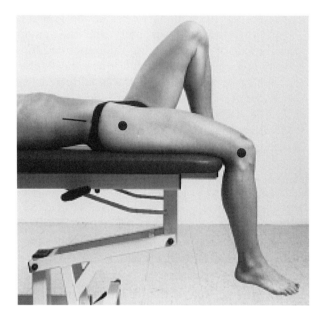

Patient position:	Supine, with hip of lower extremity to be measured extended. Buttock should be toward edge of support surface so knees extend just past the edge (Fig. 14–2).
Examiner action:	After instructing patient in motion desired, flex contralateral hip, bringing knee toward chest. Knee is allowed to flex fully. The contralateral hip should be flexed only enough to flatten lumbar spine against support surface (Fig. 14–3). (Note: Extremity *not* being flexed is extremity to be measured with goniometer and is referred to as the "tested" extremity.)
Patient action:	Patient is instructed to grasp knee to chest, only enough to flatten lumbar spine against support surface (Fig. 14–4).

Fig. 14–3. End of ROM for Thomas test. Bony landmarks for goniometer alignment (lateral midline of trunk, greater trochanter, lateral femoral epicondyle) indicated by orange line and dots.

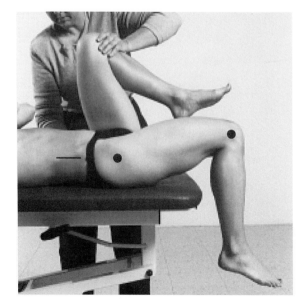

Fig. 14–4. Patient position for measurement of iliopsoas muscle length using Thomas test. Bony landmarks for goniometer alignment (lateral midline of trunk, greater trochanter, lateral femoral epicondyle) indicated by orange line and dots.

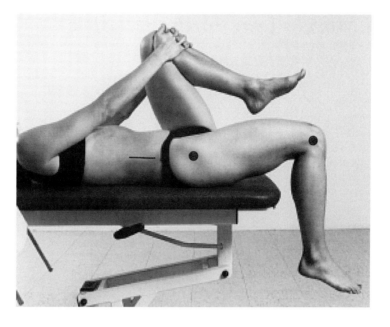

Goniometer alignment:	Palpate following bony landmarks on tested lower extremity (shown in Fig. 14–2) and align goniometer accordingly (Fig. 14–5).
Stationary arm:	Lateral midline of trunk.
Axis:	Greater trochanter of femur.
Moving arm:	Lateral epicondyle of femur.

If muscle length of iliopsoas is within normal limits, thigh of lower extremity being measured remains on examining table. No measurement is needed. If decreased muscle length of iliopsoas is present, patient's thigh being measured will rise off examining table. Maintaining proper goniometer alignment, read scale of goniometer for amount of hip flexion (Fig. 14–5). (Note: If flexion of contralateral lower extremity to chest causes tested extremity to abduct rather than lift off support surface, patient may have tight iliotibial band.)

Documentation:	Record amount of hip flexion in tested extremity.
Precaution:	Contralateral hip should be flexed by patient only enough to flatten lumbar spine against support surface. Pulling hip to chest and allowing inappropriate rotation of pelvis causes inaccurate measurement and should be avoided.

Fig. 14–5. Goniometer alignment at hip to examine iliopsoas muscle length using Thomas test.

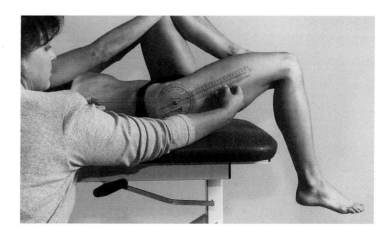

Iliopsoas Muscle Length: Prone Hip Extension Test

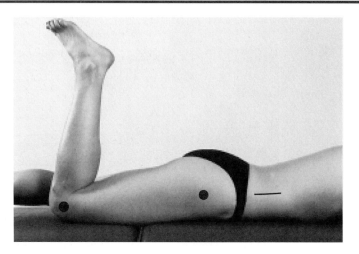

Fig. 14–6. Starting position for measurement of iliopsoas muscle length using prone extension test. Bony landmarks for goniometer alignment (lateral midline of trunk, greater trochanter, lateral femoral epicondyle) indicated by orange line and dots.

An assistant is needed to perform this measurement correctly.

Patient position:	Prone; knee flexed to 90 degrees (Fig. 14–6).
Examiner action (Examiner #1):	After instructing the patient in motion desired, stabilize pelvis by placing one hand on ipsilateral side. With other hand, extend patient's hip maximally (indicated by pelvis beginning to rise), keeping knee flexed to 90 degrees (Fig. 14–7).

Fig. 14–7. End of ROM for prone extension test. Bony landmarks for goniometer alignment (lateral midline of trunk, greater trochanter, lateral femoral epicondyle) indicated by orange line and dot.

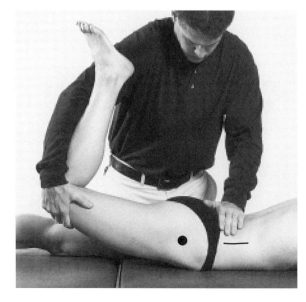

Fig. 14–8. Goniometer alignment to examine iliopsoas muscle length using prone extension test.

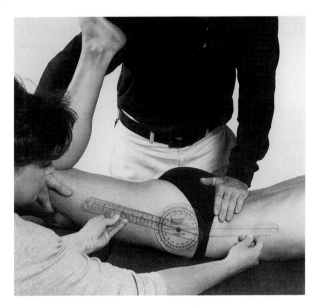

Goniometer alignment (Examiner #2):	Examiner #2 palpates following bony landmarks (shown in Fig. 14–6) and aligns goniometer accordingly (Fig. 14–8).
Stationary arm:	Lateral midline of trunk.
Axis:	Greater trochanter of femur.
Moving arm:	Lateral epicondyle of femur.

Maintaining goniometer alignment, Examiner #2 reads scale of goniometer (Fig. 14–8).

Documentation: Record patient's hip extension measurement.

Rectus Femoris Muscle Length: Thomas Test

Fig. 14–9. Starting position for measurement of rectus femoris muscle length using Thomas test. Bony landmarks for goniometer alignment (greater trochanter, lateral femoral epicondyle, lateral malleolus) indicated by orange dots.

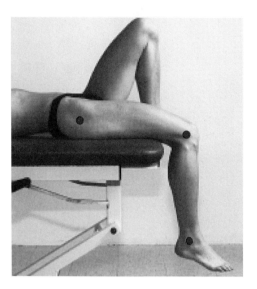

Patient position:	Supine, with hip of lower extremity to be measured extended. Buttock should be toward edge of support surface so knees extend just past the edge (Fig. 14–9).
Examiner action:	After instructing patient in motion desired, flex contralateral hip, bringing knee toward chest. Knee is allowed to flex fully. The contralateral hip should be flexed only enough to flatten lumbar spine against support surface (Fig. 14–10). (Note: Extremity *not* being flexed is extremity to be measured with the goniometer and is referred to as the "tested" extremity.)
Patient action:	Patient is instructed to grasp knee to chest, only enough to flatten lumbar spine against support surface (Fig. 14–11).

Fig. 14–10. End of ROM for Thomas test. Bony landmarks for goniometer alignment (lateral midline of trunk, greater trochanter, lateral femoral epicondyle) indicated by orange dots.

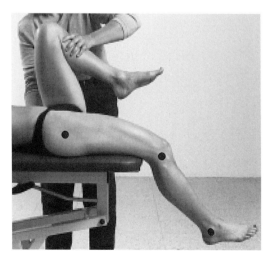

Fig. 14–11. Patient position for measurement of rectus femoris muscle length using Thomas test. Bony landmarks for goniometer alignment (lateral midline of trunk, greater trochanter, lateral femoral epicondyle) indicated by orange dots.

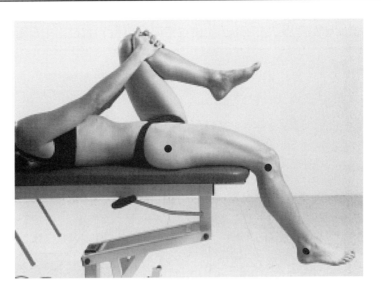

Goniometer alignment: Palpate following bony landmarks on tested lower extremity (shown in Fig. 14–9) and align goniometer accordingly (Fig. 14–12).

Stationary arm: Greater trochanter of femur.
Axis: Lateral epicondyle of femur.
Moving arm: Lateral malleolus.

If muscle length of rectus femoris is within normal limits, knee being measured remains at 90 degrees of flexion. No measurement is needed. If decreased muscle length of rectus femoris is present, patient's knee being measured will extend slightly. Maintaining proper goniometer alignment, read scale of goniometer for amount of knee flexion (Fig. 14–12).

Documentation: Record knee flexion in tested extremity.

Precaution: Contralateral hip should be flexed by patient only enough to flatten lumbar spine against support surface. Pulling hip to chest and allowing inappropriate rotation of pelvis causes inaccurate measurement and should be avoided.

Fig. 14–12. Goniometer alignment at knee to examine rectus femoris muscle length using Thomas test.

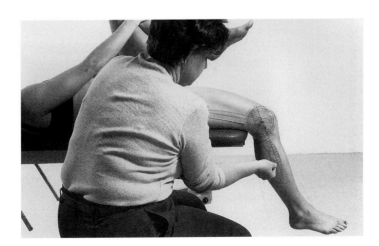

Rectus Femoris Muscle Length: Prone Technique

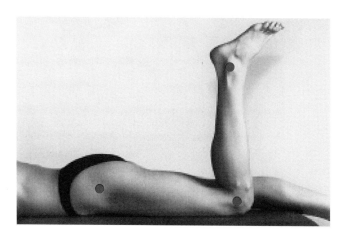

Fig. 14–13. Starting position for measurement of rectus femoris muscle length using prone technique. Bony landmarks for goniometer alignment (greater trochanter, lateral femoral epicondyle, lateral malleolus) indicated by orange dots.

Patient position:	Prone; knee flexed to 90 degrees (Fig. 14–13).
Examiner action:	After instructing patient in motion desired, flex patient's knee through full available ROM while maintaining the ipsilateral hip in full extension (Fig. 14–14).

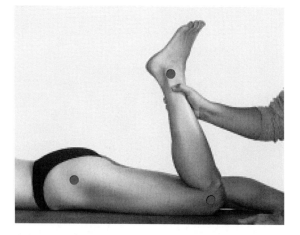

Fig. 14–14. End of ROM for rectus femoris muscle length test using prone technique. Bony landmarks for goniometer alignment (greater trochanter, lateral femoral epicondyle, lateral malleolus) indicated by orange dots.

Fig. 14–15. Patient position and goniometer alignment to examine rectus femoris muscle length using prone technique.

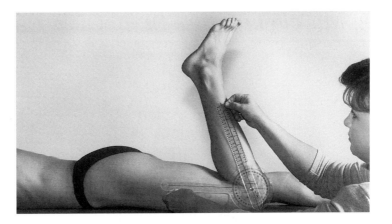

Goniometer alignment:	Palpate following bony landmarks (shown in Fig. 14–13) and align goniometer accordingly (Fig. 14–15).
Stationary arm:	Greater trochanter of femur.
Axis:	Lateral epicondyle of femur.
Moving arm:	Lateral malleolus.

Maintaining proper goniometer alignment, read scale of goniometer (Fig. 14–15).

Documentation: Record patient's maximum amount of knee flexion.

Note: The point at which the ipsilateral hip begins to flex during knee flexion marks the limit of rectus femoris muscle length. No further knee flexion should be attempted, and goniometric measurement of knee flexion should occur at that point. Figure 14–16 illustrates inaccurate positioning for measurement due to hip flexion of ipsilateral limb.

Fig. 14–16. Inaccurate positioning during prone technique allowing flexion of ipsilateral hip.

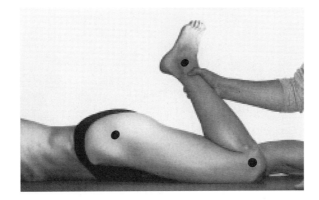

Hamstring Muscle Length: Straight Leg Raise Test

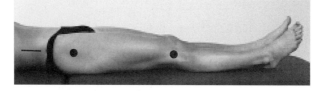

Fig. 14–17. Starting position for measurement of hamstring muscle length using straight leg raise. Bony landmarks for goniometer alignment (lateral midline of trunk, greater trochanter, lateral femoral epicondyle) indicated by orange line and dots.

An assistant is needed to perform this measurement correctly.

Patient position:

Supine, with hip and knee extended (Fig. 14–17).

Examiner action (Examiner #1):

After instructing patient in motion desired, flex patient's hip through full available ROM, while maintaining knee in full extension. One hand is placed over anterior thigh to ensure knee is maintained in full extension during movement, and hip is flexed until firm muscular resistance to further motion is felt (Fig. 14–18).

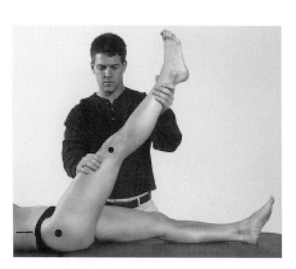

Fig. 14–18. End of ROM for straight leg raise test. Bony landmarks for goniometer alignment (lateral midline of trunk, greater trochanter, lateral femoral epicondyle) indicated by orange line and dots.

Fig. 14–19. Patient position and goniometer alignment at the end of straight leg raise test.

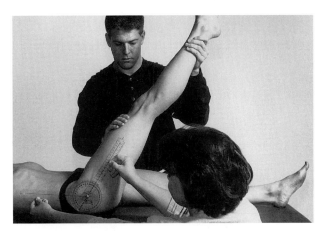

Goniometer alignment (Examiner #2):	Examiner #2 palpates following bony landmarks (shown in Fig. 14–17) and aligns goniometer accordingly (Fig. 14–19).
Stationary arm:	Lateral midline of trunk.
Axis:	Greater trochanter of femur.
Moving arm:	Lateral epicondyle of femur.

Maintaining proper goniometer alignment, Examiner #2 reads scale of goniometer (Fig. 14–19).

Documentation: Record patient's maximum amount of hip flexion.

Precaution: Contralateral lower extremity should be maintained on support surface with knee fully extended to avoid inaccurate measurement due to pelvic motion. Figure 14–20 illustrates inaccurate positioning for measurement due to hip flexion of contralateral limb.

Fig. 14–20. Incorrect positioning during the straight leg raise test allowing hip and knee flexion of contralateral extremity.

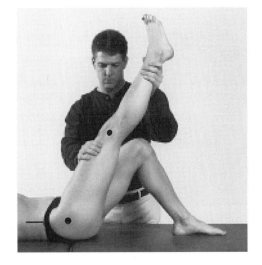

Hamstring Muscle Length: Knee Extension Test

Fig. 14–21. Starting position for measurement of hamstring muscle length using knee extension test. Bony landmarks for goniometer alignment (greater trochanter, lateral femoral epicondyle, lateral malleolus) indicated by orange dots.

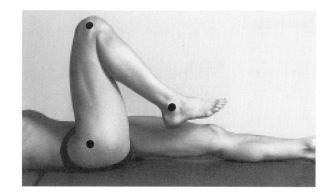

An assistant is needed to perform Option #2 of this measurement correctly.

Patient position: Supine, with hip flexed to 90 degrees. Contralateral lower extremity should be placed on support surface with knee fully extended. It is imperative that contralateral lower extremity be maintained in this position throughout testing (Fig. 14–21).

Examiner action: After instructing patient in motion desired, extend patient's knee through full available ROM while maintaining hip in 90 degrees of flexion. This passive movement allows an estimate of ROM available and demonstrates to patient exact movement desired (Fig. 14–22).

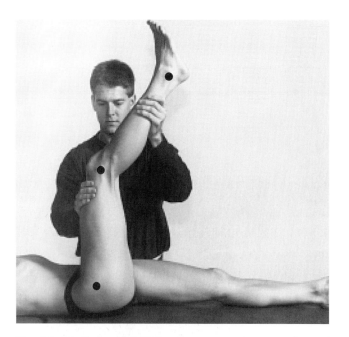

Fig. 14–22. End of ROM for knee extension test. Bony landmarks for goniometer alignment (greater trochanter, lateral femoral epicondyle, lateral malleolus) indicated by orange dots.

Fig. 14–23. Patient position and goniometer alignment at the end of *active* knee extension test.

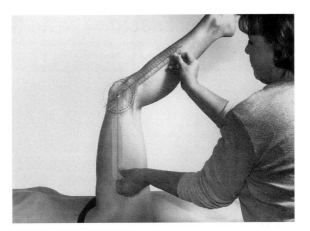

Patient/Examiner action:	**Option #1 (Fig. 14–23)**—Have patient perform active extension of knee until myoclonus is observed in hamstring muscles.
	Option #2 (Fig. 14–24)—Examiner #1 passively extends knee until firm muscular resistance to further motion is felt.
Goniometer alignment:	Palpate following bony landmarks (shown in Fig. 14–21) and align goniometer accordingly (see Figs. 14–23 and 14–24).
Stationary arm:	Greater trochanter of femur.
Axis:	Lateral epicondyle of femur.
Moving arm:	Lateral malleolus.
	Maintaining proper goniometer alignment, read scale of goniometer (see Figs. 14–23 and 14–24). For Option #2, a second examiner is needed to align goniometer and read scale.
Documentation:	Record patient's maximum amount of knee extension and which option was used.
Precaution:	Contralateral lower extremity should be maintained on support surface with knee fully extended to avoid inaccurate measurement due to pelvic motion.

Fig. 14–24. Patient position and goniometer alignment at the end of *passive* knee extension test.

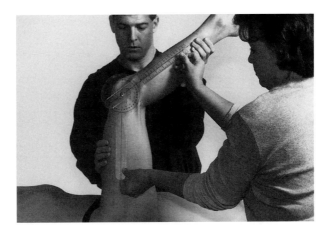

Iliotibial Band and Tensor Fasciae Latae Muscle Length: Ober Test and Modified Ober Test

Fig. 14–25. Starting position for measurement of iliotibial band and tensor fasciae latae muscle length using Ober test.

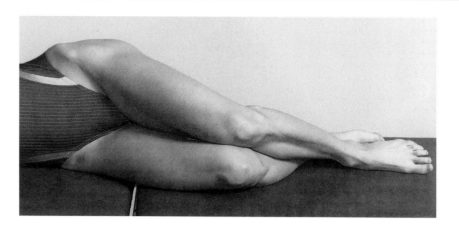

Patient position: Sidelying, with hip and knee of lowermost extremity flexed to 45 degrees to stabilize pelvis (Fig. 14–25).

Examiner action: After instructing patient in movement required, examiner places one hand on ipsilateral pelvis to stabilize it and maintain neutral pelvic alignment. Examiner uses other hand to, first, passively abduct hip and, second, extend patient's hip on upper side in line with trunk, thereby, bringing tensor fasciae latae over greater trochanter (see Figs. 14–26 and 14–27).

Patient/Examiner action: Examiner asks patient to relax muscles of lower extremity while allowing uppermost limb to drop into adduction toward table through available ROM. As limb drops toward table, examiner prevents flexion and internal rotation of hip. If hip is allowed to internally rotate and flex, tensor fasciae latae and iliotibial band are no longer in lengthened position and are not accurately tested (see Figs. 14–26 and 14–27).

Fig. 14–26. Position for performing Ober test.

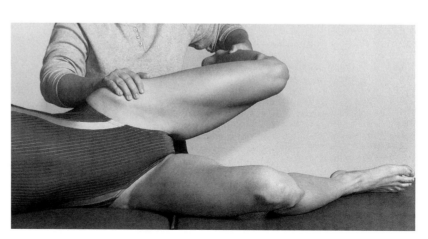

Fig. 14–27. Patient position when performing Modified Ober test.

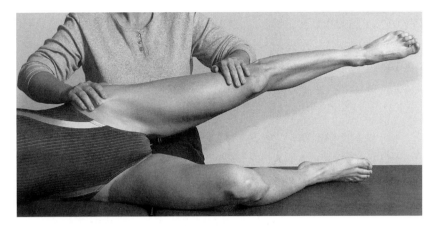

Ober Test—During performance of test, examiner maintains patient's knee in 90 degrees of flexion (Fig. 14–26).

Modified Ober Test—During performance of test, examiner maintains patient's knee in full extension (Fig. 14–27).

Measurement: Review of literature yields very few reports of using goniometers, tape measures, or any other device for measurement when performing Ober and Modified Ober tests. Traditionally, this test is performed in an "all or none" fashion. Test is either positive and patient has tight tensor fasciae latae and iliotibial band, or test is negative and patient has ideal muscle length.

Positive test: For both Ober and Modified Ober, test is considered positive for tight tensor fasciae latae and iliotibial band if relaxed hip remains abducted and does not fall below horizontal. Test is considered negative for tight tensor fasciae latae and iliotibial band if relaxed and extended hip falls below horizontal.

Precaution: Extremity being measured should not be allowed to flex and internally rotate at the hip. Figure 14–28 illustrates incorrect positioning for Ober test.

Fig. 14–28. Incorrect patient positioning for performing Ober test allowing flexion and internal rotation of the hip being tested.

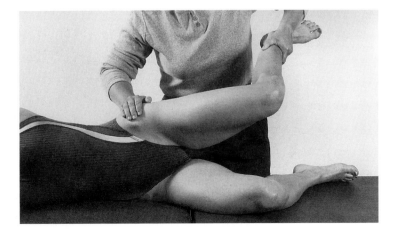

Iliotibial Band and Tensor Fasciae Latae Muscle Length: Prone Technique

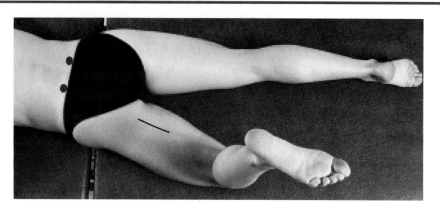

Fig. 14–29. Starting position for measurement of iliotibial band and tensor fasciae latae muscle length using the prone technique. Bony landmarks for goniometer alignment (contralateral PSIS, ipsilateral PSIS, posterior midline of ipsilateral femur) indicated by orange line and dots..

Patient position:	Prone; hip abducted and knee flexed to 90 degrees (Fig. 14–29).
Examiner action:	After instructing patient in movement required, examiner stabilizes pelvis with one hand, and adducts hip (maintaining 90-degree knee flexion) until movement of the pelvis is palpated. End point is defined as point at which initial pelvic movement is detected (Fig. 14–30).

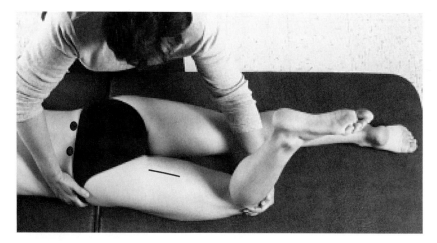

Fig. 14–30. End of ROM for prone technique for measurement of iliotibial band and tensor fasciae latae muscle length. Bony landmarks for goniometer alignment (contralateral PSIS, ipsilateral PSIS, posterior midline of ipsilateral femur) indicated by orange line and dots.

Fig. 14-31. Goniometer alignment to examine iliotibial band and tensor fasciae latae muscle length using prone technique.

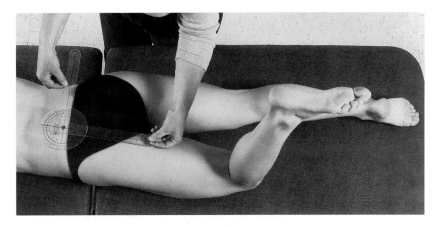

Goniometer alignment:	Palpate following bony landmarks (shown in Fig. 14–29) and align goniometer accordingly (Fig. 14–31).
Stationary arm:	Contralateral posterior superior iliac spine (PSIS).
Axis:	Ipsilateral PSIS.
Moving arm:	Posterior midline of ipsilateral femur.
	Maintaining goniometer alignment, read scale of goniometer (Fig. 14–31).
Documentation:	Record patient's hip abduction/adduction measurement.

Gastrocnemius Muscle Length Test

Fig. 14–32. Starting position for measurement of gastrocnemius muscle length. Bony landmarks for goniometer alignment (fibular head, lateral malleolus, parallel to fifth metatarsal) indicated by orange line and dots.

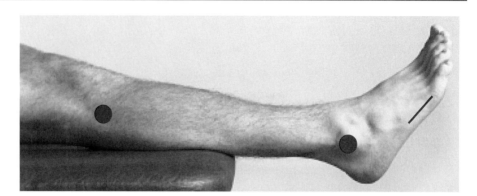

Patient position:	Supine, with hip and knee extended (Fig. 14–32).
Examiner action:	After instructing patient in motion desired, dorsiflex patient's ankle through full available ROM while maintaining knee in full extension. This passive movement allows an estimate of ROM available and demonstrates to patient exact movement desired (Fig. 14–33).
Patient/Examiner action:	Maintaining full knee extension, perform passive, or have patient perform active, dorsiflexion of ankle (Fig. 14–33).
Goniometer alignment:	Palpate following bony landmarks (shown in Fig. 14–32) and align goniometer accordingly (Fig. 14–34).
Stationary arm:	Head of fibula.
Axis:	Lateral malleolus.
Moving arm:	Parallel to fifth metatarsal.
	Maintaining proper goniometer alignment, read scale of goniometer (Fig. 14–34).

Fig. 14–33. End of ROM for gastrocnemius muscle length test. Bony landmarks for goniometer alignment (fibular head, lateral malleolus, parallel to fifth metatarsal) indicated by orange dots.

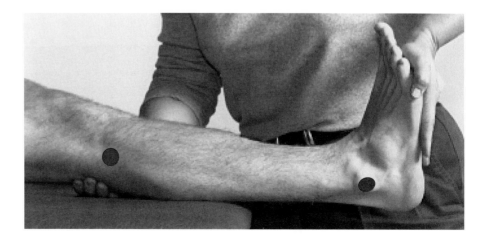

Fig. 14-34. Patient position and goniometer alignment at the end of gastrocnemius muscle length test.

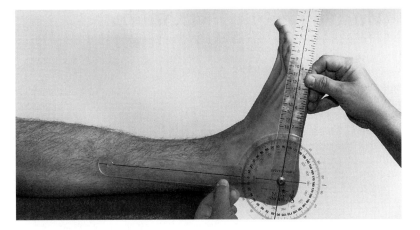

Documentation: Record patient's maximum amount of dorsiflexion.

Precaution: Examiner must ensure that knee remains in full extension during dorsiflexion movement.

Note: A suggested procedure for measuring dorsiflexion involves maintaining the subtalar joint in neutral position while dorsiflexing the patient's ankle. It is thought that in this way pronation and supination are avoided and pure dorsiflexion is measured. The procedure for maintaining neutral position of subtalar joint is described in Chapter 13 (see Fig. 13–10).

Soleus Muscle Length Test: Supine

Fig. 14–35. Starting position for measurement of soleus muscle length with patient supine. Bony landmarks for goniometer alignment (fibular head, lateral malleolus, parallel to fifth metatarsal) indicated by orange line and dots.

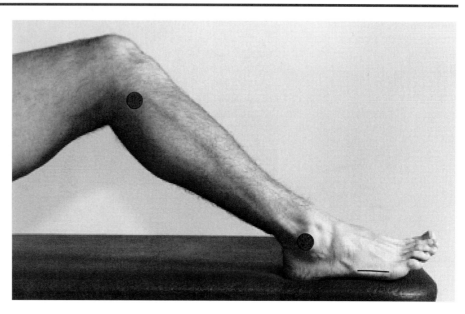

Patient position: Supine, with hip and knee flexed to 45 degrees. Placing knee in flexion relaxes gastrocnemius muscle and allows measurement of soleus muscle. Opposite lower extremity should be placed on support surface with knee fully extended (Fig. 14–35).

Examiner action: After instructing patient in motion desired, dorsiflex patient's ankle through full available ROM while maintaining hip and knee in 45 degrees of flexion. This passive movement allows an estimate of ROM available and demonstrates to patient exact movement desired (Fig. 14–36).

Patient/Examiner action: Maintaining hip and knee in 45 degrees of flexion, perform passive, or have patient perform active, dorsiflexion of ankle (Fig. 14–36).

Fig. 14–36. End of ROM for soleus muscle length test—supine. Bony landmarks for goniometer alignment (fibular head, lateral malleolus, parallel to fifth metatarsal) indicated by orange line and dots.

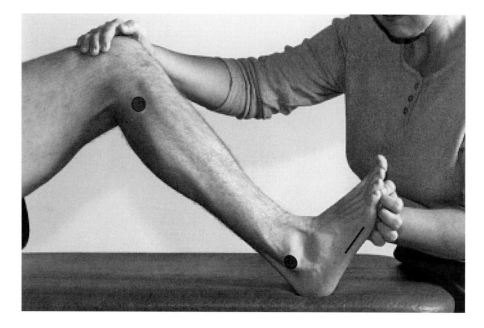

Fig. 14–37. Patient position and goniometer alignment at the end of soleus muscle length test—supine

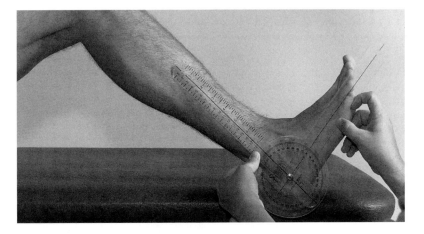

Goniometer alignment:	Palpate following bony landmarks (shown in Fig. 14–35) and align goniometer accordingly (Fig. 14–37).
Stationary arm:	Head of fibula.
Axis:	Lateral malleolus.
Moving arm:	Parallel to fifth metatarsal.

Maintaining proper goniometer alignment, read scale of goniometer (Fig. 14–37).

Documentation:	Record patient's maximum amount of dorsiflexion.

Note:	A suggested procedure for measuring dorsiflexion involves maintaining the subtalar joint in neutral position while dorsiflexing the patient's ankle. It is thought that in this way pronation and supination are avoided and pure dorsiflexion is measured. The procedure for maintaining neutral position of subtalar joint is described in Chapter 13 (see Fig. 13–10).

Soleus Muscle Length Test: Prone

Fig. 14–38. Starting position for measurement of soleus muscle length with patient prone. Bony landmarks for goniometer alignment (fibular head, lateral malleolus, parallel to fifth metatarsal) indicated by orange line and dots.

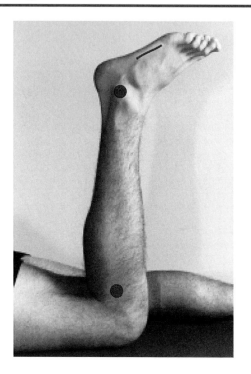

Patient position: Prone, with knee flexed to 90 degrees. Placing knee in flexion relaxes gastrocnemius muscle and allows measurement of soleus muscle. Opposite lower extremity should be placed on support surface with knee fully extended (Fig. 14–38).

Examiner action: After instructing patient in motion desired, dorsiflex patient's ankle through full available ROM while maintaining knee in 90 degrees of flexion. This passive movement allows an estimate of ROM available and demonstrates to patient exact movement desired (Fig. 14–39).

Fig. 14–39. End of ROM for soleus muscle length— prone. Bony landmarks for goniometer alignment (fibular head, lateral malleolus, parallel to fifth metatarsal) indicated by orange line and dots.

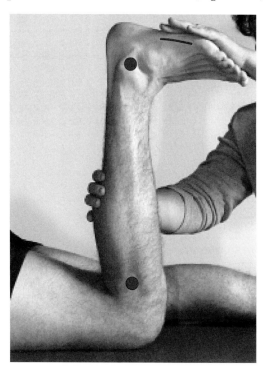

Fig. 14–40. Patient position and goniometer alignment at the end of soleus muscle length test—prone.

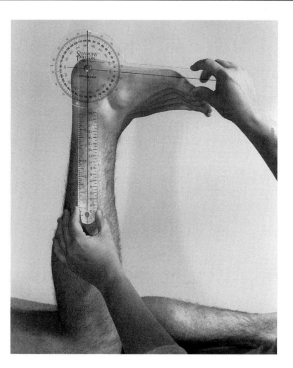

Patient/Examiner action:	Maintaining hip and knee in 90 degrees of flexion, perform passive, or have patient perform active, dorsiflexion of ankle (Fig. 14–39).
Goniometer alignment:	Palpate following bony landmarks (shown in Fig. 14–38) and align goniometer accordingly (Fig. 14–40).
Stationary arm:	Head of fibula.
Axis:	Lateral malleolus.
Moving arm:	Parallel to fifth metatarsal.
	Maintaining proper goniometer alignment, read scale of goniometer (Fig. 14–40).
Documentation:	Record patient's maximum amount of dorsiflexion.
Note:	A suggested procedure for measuring dorsiflexion involves maintaining the subtalar joint in neutral position while dorsiflexing the patient's ankle. It is thought that in this way pronation and supination are avoided and pure dorsiflexion is measured. The procedure for maintaining neutral position of subtalar joint is described in Chapter 13 (see Fig. 13–10).

References

1. Cornbleet SL, Woolsey NB: Assessment of hamstring muscle length in school-aged children using the sit-and-reach test and the inclinometer measure of hip joint angle. Phys Ther 1996;76:850–855.
2. Doucette SA, Goble EM: The effect of exercise on patellar tracking in lateral patellar compression syndrome. Am J Sports Med 1992;20:434–440.
3. Ekman EF, Pope T, Martin DF, et al.: Magnetic resonance imaging of iliotibial band syndrome. Am J Sports Med 1994;22:851–854.
4. Gajdosik RL, Rieck MA, Sullivan DK, et al.: Comparison of four clinical tests for assessing hamstring muscle length. J Orthop Sports Phys Ther 1993;18:614–618.
5. Gose JC, Schweizer P: Iliotibial band tightness. J Orthop Sports Phys Ther 1989;10:399–407.
6. Grady JF, Saxena A: Effects of stretching the gastrocnemius muscle. J Foot Surg 1991;30:465–469.
7. Greene WB, Heckman JD: The Clinical Measurement of Joint Motion. Rosemont, Ill, American Academy of Orthopaedic Surgeons, 1994.
8. Gautam VK, Anand S: A new test for estimating iliotibial band contracture. J Bone Joint Surg Br 1998;80:474–475.
9. Hilyard A: Recent developments in the management of patellofemoral pain: The McConnell programme. Physiotherapy 1990;76:559–565.
10. Hoppenfeld S: Physical Examination of the Spine and Extremities. Norwalk, Conn, Appleton & Lange, 1976.
11. Jackson A, Langford NJ: The criterion-related validity of the sit-and-reach test: Replication and extension of previous findings. Res Q Exerc Sport 1989;60:384–387.
12. Katz K, Rosenthal A, Yosipovitch Z: Normal ranges of popliteal angle in children. J Pediatr Orthop 1992;12:229–231.
13. Kendall FP, McCreary EK: Muscles: Testing and Function, 4th ed. Baltimore, Williams & Wilkins, 1994.
14. Kendall HO, Kendall FP, Boynton DA: Posture and Pain. Baltimore, Williams & Wilkins, 1952.
15. Lee LW, Kerrigan C, Croce UD: Dynamic implications of hip flexion contractures. Am J Phys Med Rehabil 1997;76:502–508.
16. Magee, DJ: Orthopedic Physical Assessment, 3rd ed. Philadelphia, WB Saunders, 1997.
17. Melchione WE, Sullivan MS: Reliability of measurements obtained by use of an instrument designed to indirectly measure iliotibial band length. J Orthop Sports Phys Ther 1993;18:511–515.
18. Ober FR: Back strain and sciatica. JAMA 1935;104:1580–1581.
19. Pandya S, Florence JM, King WM, et al.: Reliability of goniometric measurements in patients with Duchenne muscular dystrophy. Phys Ther 1985;65:1339–1342.
20. Reade E, Hom L, Hallum A, et al.: Changes in popliteal angle measurement in infants up to one year of age. Dev Med Child Neurol 1984;26:774–780.
21. Reid DC, Burnham RS, Saboe LA, et al.: Lower extremity flexibility patterns in classical ballet dancers and their correlation to lateral hip and knee injuries. Am J Sports Med 1987;15:347–352.
22. Shephard RJ, Berridge M, Montelpare W: On the generality of the "sit and reach" test: An analysis of flexibility data for an aging population. Res Q Exerc Sport 1990;61:326–330.
23. Wang SS, Whitney SL, Burdett RG, Janosky JE: Lower extremity muscular flexibility in long distance runners. J Orthop Sports Phys Ther 1993;17:102–107.

15

RELIABILITY and VALIDITY of MEASUREMENTS of RANGE of MOTION and MUSCLE LENGTH TESTING of the LOWER EXTREMITY

RELIABILITY AND VALIDITY OF LOWER EXTREMITY GONIOMETRY

Chapters 11 through 14 presented techniques for measuring range of motion of joints and length of muscles in the lower extremities. When selecting appropriate techniques for measuring range of motion and muscle length, one must consider whether the technique selected has been shown to be reliable and valid.[11] This chapter presents information regarding the reliability and validity (when available) of techniques for measuring lower extremity range of motion and muscle length. In accordance with the discussion of the preferred methods of analyzing reliability presented in Chapter 2, only those studies that examined reliability using the intraclass correlation coefficient (ICC), or Pearson product moment correlation coefficient (Pearson's r) with a follow-up test are included.

As is apparent from the information and tables that follow, seldom is one method of goniometry or muscle length testing shown to be clearly preferable in terms of reliability as demonstrated by more than one investigator. In fact, many studies are so vaguely described as to be unrepeatable by others, and studies that are repeated in some form often produce conflicting results. Therefore, unless obvious conclusions can be made regarding the efficacy of one technique over another, no interpretive comments are made regarding the information presented in this chapter. Rather, the chapter serves as a reference to the reader and, it is hoped, makes obvious the areas of research in lower extremity goniometry and muscle length testing that have yet to be addressed.

Hip Flexion/Extension

Several studies that examine the reliability of hip flexion and extension range of motion have been published. Using a combination of the Thomas and Mundale techniques (see Chapters 11 and 14 for a description of the Mundale and Thomas techniques), Stuberg and colleagues[33] measured the reliability of measurements of passive hip flexion with the knee extended (straight leg raise) and passive hip extension in 20 children, aged 5 to 21 years, with moderate to severe hypertonicity. To examine inter-rater reliability, three pediatric physical therapists repeated each of the measurements three times on each child in one testing session, using a blinded goniometer. The measurements were repeated 5 to 7 days later on five of the subjects to determine intrarater reliability. A two-way analysis of variance (ANOVA) for repeated measures was used to determine intrarater and inter-rater reliability for each motion. Analysis of intrarater reliability showed no significant difference between the three measures taken by a single examiner in one session, and intrarater error was calculated at less than or equal to 5 degrees for the majority of measurements, based on the 95% confidence interval. Conversely, significant inter-rater variation was found for both hip flexion and extension measurements.

Active hip flexion and extension, along with 26 other motions of the upper and lower extremities, were measured in 60 adults, aged 60 to 84 years, by Walker and colleagues.[35] Techniques recommended by the American Academy of Orthopaedic Surgeons (AAOS)[2] were used for all measurements. Prior to data collection, intrarater reliability was determined using four subjects. Although the exact number of motions measured to determine reliability is unclear from the procedure, the authors reported a Pearson's r for intrarater reliability greater than .81 for all hip motions (Table 15–1). Mean error between measurements was calculated to be 5 degrees ±1 degree.

In a study designed to compare reliability of the Orthoranger (an electronic, computerized goniometer) and the universal goniometer, Clapper and Wolf[9] examined intrarater reliability of active hip flexion and extension goniometry, in addition to eight other motions of the lower extremities. Twenty healthy adults were included in the examination of reliability. The specific technique for measuring hip flexion and extension was not delineated in the article, so comparison to other studies is difficult. Intraclass correlation coefficients (ICC) reported for hip flexion and extension were .95 and .83, respectively (see Table 15–1).

Two additional studies examined the reliability of measuring the range of motion of hip extension but not of hip flexion. Both of these studies focused

Table 15–1. INTRARATER RELIABILITY: HIP FLEXION/EXTENSION RANGE OF MOTION

HIP FLEXION

Study	Technique	n	Sample	r*	ICC†
Walker et al.[35]	AAOS	4	Healthy adults (ages not provided)	>.81	
Clapper & Wolf[9]	Unknown	20	Healthy adults 10 females—mean age 28.3 yr 10 males—mean age 30.0 yr	.75	.95

HIP EXTENSION

Study	Technique	n	Sample	r	ICC
Bartlett et al.[5]	AAOS (contralateral hip flexed)	14	Myelomeningocele (4–19 yr)	.93	
		14	Spastic diplegia (6–20 yr)	.82	
Bartlett et al.[5]	Mundale	14	Myelomeningocele (4–19 yr)	.91	
		14	Spastic diplegia (6–20 yr)	.63	
Bartlett et al.[5]	Pelvifemoral angle	14	Myelomeningocele (4–19 yr)	.92	
		14	Spastic diplegia (6–20 yr)	.78	
Bartlett et al.[5]	Thomas test	14	Myelomeningocele (4–19 yr)	.93	
		14	Spastic diplegia (6–20 yr)	.89	
Clapper & Wolf[9]	Unknown	20	Healthy adults 10 females—mean age 28.3 yr 10 males—mean age 30.0 yr		.83
Pandya et al.[27]	Thomas test	150	Duchenne's muscular dystrophy (<1–20 yr)		.85
Walker et al.[35]	AAOS	4	Healthy adults (ages not provided)	>.81	

* Pearson's r
† Intraclass correlation
AAOS, American Academy of Orthopaedic Surgeons

Table 15–2. INTER-RATER RELIABILITY: HIP FLEXION/EXTENSION RANGE OF MOTION

HIP FLEXION

Study	Technique	*n*	Sample	*r**	ICC[†]
Ahlback & Lindahl[1]	Pelvifemoral angle	20	Healthy adults (ages not provided)		.56
Ahlback & Lindahl[1]	AAOS (contralateral hip flexed)	20	Healthy adults (ages not provided)		.74

HIP EXTENSION

Study	Technique	*n*	Sample	*r*	ICC
Ahlback & Lindahl[1]	Pelvifemoral angle	20	Healthy adults (ages not provided)		.55
Bartlett et al.[5]	AAOS (contralateral hip flexed)	14	Myelomeningocele (4–19 yr)	.92	
		14	Spastic diplegia (6–20 yr)	.80	
Bartlett et al.[5]	Mundale	14	Myelomeningocele (4–19 yr)	.79	
		14	Spastic diplegia (6–20 yr)	.84	
Bartlett et al.[5]	Pelvifemoral angle	14	Myelomeningocele (4–19 yr)	.73	
		14	Spastic diplegia (6–20 yr)	.77	
Bartlett et al.[5]	Thomas test	14	Myelomeningocele (4–19 yr)	.90	
		14	Spastic diplegia (6–20 yr)	.70	
Drews et al.[12]	Thomas test (sidelying)	9	Healthy infants (12 hr to 6 days)	.56 (left) .74 (right)	
Pandya et al.[27]	Thomas test	21	Duchenne's muscular dystrophy (<1–20 yr)		.74

* Pearson's *r*
† Intraclass correlation
AAOS, American Academy of Orthopaedic Surgeons

on the measurement of hip extension in children who either were healthy[12] or had a diagnosis of Duchenne's muscular dystrophy.[27] The Thomas test position was used to measure hip extension in both of the studies, although investigators in the Drews et al.[12] study modified the Thomas test position by placing the infant (aged 12 hours to 6 days) in sidelying position for the measurement. Intrarater reliability was reported for only the Pandya et al.[27] study, in which 150 children, aged 1 to 20 years, were examined, and a correlation of .85 was obtained (ICC) (see Table 15–1). Both the Pandya et al.[27] and Drews et al.[12] studies examined inter-rater reliability, which was calculated on 21 and 9 subjects, respectively. Pandya et al.[27] reported an inter-rater ICC of .74 for hip extension, whereas Drews et al.[12] reported values of .56 for the left hip and .74 for the right (Pearson's *r*) (Table 15–2). The standard error of measurement (SEMm) from the Drews et al.[12] study (calculated by the author of this text from data provided) was 3.1 degrees for the right hip and 4 degrees for the left hip.

Owing to the variation in measuring techniques for hip flexion and extension, reliability of measurement of these two motions would be expected to vary, depending on the technique used. Two different groups of investigators compared reliability characteristics of different methods of measuring hip flexion or extension. Bartlett et al.[5] measured hip extension in healthy children and in children with meningomyelocele or spastic diplegia. All subjects were between the ages of 4 and 20 years. Four different positioning techniques were compared: AAOS (contralateral hip flexed), Mundale, pelvifemoral angle, and Thomas (see Chapters 11 and 14 for a description of techniques). Both intrarater and inter-rater reliability were reported using Pearson's *r*. Values for intrarater reliability ranged from .63 for the Mundale test in the group with spastic diplegia to .93 for the AAOS test in the group with meningomyelocele (see Table 15–1). Single-rater error in the group of healthy children was reported as 5 degrees when using the AAOS and Thomas techniques, and 10 degrees when using the Mundale and pelvifemoral angle techniques. Inter-rater reliability was generally lower than intrarater reliability, and correlation values ranged from .70 for the Thomas test in patients with spastic diplegia to .92 for the AAOS technique in patients with meningomyelocele (see Table 15–2). Rater error was calculated based on the 95% confidence interval for the mean difference between raters, and was reported as 10 degrees for all techniques except the Mundale (14 degrees) in children with meningomyelocele; 10 degrees for the Mundale and pelvifemoral angle techniques in healthy children, 3 degrees for the AAOS and Thomas techniques in healthy children, and 11.5 degrees and 12.2 degrees, respectively, for the AAOS and Thomas techniques in patients with spastic diplegia.

A second group of investigators[1] measured hip flexion in 20 healthy adults of unstated age using both the AAOS technique (but with the contralateral hip extended) and the pelvifemoral angle technique, and hip extension in the same 20 healthy adults using the pelvifemoral angle technique. Two examiners performed the same measurements in each subject in order to examine variability between raters (intrarater reliability was not considered). Although the investigators did not use inferential statistics to report inter-rater reliability, the raw data were reported, allowing the reader to calculate the ICCs for inter-rater reliability for each test. Intraclass correlation coefficients and the SEMm were calculated by the author of this text for each set of data (hip flexion, AAOS technique with contralateral hip extended; hip flexion, pelvifemoral angle technique; hip extension, pelvifemoral angle technique). Intraclass correlation coefficients (ICCs) were calculated using a two-way random effects model with absolute agreement. The ICCs are reported in Table 15–2 and indicate higher inter-rater reliability for measuring hip flexion when using the Thomas technique than when using the pelvifemoral angle technique in this group of examiners. Reliabilities for measuring hip extension using the pelvifemoral angle technique were similar to those obtained in measuring hip flexion using the same technique. The SEMm for hip flexion was 4.2 degrees using the pelvifemoral angle technique and 5.2 degrees using the AAOS technique with the contralateral hip extended. When hip extension was performed using the pelvifemoral angle technique, the SEMm was 1.9 degrees.

Hip Abduction/Adduction

As was true in the case of hip flexion and extension, few studies have examined the reliability of hip abduction and adduction range of motion measurements. Both intrarater and inter-rater reliability of hip abduction measurement, along with five other motions of the upper and lower extremities, was examined in a group of 12 healthy adult males aged 26 to 54 years.[7] All motions were measured in each subject three times per session by each of four different physical therapists. Values for intra- and inter-rater reliability were reported as .75 for intrarater reliability and .55 for inter-rater reliability (ICC) (Tables 15–3 and 15–4). Repeated measures analysis of variance (ANOVA) revealed significant intrarater variation for two of the four examiners, and significant inter-rater variation among all four examiners, for measurements of hip abduction.

Inter-rater reliability was examined for hip abduction and adduction measurements in a subgroup of 54 healthy infants aged 12 hours to 6 days old.[12] The subgroup consisted of 9 infants in whom passive hip abduction and adduction were measured. Abduction was measured twice, once with the hip in 0 degrees of extension, and once with the hip flexed to 90 degrees. Adduction was measured with the hip in 0 degrees of extension. Seven other motions of the lower extremities also were examined in this study (see the remainder of this chapter for other motions of the lower extremity). Specific

Table 15–3. INTRARATER RELIABILITY FOR HIP AB/ADDUCTION RANGE OF MOTION

HIP ABDUCTION

Study	Technique	n	Sample	r*	ICC[†]
Boone et al.[7]	AROM	12	Healthy males (26–54 yr)		.75
Clapper & Wolf[9]	AROM	20	Healthy adults 10 females—mean age 28.3 yr 10 males—mean age 30.0 yr		.86
Walker et al.[35]	AROM	4	Healthy adults (ages not provided)	>.81	

HIP ADDUCTION

Study	Technique	n	Sample	r	ICC
Clapper & Wolf[9]	AROM	20	Healthy adults 10 females—mean age 28.3 yr 10 males—mean age 30.0 yr		.80
Walker et al.[35]	AROM	4	Healthy adults (ages not provided)	>.81	

* Pearson's r
† Intraclass correlation
AROM, active range of motion

goniometric alignment and techniques were difficult to discern from the description of the study. Inter-rater reliabilities (Pearson's r) ranged from a high of .97 for hip abduction with the hip extended in the left lower extremity, to a low of .57 for hip abduction with the hip flexed in the same extremity (see Table 15–4). The SEMm from the Drews et al.[12] study (calculated by the author of this text from data provided) ranged from 1.7 degrees for left hip abduction with the hip extended to 6.4 degrees for left hip abduction with the hip flexed.

Other investigators who have examined reliability of hip abduction and adduction include Clapper and Wolf,[9] Stuberg et al.,[33] and Walker et al.[35] These studies have been described previously, and each used a different statistical method for reporting reliability. Two of the studies[9, 35] reported data only on intrarater reliability. Clapper and Wolf[9] reported ICC levels of .86 and .80 for hip abduction and adduction, respectively, whereas Walker et al.[35] used Pearson's r and reported values "greater than .81" for both hip abduction and hip adduction (see Table 15–3) and a mean error between repeated measures of 5 degrees. Stuberg et al.[33] examined both intrarater and inter-rater reliability for hip abduction and adduction using a two-way ANOVA for repeated measures (see the Hip Flexion/Extension Reliability section of this chapter). No significant difference was found between the three measures of hip abduction or adduction taken by a single examiner, and intrarater error was calculated at less than or equal to 5 degrees for the majority of measurements, based on the 95% confidence interval. Significant

Table 15–4. INTER-RATER RELIABILITY FOR HIP AB/ADDUCTION RANGE OF MOTION

HIP ABDUCTION

Study	Technique	n	Sample	r*	ICC[†]
Boone et al.[7]	AROM	12	Healthy males (26–54 yr)		.55
Drews et al.[12]	PROM (hip extended) (hip flexed)	9	Infants (12 hr–6 days)	 .87 (R) .97 (L) .59 (R) .57 (L)	

HIP ADDUCTION

Study	Technique	n	Sample	r
Drews et al.[12]	PROM	9	Infants (12 hr–6 days)	.62 (R) .70 (L)

* Pearson's r
† Intraclass correlation
AROM, active range of motion; PROM, passive range of motion; R, right; L, left

within-session inter-rater variation was found for hip adduction but not for abduction, although across-session inter-rater variation was significant for both measures.

Hip Medial/Lateral Rotation

Intrarater reliability of hip rotation measurements has been reported by two groups of investigators whose studies have been described previously (see the Hip Flexion/Extension and Hip Abduction/Adduction sections of this chapter).[9, 35] One of the studies indicated that goniometric measurements were performed as described by the AAOS,[35] while the second study did not describe the goniometric techniques used.[9] However, in neither of the above studies can the relative flexed or extended position of the hip be determined, as the AAOS guidelines describe techniques for measuring hip rotation with the hip flexed or extended.[2, 19] Intrarater reliability of both hip medial and lateral rotation measurements was reported as "greater than .81" by Walker et al.,[35] with a mean error between repeated measures of 5 degrees. The study by Clapper and Wolf[9] demonstrated lower reliability for hip lateral rotation measurements (.80) than for measurements of hip medial rotation (.92) (Table 15–5).

Two studies that investigated inter-rater reliability of hip rotation included detailed descriptions of patient positioning used during hip rotation measurements.[12, 31] Drews et al.,[12] whose study has been described previously (see the Hip Abduction/Adduction section), measured passive hip rotation with the hip and knee flexed to 90 degrees and the patient in the supine position. These investigators reported correlation values (Pearson's r) for inter-rater reliability of hip medial rotation as .78 on the right and .91 on the left, and for hip lateral rotation as .63 on the right and .79 on the left[12] (Table 15–6). The SEMm from the Drews et al.[12] study (calculated by the author of this text from data provided) ranged from 2.8 degrees for medial rotation of the left hip to 7.0 degrees for lateral rotation of the right hip.

Simoneau et al.[31] compared the influence of hip position and sex on active hip rotation in 60 college-age individuals. Hip medial and lateral rotation were measured in each individual by two examiners with the subject in both the seated and the prone position. Inter-rater reliabilities were calculated using ICCs and were reported to range from .90 to .94 for all measurements of

Table 15–5. INTRARATER RELIABILITY FOR HIP MEDIAL/LATERAL ROTATION RANGE OF MOTION

HIP MEDIAL ROTATION

Study	Technique	n	Sample	r*	ICC†
Clapper & Wolf[9]	AROM	20	Healthy adults 10 females—mean age 28.3 yr 10 males—mean age 30.0 yr		.92
Walker et al.[35]	AROM	4	Healthy adults (ages not provided)	>.81	

HIP LATERAL ROTATION

Study	Technique	n	Sample	r	ICC
Clapper & Wolf[9]	AROM	20	Healthy adults 10 females—mean age 28.3 yr 10 males—mean age 30.0 yr		.80
Walker et al.[35]	AROM	4	Healthy adults (ages not provided)	>.81	

Note: Patient position (prone, supine, or seated) and hip position (flexed or extended) during measurement were not described in any of the cited studies.
* Pearson's r
† Intraclass correlation
AROM, active range of motion

Table 15–6. INTER-RATER RELIABILITY FOR HIP MEDIAL/LATERAL ROTATION MEASUREMENT

HIP MEDIAL ROTATION

Study	Technique	n	Sample	r*	ICC†
Drews et al.[12]	PROM (patient supine; hip & knee flexed 90°)	9	Infants (12 hr–6 days)	.78 (R) .91 (L)	
Simoneau et al.[31]	AROM (patient prone, hip extended)	60	Healthy adults (18–27 yr)		.94
	(patient seated, hip flexed)				.91

HIP LATERAL ROTATION

Study	Technique	n	Sample	r	ICC
Drews et al.[12]	PROM (patient supine; hip & knee flexed 90°)	9	Infants (12 hr–6 days)	.63 (R) .79 (L)	
Simoneau et al.[31]	AROM (patient prone; hip extended)	60	Healthy adults (18–27 yr)		.94
	(patient seated; hip flexed)				.90

* Pearson's r
† Intraclass correlation
PROM, passive range of motion; AROM, active range of motion; R, right; L, left

hip rotation (see Table 15–6), regardless of whether the hip was flexed or extended when the measurement was taken. Calculation of the SEMm from the data provided in the Simoneau et al.[31] study revealed SEMm values between 2.1 degrees and 2.6 degrees for all measurements of hip rotation, again regardless of whether the hip was flexed or extended during the measurement.

Both intrarater and inter-rater reliability of hip rotation measurements also have been reported by a group of investigators using the inclinometer. Ellison et al.[13] examined hip rotation range of motion in a group of 100 healthy subjects, aged 20 to 41 years, and in a group of 50 patients with low back pain, aged 23 to 61 years. For the reliability study, measurements were taken on a subgroup of 22 of the healthy subjects. Each of the 22 subjects was measured for hip medial and lateral rotation by three examiners with the subject positioned in both the prone and seated positions. Measurements were taken with both the universal goniometer and with the inclinometer, but only reliability data on the inclinometer was reported in the study. Intraclass correlation coefficients were used to report reliabilities that ranged from .96 to .99 both within the same rater and between raters.

Knee Flexion/Extension

Various investigators have examined the reliability of goniometric measurement of knee flexion and extension. Intrarater reliability of active knee flexion and extension range of motion was examined by several groups,[7–9, 35] some of whose studies have been described previously (see the Hip section of this chapter). Brosseau et al.[8] compared the reliability of the universal goniometer with that of the parallelogram goniometer for measuring active knee flexion in 60 healthy college-age adults. Measurements were made with the universal goniometer using standard landmarks with the subjects positioned supine and with the knee in two separate positions, slightly flexed and flexed at a larger angle. Intraclass correlation coefficients for intrarater reliability for the two positions of knee flexion ranged from a low of .86 to a high of .97 (Table 15–7), while inter-rater reliability ranged from a low of .62 to a high of .94 (Table 15–8). Intrarater error ranged from 3.8 degrees to 5.5 degrees, and inter-rater error ranged from 7.3 degrees to 18.1 degrees. The actual level of reliability and the measurement error obtained depended on

Table 15–7. INTRARATER RELIABILITY: KNEE RANGE OF MOTION

KNEE FLEXION

Study	Technique	n	Sample	r*	ICC†
Boone et al.[7]	AROM	12	Healthy males (25–54 yr)		.87
Clapper & Wolf[9]	AROM	20	10 males—mean age 28.3 yr 10 females—mean age 30.0 yr		.95
Walker et al.[35]	AROM	4	Healthy adults (ages not provided)	>.81	
Brosseau et al.[8]	AROM	60	Healthy adults (mean age 20.6 yr)		.86–.97‡
Rothstein et al.[30]	PROM	12	Patients; no ages or diagnoses supplied	.97–.99§	.97–.99§
Watkins et al.[37]	PROM	43	Patients (18–80 yr) (mean age 39.5 yr)		.99

KNEE EXTENSION

Study	Technique	n	Sample	r	ICC
Clapper & Wolf[9]	AROM	20	Healthy adults 10 males—mean age 28.3 yr 10 females—mean age 30.0 yr		.85
Walker et al.[35]	AROM	4	Healthy adults (ages not provided)	>.81	
Rothstein et al.[30]	PROM	12	Patients; no ages or diagnoses supplied	.91–.96§	.91–.97§
Watkins et al.[37]	PROM	43	Patients (18–80 yr) (mean age 39.5 yr)		.98
Pandya et al.[27]	PROM	150	Duchenne's muscular dystrophy; (<1–20 yr)		.93

* Pearson's r
† Intraclass correlation
‡ Dependent upon patient position and tester performing measurement
§ Dependent upon type of goniometer used
AROM, active range of motion; PROM, passive range of motion

the examiner performing the measurement, which measurement was used for the analysis, and the position of the knee (less or more flexed). Both intrarater and inter-rater reliability levels were higher with the knee more flexed and lower with the knee in the less flexed position.

Boone et al.,[7] Clapper and Wolf,[9] and Walker et al.[35] also have examined intrarater reliability of active knee flexion range of motion using the universal goniometer. Exact positioning of the subjects in the Clapper and Wolf[9] and Walker et al.[35] studies was not described in sufficient detail to determine whether the subjects were positioned prone or supine, nor were the landmarks that were used listed. Subjects in the Boone et al.[7] study were positioned supine for knee measurement, but the distal arm of the goniometer was aligned with the tibia rather than with the fibula. Other details of each of these studies have been described previously (see the Hip section of this chapter). Two of these groups of investigators used ICCs for determining reliability and obtained values ranging from .85 for knee extension to .95 for knee flexion.[7, 9] Repeated measures ANOVA performed on data for measurements of knee flexion in the Boone et al.[7] study revealed significant intrarater variation for one of the four examiners and significant inter-rater variation among all four examiners. Walker et al.[35] calculated reliability using Pearson's r and obtained values for intrarater reliability of greater than .81 (see Table 15–7) and a mean error between repeated measures of 5 degrees.

Other groups of investigators have examined the reliability of measuring passive, rather than active, knee flexion range of motion. Both Rothstein et al.[30] and Watkins et al.[37] examined the reliability of passive knee flexion and extension measurements on patients in a clinical setting. The two groups of 12 (Rothstein et al.[30]) and 43 (Watkins et al.[37]) patients possessed a variety of diagnoses. No standardization of patient positioning or landmarks was used in either study. Patients in the study conducted by Rothstein et al.[30] had measurements of knee motion taken with three different goniometers, and reliability using each instrument was compared. Data were analyzed using both Pearson's r[30] and ICCs.[30, 37] Intrarater reliability for all measurements was quite high (see Table 15–7) regardless of the type of goniometer used.[30]

Two additional groups of investigators examined the reliability of passive knee extension measurements in children. One group measured passive knee extension in a sample of 150 children with Duchenne's muscular dystrophy,[27] while the other group measured the same motion in 20 children with cerebral palsy.[33] Both studies have been described previously (see the Hip section of this chapter). Intrarater reliability for the measurement of passive knee extension in the children with Duchenne's muscular dystrophy was .93 (ICC)[27] (see Table 15–7). Stuberg et al.[33] reported no significant differences among the three measurements of passive knee extension taken by a single examiner in each of 20 children with cerebral palsy based on a two-way ANOVA for repeated measures.

Most studies of inter-rater reliability of goniometric measurement of knee motion demonstrate much higher reliability for knee flexion than for knee extension measurements (Table 15–8). Inter-rater reliabilities at or above .90

Table 15–8. INTER-RATER RELIABILITY: KNEE RANGE OF MOTION

KNEE FLEXION

Study	Technique	n	Sample	r*	ICC†
Boone et al.[7]	AROM	12	Healthy males (25–54 yr)		.50
Brosseau et al.[8]	AROM	60	Healthy adults (mean age 20.6 yr)		.62–.94‡
Gogia et al.[18]	PROM	30	Healthy adults (20–60 yr) (mean age 35 yr)	.98	.99
Mitchell et al.[26]	AROM	20	Healthy adults & adults with arthritis (ages not provided)	.96	
Rothstein et al.[30]	PROM	12	Patients; no ages or diagnoses supplied	.88–.91§	.91–.99§
Watkins et al.[37]	PROM	43	Patients (18–80 yr) (mean age 39.5 yr)		.90
Rheault et al.[28]	AROM	20	Healthy adults (mean age 24.8 yr)	.87	

KNEE EXTENSION

Study	Technique	n	Sample	r	ICC
Drews et al.[12]	PROM	9	Healthy infants (12 hr–6 days)	.69 (left) .89 (right)	
Rothstein et al.[30]	PROM	12	Patients; no ages or diagnoses supplied	.63–.70§	.64–.71§
Watkins et al.[37]	PROM	43	Patients (18–80 yr) (mean age 39.5 yr)		.86
Pandya et al.[27]	PROM	21	Duchenne's muscular dystrophy (4–20 yr)		.58

* Pearson's r
† Intraclass correlation
‡ Dependent upon patient position and tester performing measurement
§ Dependent upon type of goniometer used
AROM, active range of motion; PROM, passive range of motion

(ICC) were obtained in three studies measuring knee flexion range of motion, all of which have been described previously.[8, 30, 37] These studies included measurement of both passive and active knee flexion in healthy adults and in adult patients with varied diagnoses.

Gogia et al.[18] examined both inter-rater reliability and validity of flexion and extension measurements of the knee joint in 30 healthy adults between the ages of 20 and 60 years. Subjects were positioned passively in some arbitrarily determined degree of knee flexion, then goniometric measurement of the knee position was taken separately by two examiners. An x-ray was taken of each subject's knee prior to allowing the subject to move. Inter-rater reliability and validity of goniometric measurements were calculated using both the ICC and Pearson's r. Reliabilities ranged from .98 (Pearson's r) to .99 (ICC) for inter-rater reliability and from .97 (Pearson's r) to .99 (ICC) for validity, providing support for the reliability and validity of goniometric measurements of knee flexion (see Table 15–8).

High inter-rater reliability for knee flexion measurements using a universal goniometer also was obtained by Mitchell and colleagues.[26] This group of investigators measured active knee flexion in a group of 20 adults who either were healthy or had a diagnosis of rheumatoid arthritis. A standardized technique was used for aligning the goniometer that involved positioning the proximal and distal arms of the instrument parallel to the anterior aspect of the thigh and the tibia and the axis parallel to the lateral knee joint line. Despite the fact that neither examiner had previous clinical experience in using a goniometer, inter-rater reliabilities (Pearson's r) were quite high (.96) with a standard error reported of 0.16 degrees (see Table 15–8).

Only two studies were found in which inter-rater reliability levels for knee flexion fell below .90. One study involved examination of inter-rater reliability of knee flexion range of motion in a group of 20 healthy adults.[28] Data were analyzed using Pearson's r to determine correlation and paired t tests to determine whether a significant difference existed between the data obtained by the two examiners. Although a Pearson's r value of .87 was obtained, indicating good reliability, the paired t tests demonstrated a significant difference between examiners.[28] The other study, in which inter-rater reliability of knee flexion measurements was low, involved the measurement of active knee flexion in a group of 12 healthy adult males aged 25 to 54 years.[7] Standardized patient positioning and landmarks for goniometry were used. Inter-rater reliability was calculated using ICCs, and reliability for knee flexion equaled .50 (see Table 15–8).

In general, values for inter-rater reliability for knee extension goniometry are less than those reported for knee flexion (see Table 15–8). The majority of the studies encountered in the literature have examined reliability of passive knee extension measurements.[12, 27, 30, 37] Reports of inter-rater reliability for knee extension goniometry ranged from a low of .58 to a high of .86 when ICCs were used to analyze the data regardless of whether standardized testing positions and techniques were used during measurement. In fact, the highest inter-rater reliability for knee extension measurements was obtained when examiners were allowed to use their own techniques for measurement,[37] although Rothstein et al.[30] did find that inter-rater reliability of knee extension measurements improved "dramatically" when standardized patient positioning was used. In the single study using Pearson's r to analyze the data,[12] inter-rater reliability for knee extension goniometry was reported as .69 for the left knee and .89 for the right knee. The SEMm from this study (calculated by the author of this text from data provided) was 2.2 degrees for the right knee and 3.7 degrees for the left knee.

Ankle Pronation and Supination: Dorsiflexion/Plantarflexion Components

Most reliability studies of active ankle dorsiflexion and plantarflexion range of motion measurements have been performed on healthy adult subjects. Two of these studies have been described previously (see the Hip and Knee sections of this chapter), and these investigators obtained intrarater reliabilities for ankle dorsiflexion of .92 (ICC)[9] and greater than .81 (Pearson's r)[35] and of .96 (ICC)[9] and greater than .81 (Pearson's r)[35] for ankle plantarflexion (Table 15–9). The mean error between repeated measures in the Walker et al.[35] study was 5 degrees.

A third study, which examined the reliability of measurements of ankle motion in healthy adults, compared ankle dorsiflexion measurements using various distal landmarks and various methods of dorsiflexing the ankle.[6] Ankle dorsiflexion was measured in 36 female subjects. The dorsiflexion motion was accomplished in three different ways: 1) passively to the point of notable tension; 2) passively with maximal force; and 3) passively with maximal force and active assistance by the subject. Each motion was measured three times, and the distal landmark was altered each time by using either the fifth metatarsal, the heel, or the plantar surface of the foot for alignment of the moving arm of the goniometer. An ANOVA revealed a significant

Table 15–9. INTRARATER RELIABILITY: ANKLE RANGE OF MOTION

ANKLE DORSIFLEXION

Study	Technique	n	Sample	r*	ICC†
Bohannon et al.[6]	PROM and AAROM	36	Healthy females		.80–.93‡
Clapper & Wolf[9]	AROM	20	Healthy adults (20–36 yr) 10 males—mean age 28.3 yr 10 females—mean age 30.0 yr		.92
Diamond et al.[10]	PROM, measurements taken in STJN	25	Diabetes (34–77 yr)		.89 (R) .96 (L)
Elveru et al.[14]	PROM	43 (50 ankles)	Neurologic or orthopaedic disorders (12–81 yr)		.90
Pandya et al.[27]	PROM	150	Duchenne's muscular dystrophy (4–20 yr)		.90
Walker et al.[35]	AROM	4	Healthy adults (ages not provided)	>.81	
Youdas et al.[40]	AROM	38 (45 ankles)	Orthopaedic problems (13–71 yr)		.78–.96§

ANKLE PLANTARFLEXION

Study	Technique	n	Sample	r	ICC
Clapper & Wolf[9]	AROM	20	Healthy adults 10 males—mean age 28.3 yr 20 females—mean age 30.0 yr		.96
Elveru et al.[14]	PROM	43 (50 ankles)	Neurologic or orthopaedic disorders (12–81 yr)		.86
Walker et al.[35]	AROM	4	Healthy adults (ages not provided)	>.81	
Youdas et al.[40]	AROM	38 (45 ankles)	Orthopaedic disorders (13–71 yr)		.64–.98§

* Pearson's r
† Intraclass correlation
‡ Dependent upon type of measurement and distal landmark used
§ 10 testers performed measurement
PROM, passive range of motion; AAROM, active assisted range of motion; AROM, active range of motion; STJN, subtalar joint neutral; R, right; L, left

difference in the ankle dorsiflexion measurements under the three conditions and when the different landmarks were used. The amount of ankle dorsiflexion obtained was greatest when the examiner passively dorsiflexed the ankle with maximal force and was actively assisted by the subject. The least amount of dorsiflexion was obtained when the examiner performed passive ankle dorsiflexion to notable tension. Variations in the landmark used also influenced the amount of dorsiflexion obtained. Dorsiflexion measurements were highest when the heel was used as the distal landmark and lowest when the fifth metatarsal was used. Intrarater reliability of each measurement was calculated using ICCs, and all measurements were found to be reliable (range .80 to .93). However, measurements of ankle dorsiflexion that involved using the heel as the distal landmark or passive dorsiflexion to notable tension were the least reliable[6] (see Table 15–9).

One group of investigators compared visual estimation and goniometric measurements of active ankle dorsiflexion and plantarflexion range of motion in 45 ankles of a group of 38 patients with orthopaedic disorders aged 13 to 71 years.[40] No standardized method was used for either patient positioning or goniometric measurement. Measurements were made by 10 examiners, and intrarater reliability was determined for each examiner. Intrarater reliabilities were calculated using ICCs only for measurements of ankle motion made with the universal goniometer and ranged from .78 to .96 for ankle dorsiflexion and from .64 to .98 for ankle plantarflexion[40] (see Table 15–9). However, inter-rater reliabilities for ankle dorsiflexion and plantarflexion were quite poor, whether goniometric measurement or visual estimation was used (Table 15–10). The lack of a standardized measurement procedure and standardized patient positioning probably contributed to these poor reliabilities. The authors of this study concluded that the same therapist should perform any repeated measurements of ankle range of motion because of the poor inter-rater reliabilities found in this study.

Some investigators who have examined the reliability of measurements of passive motion of the ankle joint have done so within the pediatric

Table 15–10. INTER-RATER RELIABILITY: ANKLE RANGE OF MOTION

ANKLE DORSIFLEXION

Study	Technique	n	Sample	r*	ICC†
Diamond et al.[10]	PROM, measurements taken in STJN	31	Diabetes (34–77 yr)		.74(R) .87(L)
Elveru et al.[14]	PROM	43 (50 ankles)	Orthopaedic & neurologic disorders (12–81 yr)		.50
Pandya et al.[27]	PROM	21	Duchenne's muscular dystrophy (<1–20 yr)		.73
Youdas et al.[40]	AROM	38 (45 ankles)	Orthopaedic disorders (13–71 yr)		.28

ANKLE PLANTARFLEXION

Study	Technique	n	Sample	r	ICC
Drews et al.[12]	PROM	9	Healthy infants (12 hr–6 days)	.84(L) .89(R)	
Elveru et al.[14]	PROM	43 (50 ankles)	Orthopaedic & neurologic disorders (12–81 yr)		.72
Youdas et al.[40]	AROM	38 (45 ankles)	Orthopaedic disorders (13–71 yr)		.25

* Pearson's r
† Intraclass correlation
PROM, passive range of motion; STJN, subtalar joint neutral; AROM, active range of motion; R, right; L, left

population. Three of these studies have been described previously (see the Hip and Knee sections of this chapter) and involve reliability of measuring passive ankle joint motion in healthy infants and in children with a variety of diagnoses.[12, 27, 33] Passive ankle plantarflexion was measured by two examiners in a group of 54 healthy infants between the ages of 12 hours and 6 days.[12] A subgroup of nine of the infants was used to examine inter-rater reliability of passive ankle plantarflexion measurements using Pearson's *r*. Values for inter-rater reliability reported in this study were .84 for the left ankle and .89 for the right ankle (see Table 15–10). The SEMm from this study (calculated by the author of this text from data provided) was 2.6 degrees for right ankle plantarflexion and 3.1 degrees for the left ankle.

Stuberg and colleagues[33] measured the reliability of passive ankle goniometry in a group of children with cerebral palsy; however, this group of investigators examined ankle dorsiflexion measurements. Specifics about the study's protocol have been described previously (see the Hip section of this chapter). A two-way ANOVA for repeated measures was used to determine intrarater and inter-rater reliability of passive ankle dorsiflexion measurement. Analysis of intrarater reliability showed no significant difference between the three measures taken by a single examiner in one session, and intrarater error was calculated at less than or equal to 5 degrees. Conversely, significant inter-rater variation was found.

Both inter-rater and intrarater reliability of passive ankle dorsiflexion measurement was examined in a third group of children, all of whom had a diagnosis of Duchenne's muscular dystrophy.[27] Goniometric measurements were performed using standardized procedures and positioning. Inter-rater and intrarater reliabilities were calculated on 21 and 150 patients, respectively, using ICCs. Reliabilities were .73 for inter-rater and .90 for intrarater reliability of passive ankle dorsiflexion measurement (see Tables 15–9 and 15–10).

Two groups of investigators have examined the reliability of passive ankle dorsiflexion measurements in the adult population.[10, 14] Elveru et al.[14] measured passive ankle dorsiflexion and plantarflexion in 50 ankles of 43 patients with neurologic or orthopaedic disorders. No standardized patient positioning or goniometric technique was used in the study. Two measurements of ankle plantarflexion and dorsiflexion were taken on each patient by two examiners using a blinded goniometer. The first measurement of each pair of measurements was used to calculate intertester reliability. Intraclass correlation coefficients were used to determine both intrarater and inter-rater reliability. Intrarater reliability for ankle motions equaled .90 for dorsiflexion and .86 for plantarflexion, while inter-rater reliability was .50 for dorsiflexion and .72 for plantarflexion (see Tables 15–9 and 15–10).

Reliability of passive ankle dorsiflexion but not of plantarflexion was examined by Diamond et al.[10] in a group of 31 patients with diabetes mellitus. Two examiners measured passive ankle dorsiflexion range of motion using a standardized procedure that involved maintaining the subtalar joint in a neutral position during the measurement. Extensive training (20 training sessions over 18 months) was undertaken by each examiner prior to the period of data collection. Both intrarater and inter-rater reliability were assessed using ICCs. Values reported for reliability of ankle dorsiflexion were .89 (right ankle) and .96 (left ankle) for intrarater, and .74 (right ankle) and .87 (left ankle) for inter-rater (see Tables 15–9 and 15–10). The SEMm also was reported for all goniometric data. Values for SEMm were 1 degree (left ankle) and 3 degrees (right ankle) for repeated measurements taken by the same examiner, and 2 degrees (left ankle) and 3 degrees (right ankle) for measurements taken by different examiners.[10]

Subtalar Supination and Pronation: Inversion/Eversion Components

Reliability of goniometric inversion and eversion measurements varies widely depending on the technique employed to perform the measurement. Elveru et al.[14] measured passive inversion and eversion of the subtalar joint in 43 patients (50 ankles) with neurologic and orthopaedic disorders. Examiners measured subtalar inversion and eversion motion and the neutral position of the subtalar joint using a universal goniometer with the patient in a prone, non–weight-bearing position. The neutral subtalar position was determined through palpation. Measurements of inversion and eversion were taken without referencing them to the neutral position of the subtalar joint, but later the measurements were recalculated based on the subtalar neutral position. Each examiner was provided with standardized written instructions detailing the techniques for determining the neutral position of the subtalar joint and for measuring passive inversion and eversion. Range of motion measurements were taken by placing the goniometer on the posterior aspect of the joint with the proximal arm aligned along the midline of the calf and the distal arm aligned with the posterior midline of the calcaneus. Both intrarater and inter-rater reliabilities were calculated using ICCs. In the case of both intrarater and inter-rater reliability, ICC levels were lower when the measurement was referenced to the neutral position of the subtalar joint as compared with measurements taken with no reference used (Tables 15–11 and 15–12). The authors attributed this decreased reliability to the error associated with determining the subtalar neutral position.[14]

Table 15–11. INTRARATER RELIABILITY: SUBTALAR JOINT RANGE OF MOTION

SUBTALAR INVERSION

Study	Technique	*n*	Sample	*r**	ICC[†]
Boone et al.[7]	AROM	12	Healthy adult males (26–54 yr)		.80
Diamond et al.[10]	PROM, referenced from anatomical zero	25	Diabetes (34–77 yr)		.92(R) .96(L)
Elveru et al.[14]	PROM	43 (50 ankles)	Orthopaedic & neurologic disorders (12–81 yr)		.62, referenced to STJN .74, not referenced to STJN
Walker et al.[35]	AROM	4	Healthy adults (ages not provided)	>.81	

SUBTALAR EVERSION

Study	Technique	*n*	Sample	*r*	ICC
Diamond et al.[10]	PROM, referenced from anatomical zero	25	Diabetes (ages 34–77 yr)		.96(R) .96(L)
Elveru et al.[14]	PROM	43 (50 ankles)	Orthopaedic & neurologic disorders (12–81 yr)		.59, referenced to STJN .75, not referenced to STJN
Walker et al.[35]	AROM	4	Healthy adults (ages not provided)	>.81	

* Pearson's *r*
† Intraclass correlation
AROM, active range of motion; PROM, passive range of motion; STJN, subtalar joint neutral; R, right; L, left

Table 15–12. INTER-RATER RELIABILITY: SUBTALAR JOINT RANGE OF MOTION

SUBTALAR INVERSION

Study	Technique	n	Sample	r*	ICC†
Boone et al.[7]	AROM	12	Healthy adult males (26–54 yr)		.69
Diamond et al.[10]	PROM, referenced from anatomical zero	31	Diabetes (34–77 yr)		.86(R) .89(L)
Drews et al.[12]	PROM	9	Healthy infants (12 hr–6 days)	.56 (L) .71 (R)	
Elveru et al.[14]	PROM	43 (50 ankles)	Orthopaedic & neurologic disorders (12–81 yr)		.15, referenced to STJN .32, not referenced to STJN
Smith-Oricchio & Harris[32]	PROM, referenced to STJN	20	Ankle pathology (18–53 yr)		.42

SUBTALAR EVERSION

Study	Technique	n	Sample	r	ICC
Diamond et al.[10]	PROM, referenced from anatomical zero	31	Diabetes (34–77 yr)		.79(R) .78(L)
Drews et al.[12]	PROM	9	Healthy infants (12 hr–6 days)	.33(L) .62(R)	.
Elveru et al.[14]	PROM	43 (50 ankles)	Orthopaedic & neurologic disorders (12–81 yr)		.12, referenced to STJN; .17, not referenced to STJN
Smith-Oricchio & Harris[32]	PROM, referenced to STJN	20	Ankle pathology (18–53 yr)		.60

* Pearson's *r*
† Intraclass correlation
AROM, active range of motion; PROM, passive range of motion; STJN, subtalar joint neutral; R, right; L, left

Low inter-rater reliabilities for subtalar inversion and eversion measurements also were found by a group of investigators who used a similar technique to that used by Elveru et al.[14] Smith-Oricchio and Harris[32] measured subtalar inversion and eversion in reference to the subtalar neutral position in 20 patients with recent ankle pathology. Patients were measured in the prone, non–weight-bearing position as well as in a standing, weight-bearing position. Goniometric alignment was along the posterior aspect of the joint, as described in the previous study.[14] Inter-rater reliability was calculated using ICCs. Low inter-rater reliability was found for both calcaneal inversion and eversion measurements taken in the prone, non–weight-bearing position (see Table 15–12). However, inter-rater reliability of subtalar eversion measurements taken with the patient standing on both feet was high (ICC = .91). The authors attributed this difference to the fact that the subtalar motion measured with the patient in the prone position was passive, whereas the motion measured with the patient in the standing position was active eversion, removing a variable and a potential source of error from the examiner.[32]

Yet a third group of investigators examined reliability of measurements of subtalar inversion and eversion by using similar goniometric techniques to those described in the studies by Elveru et al.[14] and Smith-Oricchio and Harris.[32] Subtalar inversion and eversion range of motion was measured in a group of 31 patients with diabetes mellitus.[10] Measurements were taken with the goniometer placed along the posterior aspect of the joint and the arms of the goniometer aligned as described in the previous studies.[14, 32] No attempt was made by these examiners to reference subtalar measurements to the subtalar neutral position. Instead, motion of the subtalar joint was referenced to "anatomical zero."[10] Unlike examiners in the previous two studies, the examiners in this study underwent a period of extensive training (18 months) prior to data collection. Both intrarater and inter-rater reliabilities were calculated using ICCs. For calcaneal inversion, intrarater reliability (calculated on data from 25 patients) was .96, for the left and .92, for the right, and for calcaneal eversion it equaled .96 in both extremities (see Table 15–11). Inter-rater reliability (calculated on data from 31 patients) ranged from a low of .78 for calcaneal eversion on the left to a high of .89 for calcaneal inversion on the left (see Table 15–12). The SEMm was reported as 2 degrees for measurements of calcaneal inversion taken by the same examiner and 3 degrees for measurements taken by two different examiners, regardless of the side (right or left) measured. For calcaneal eversion, the SEMm for measurements taken by the same examiner was 1 degree, regardless of side measured, and the SEMm for measurements taken by two different examiners was 2 degrees on the right and 4 degrees on the left. The higher levels of reliability obtained in this study as compared to other investigations were attributed by the authors to the extensive period of training undertaken by the examiners prior to data collection.[10]

Other investigators have used different methods of measuring eversion and inversion range of motion in their studies of reliability. Walker and colleagues[35] measured inversion and eversion on a group of four healthy adults using the anterior approach described by the AAOS in its 1965 publication.[2] Only inversion motion was measured by Boone and colleagues[7] on a group of 12 healthy adult males using the same technique used by the investigators in the Walker et al.[35] study. Since both groups measured active range of motion, presumably the motion measured was combined forefoot and hindfoot motion, although that fact could not be clearly discerned from either study. Boone et al.[7] calculated reliability using the ICC and reported intrarater reliability for inversion measurements of .80 (see Table 15–11). Intrarater reliabilities for both inversion and eversion measurements were reported as greater than .81 (Pearson's r) by Walker and colleagues,[35] with a mean error between repeated measures of 5 degrees. Inter-rater reliability, which was calculated by only one group[7] and only for inversion, equaled .69 (ICC) (see Table 15–12).

Finally, inter-rater reliability of inversion and eversion measurements of the foot were calculated in a study based on results obtained in nine healthy infants aged 12 hours to 6 days.[12] The investigators used a unique and rather vaguely described technique for measuring inversion and eversion, in which the measurements were taken by aligning the moving arm of the goniometer along the midline of the plantar surface of the foot. The alignment of the stationary arm was not provided in the published report, nor was the reference position against which the measurement was taken explained. Inter-rater reliability was calculated using Pearson's r, and values ranged from a low of .33 for eversion of the left foot to a high of .71 for inversion of the right foot (see Table 15–12). The SEMm for this study (calculated by the author of this text from data provided) ranged from 3.8 degrees for measurements of inversion on the right foot to 7.0 degrees for measurements of eversion on the left foot.

Metatarsophalangeal Flexion/Extension

Only a single study that used inferential statistics to examine reliability of goniometric measurements of extension of the first metatarsophalangeal (MTP) joint was found. Hopson and colleagues[23] calculated the intrarater reliability of four different methods of measuring extension of the first MTP joint in a group of 20 healthy adults aged 21 to 43 years. The methods

Table 15–13. INTRARATER RELIABILITY: FIRST MTP JOINT EXTENSION

Study	Technique	n	Sample	ICC*
Hopson et al.[23]	PROM	20	Healthy adults (21–43 yr)	.95, medial side NWB .91, dorsum NWB .95, partial WB .98, full WB

* Intraclass correlation
PROM, passive range of motion; NWB, non–weight-bearing; WB, weight-bearing

compared included: 1) measuring from the medial side of the joint with the subject in a non–weight-bearing position; 2) measuring from the dorsal surface of the joint with the subject in a non–weight-bearing position; 3) measuring from the medial side of the joint with the subject seated in a partial weight-bearing position; and 4) measuring from the medial side of the joint with the subject standing in a full weight-bearing position. Intrarater reliability of each method was calculated using ICC. Reliabilities ranged from a low of .91 for method #2 to a high of .98 for method #4 (Table 15–13). The authors concluded that all four methods of measuring extension of the first MTP were reliable but should not be considered interchangeable measurements.[23]

RELIABILITY OF MUSCLE LENGTH TESTING

Tests for Iliopsoas Muscle Length

Wang et al.[36] performed intrarater reliability measurements on 10 subjects using the Thomas test (described in Chapter 14) to examine the length of the iliopsoas muscle. Results indicated reliability correlations (ICC) for both the dominant and the non-dominant iliopsoas equal to .97. During the flexibility examination of 117 elite athletes, Harvey[22] included the Thomas test for examination of muscle length of both the iliopsoas and the rectus femoris. Harvey[22] reported intratester reliability correlations (ICC) for all flexibility tests performed in the study as ranging from .91 to .94, not specifying which test yielded which correlation. Table 15–14 provides a summary of studies related to intratester reliability of the measurement of iliopsoas muscle length.

Tests for Rectus Femoris Muscle Length

In studies previously presented in which the Thomas test was used to measure test-retest reliability of iliopsoas muscle length measurement, the two investigations also used the Thomas test to measure rectus femoris muscle

Table 15–14. INTRATESTER RELIABILITY OF TESTS FOR ILIOPSOAS MUSCLE LENGTH

Study	Technique	n	Sample	ICC*
Wang et al.[36]	Thomas	10	Healthy adults (18–37 yr)	.97 (dominant) .97 (nondominant)
Harvey[22]	Thomas	117	Elite athletes	.91–.94[†]

* Intraclass correlation
† Refer to text for explanation.

length by taking measurements at the knee (the technique is described in Chapter 14). Wang et al.[36] reported intrarater reliability coefficients for the dominant rectus femoris equal to .97 and non-dominant rectus femoris equal to .96 (ICC). As indicated previously, Harvey[22] reported intrarater reliability correlations for measurements of muscle length of both the iliopsoas and the rectus femoris as ranging from .91 to .94, not specifying which test resulted in which correlation. Table 15–15 provides a summary of studies related to intrarater reliability of rectus femoris muscle length measurement.

Tests for Hamstring Muscle Length

Review of the literature indicates that of all research on muscle length tests for the extremities (upper and lower), the majority has been conducted on the reliability of hamstring muscle length testing. Three tests have been presented in the literature as a means to measure the length of the hamstring muscles: straight leg raise, knee extension test—active, and knee extension test—passive. These tests are described in detail in Chapter 14.

Straight Leg Raise

As part of a larger reliability study, Hsieh et al.[24] evaluated the reliability of the straight leg raise test on 10 subjects using a test-retest design. Results indicated an intrarater correlation coefficient (Pearson's r) of .95 (SEMm was 1.8 degrees). Rose[29] investigated the reliability of the straight leg raise test as a part of a larger study examining other clinical range of motion measurements. Each lower extremity of 18 subjects was measured twice, resulting in intrarater reliability coefficients (Pearson's r) of .86 and .83 for the right and left lower extremity, respectively. The author reported the least significant difference as 17.4 degrees for the right lower extremity and 18.9 degrees for the left lower extremity.

Prior to examining the muscle flexibility of the lower extremity of long distance runners, Wang et al.[36] established the intrarater reliability of the straight leg raise in 10 subjects. Results indicated correlation coefficients (ICC) of .90 for the dominant limb and .91 for the non-dominant limb. In a study intended to determine the appropriate method for increasing hamstring flexibility, Hanten and Chandler[21] measured the left leg of 75 females two times in order to establish the reliability of the straight leg raise test. The intrarater reliability coefficient (ICC) was reported to be .91.

Knee Extension Test — Active

The earliest reported study on the reliability of the active knee extension test was by Gajdosik and Lusin.[16] These authors suggested that the straight leg

Study	Technique	n	Sample	ICC*
Wang et al.[36]	Thomas	10	Healthy adults (18–37 yr)	.97 (dominant) .96 (nondominant)
Harvey[22]	Thomas	117	Elite athletes	.91–.94[†]

Table 15–15. INTRATESTER RELIABILITY OF TESTS FOR RECTUS FEMORIS MUSCLE LENGTH

* Intraclass correlation
† Refer to text for explanation.

raise was not a valid test for measuring hamstring muscle length because of difficulty in controlling movement at the pelvis, as well as because the straight leg raise was primarily a test to examine neurologic tissue (sciatic nerve), not muscle length. Therefore, Gajdosik and Lusin[16] introduced the active knee extension test (described in Chapter 14) and examined intratester reliability on 15 males using a test-retest design. Reported correlation coefficients (Pearson's r) were .99 for both the right and the left lower extremity. However, appropriate follow-up testing to analyze for random and systematic error was not included (refer to Chapter 2). This study is included in this chapter because it is one of the first investigations to use the active 90/90 test.

Establishing reliability of the active knee extension test for measurement of hamstring muscle length on 12 subjects as part of a study intended to determine the most efficient muscle stretching technique, Sullivan et al.[34] examined both the intratester reliability of, and the intertester reliability between, two testers. The authors reported the intratester reliability (ICC) on the active knee extension test as .99 for both testers and the intertester reliability (ICC) between the two testers as .93.

In a study to determine the effects of increasing the length of the hamstrings on the strength of those muscles, Worrell et al.[39] examined the intratester reliability of the active knee extension test in 10 subjects measured twice. The authors reported a correlation coefficient (ICC) of .93 (SEMm = 2.91 degrees). In another study comparing two types of stretching techniques for increasing hamstring flexibility, Webright et al.[38] reported on the intratester and intertester reliability of the active knee extension test using two examiners. Using a test-retest design on 12 subjects, both examiners achieved intrarater reliability coefficients (ICC) of .98 (SEMm = 1.68 degrees); intertester reliability (ICC) between the examiners also was reported as .98 (SEMm = 1.80 degrees).

Knee Extension Test — Passive

Fredriksen et al.[15] agreed with Gajdosik and Lusin[16] that the straight leg raise was an inadequate measure of hamstring muscle length because of difficulty in controlling pelvic movement. However, these authors questioned the validity of the active knee extension test because the test depended on the strength of the quadriceps muscles as well as on the ability of the subject to simultaneously contract the quadriceps muscles and relax the hamstring muscles. Therefore, Fredriksen et al.[15] suggested that the passive knee extension test (described in Chapter 14), in which the examiner moved the leg through the available range of motion, was the most appropriate test to measure hamstring muscle length. Two testers examined the reliability of the passive knee extension test on two subjects (one male, one female) measured across 8 days. A total of 28 measurements were taken by each tester, and these measurements were analyzed with a Pearson correlation and paired t test. The authors reported intertester correlation coefficients of .99 and no significant difference between testers, concluding that "the passive knee extension test is a simple and reliable method."

Bandy and colleagues[3, 4] performed two studies attempting to determine the optimal length of time that the hamstring muscles should be placed in a sustained stretch position. As part of these studies, the authors reported reliability of the passive knee extension test, performed before and after 6 weeks on the control group. The correlation values reported for the control group's pretest and post-test measurements using the passive knee extension test were .91 (ICC) for the 15 control subjects in the first study[3] and .97 (ICC) for the 20 control subjects in the second study.[4]

Table 15–16. INTRATESTER RELIABILITY OF TESTS FOR HAMSTRING MUSCLE LENGTH

Study	Technique	n	Sample	r*	ICC†
Hsieh[24]	SLR	10	Healthy adults (26–30 yr)	.95	
Rose[29]	SLR	18	Healthy adults (mean age 19.5 yr)	.86 (R) .83 (L)	
Wang et al.[36]	SLR	10	Healthy adults (18–37 yr)		.90‡ .91§
Hanten & Chandler[21]	SLR	75	Healthy females (18–29 yr)		.91
Gajdosik & Lusin[16]	Active‖	15	Healthy males (18–26 yr)	.99 (R) .99 (L)	
Sullivan et al.[34]	Active	12	Healthy adults		.99, .99¶
Worrell et al.[39]	Active	10	Healthy adults		.93
Webright et al.[38]	Active	12	Healthy adults		.98, .98¶
Bandy & Irion[3]	Passive**	15	Healthy adults (22–36 yr)	.91	
Bandy et al[4]	Passive	20	Healthy adults (20–40 yr)	.97	
Gajdosik et al.[17]	SLR, active, passive	30	Healthy adults (18–40 yr)		.83 (SLR) .86 (active) .90 (passive)

* Pearson's r
† Intraclass correlation
‡ Dominant
§ Nondominant
‖ Active knee extension test (90/90 active)
¶ Two testers performed measurement.
** Passive knee extension test (90/90 passive)
SLR, straight leg raise; R, right; L, left

Comparison of Three Measurement Techniques

In a study intended to compare the reliability of the three previously described techniques of hamstring muscle length measurement, Gajdosik et al.[17] performed the straight leg raise test, the knee extension test—active, and the knee extension test—passive on 30 males using a test-retest design. Reported intrarater reliability coefficients (ICC) were .83 for the straight leg raise test, .86 for the knee extension test—active, and .90 for the knee extension test—passive. The authors concluded that the results of the study suggest that the tests "probably represent similar, yet indirect measurements of hamstring length."

Summary: Tests for Hamstring Muscle Length

A summary of studies that examined the reliability of tests to measure hamstring muscle length are presented in Tables 15–16 and 15–17. As indicated

Table 15–17. INTERTESTER RELIABILITY OF TESTS FOR HAMSTRING MUSCLE LENGTH

Study	Technique	n	Sample	r*	ICC†
Sullivan et al.[34]	Active‡	12	Healthy adults		.93
Webright et al.[38]	Active	12	Healthy adults		.98
Fredriksen et al.[15]	Passive§	2	Healthy adults	.99	

* Pearson's r
† Intraclass correlation
‡ Active knee extension test (90/90 active)
§ Passive knee extension test (90/90 passive)

in the tables, irrespective of the measurement test used, reliability correlations across all tests ranged from .83 to .99 for intratester reliability (see Table 15–16) and from .93 to .99 for intertester reliability (see Table 15–17).

TESTS FOR ILIOTIBIAL BAND AND TENSOR FASCIAE LATAE MUSCLE LENGTH

Examination of the reliability of any of the measurement techniques (observation, tape measure, goniometer, inclinometer) used during the Ober test or modification of the Ober test is very rare. Only one published study examining the reliability of the Ober or Modified Ober test and only one published study analyzing the reliability of the prone test could be found after extensive review of the literature (Ober tests are described in Chapter 14).

Pandya et al.[27] examined the reliability of using a goniometer to quantify the prone test for measurement of iliotibial band and tensor fasciae latae muscle length. (Note: Although Gautam and Anand[20] published their description of the prone testing procedure as a "new test" in 1998, Pandya et al.[27] had already published a reliability study on the prone test in 1985.) Intrarater reliability testing was performed on 150 children, with reported reliability coefficients (ICC) of .81; intertester reliability testing was performed on 21 children with a reliability coefficient (ICC) reported as .25.

As indicated in Chapter 14, Melchione and Sullivan[25] described using an inclinometer placed at the distal lateral thigh of the extremity on which the Modified Ober test was being performed. Both intrarater and inter-rater reliability of the technique was examined using a test-retest design on 10 subjects with anterior knee pain. Results indicated intratester reliability coefficients (ICC) of .94 (SEMm = 1 degree) and intertester reliability coefficients (ICC) of .73 (SEMm = 1 degree). The authors concluded that the "repeated measurements obtained with the described method (inclinometer) demonstrated good reliability between testers and excellent reliability within testers."

TESTS FOR GASTROCNEMIUS AND SOLEUS MUSCLE LENGTH

In a study with the ultimate purpose of examining the lower extremity flexibility of long-distance runners, Wang et al.[36] reported intratester reliability of measurements of the length of the gastrocnemius muscle (measured supine) and of the soleus muscle (measured prone) in 10 subjects. Results indicated a reliability correlation (ICC) for gastrocnemius muscle length of .98 for both the dominant and non-dominant limb; the soleus reliability correlations (ICC) were .93 for the dominant limb and .94 for the non-dominant limb.

References

1. Ahlback SO, Lindahl O: Sagittal mobility of the hip joint. Acta Orthop Scand 1964;34: 310–322.
2. American Academy of Orthopaedic Surgeons: Joint Motion: Method of Measuring and Recording. Chicago, American Academy of Orthopaedic Surgeons, 1965.
3. Bandy WD, Irion JM: The effect of time on static stretch on the flexibility of the hamstring muscles. Phys Ther 1994;74:54–61.
4. Bandy WD, Irion JM, Briggler M: The effect of time and frequency of static stretching on flexibility of the hamstring muscles. Phys Ther 1997;77:1090–1096.

5. Bartlett JD, Wolf LS, Shurtleff DB, et al.: Hip flexion contractures: A comparison of measurement methods. Arch Phys Med Rehabil 1985;66:620–625.

6. Bohannon RW, Tiberio D, Zito M: Selected measures of ankle dorsiflexion range of motion: Differences and intercorrelations. Foot Ankle Int 1989;10:99–103.

7. Boone DC, Azen SP, Lin C, et al.: Reliability of goniometric measurements. Phys Ther 1978;58:1355–1360.

8. Brosseau L, Tousignant M, Budd J, et al.: Intratester and intertester reliability and criterion validity of the parallelogram and universal goniometers for active knee flexion in healthy subjects. Physiother Res Int 1997;2:150–166.

9. Clapper MP, Wolf SL: Comparison of the reliability of the Orthoranger and the standard goniometer for assessing active lower extremity range of motion. Phys Ther 1988;68:214–218.

10. Diamond JE, Mueller MJ, Delitto A, et al.: Reliability of a diabetic foot evaluation. Phys Ther 1989;69:797–802.

11. Domholdt E: Physical Therapy Research: Principles and Applications, 2nd ed. Philadelphia, WB Saunders, 2000.

12. Drews JE, Vraciu JK, Pellino G: Range of motion of the joints of the lower extremities of newborns. Phys Occup Ther Ped 1984;4:49–62.

13. Ellison JB, Rose SJ, Sahrmann SA: Patterns of hip rotation range of motion: A comparison between healthy subjects and patients with low back pain. Phys Ther 1990;70:537–541.

14. Elveru RA, Rothstein JM, Lamb RL: Goniometric reliability in a clinical setting: Subtalar and ankle joint measurements. Phys Ther 1988;68:672–677.

15. Fredriksen H, Dagfinrud H, Jacobsen V, et al.: Passive knee extension test to measure hamstring muscle tightness. Scand J Med Sci Sports 1997;7:279–282.

16. Gajdosik R, Lusin G: Hamstring muscle tightness: Reliability of an active-knee-extension test. Phys Ther 1983;63:1085–1088.

17. Gajdosik RL, Rieck MA, Sullivan DK, et al.: Comparison of four clinical tests for assessing hamstring muscle length. J Orthop Sports Phys Ther 1993;18:614–618.

18. Gogia PP, Braatz JH, Rose SJ, et al.: Reliability and validity of goniometric measurements at the knee. Phys Ther 1987;7:192–195.

19. Greene WB, Heckman JD: The Clinical Measurement of Joint Motion. Rosemont, Ill, American Academy of Orthopaedic Surgeons, 1994.

20. Gautam VK, Anand S: A new test for estimating iliotibial band contracture. J Bone Joint Surg 1998;80-B:474–475.

21. Hanten W, Chandler S: Effects of myofascial release leg pull and sagittal plane isometric contract-relax techniques on passive straight leg raise angle. J Orthop Sports Phys Ther 1994;20:138–144.

22. Harvey D: Assessment of the flexibility of elite athletes using the modified Thomas test. Br J Sports Med 1998;32:68–70.

23. Hopson MM, McPoil TG, Cornwall MW: Motion of the first metatarsophalangeal joint: Reliability and validity of four measurement techniques. J Am Podiatr Med Assoc 1995;85:198–204.

24. Hsieh CY, Walker JM, Gillis K: Straight-leg raising test: Comparison of three instruments. Phys Ther 1983;63:1429–1433.

25. Melchione WE, Sullivan MS: Reliability of measurements obtained by use of an instrument designed to indirectly measure iliotibial band length. J Orthop Sports Phys Ther 1993;18:511–515.

26. Mitchell WS, Millar J, Sturrock RD: An evaluation of goniometry as an objective parameter for measuring joint motion. Scot Med J 1975;20:57–59.

27. Pandya S, Florence JM, King WM, et al.: Reliability of goniometric measurements in patients with Duchenne muscular dystrophy. Phys Ther 1985;65:1339–1342.

28. Rheault W, Miller M, Nothnagel P, et al.: Intertester reliability and concurrent validity of fluid-based and universal goniometers for active knee flexion. Phys Ther 1988;68:1676–1678.

29. Rose MJ: The statistical analysis of the intra-observer repeatability of four clinical measurement techniques. Physiotherapy 1991;77:89–91.

30. Rothstein JM, Miller PJ, Roettger RF: Goniometric reliability in a clinical setting: Elbow and knee measurements. Phys Ther 1983;63:1611–1615.

31. Simoneau CC, Hoenig KJ, Lepley JE, et al.: Influence of hip position and gender on active hip internal and external rotation. J Orthop Sports Physiol Ther 1998;28:158–164.

32. Smith-Oricchio K, Harris BA: Interrater reliability of subtalar neutral, calcaneal inversion and eversion. J Orthop Sports Physiol Ther 1990;12:10–15.

33. Stuberg WA, Fuchs RH, Miedaner JA: Reliability of goniometric measurements of children with cerebral palsy. Dev Med Child Neurol 1988;30:657–666.

34. Sullivan MK, Dejulia JJ, Worrell TW: Effect of pelvic position and stretching method on hamstring muscle flexibility. Med Sci Sports Exerc 1992;24:1383–1389.

35. Walker JM, Sue D, Miles-Elkousy N, et al.: Active mobility of the extremities in older subjects. Phys Ther 1984;4:919–923.

36. Wang SS, Whitney SL, Burdett RG, et al.: Lower extremity muscular flexibility in long distance runners. J Orthop Sports Phys Ther 1993;17:102–107.

37. Watkins MA, Riddle DL, Lamb RL, et al.: Reliability of goniometric measurements and visual estimates of knee range of motion obtained in a clinical setting. Phys Ther 1991;71: 90–97.
38. Webright W, Randolph BJ, Perrin D: Comparison of nonballistic active knee extension in neural slump position and static stretch techniques of hamstring flexibility. J Orthop Sports Phys Ther 1997;26:7–13.
39. Worrell TW, Smith TL, Winegardner J: Effect of hamstring stretching on hamstring muscle performance. J Orthop Sports Phys Ther 1994;20:154–159.
40. Youdas JW, Bogard CL, Suman VJ: Reliability of goniometric measurements and visual estimates of ankle joint active range of motion obtained in a clinical setting. Arch Phys Med Rehabil 1993;74:1113–1118.

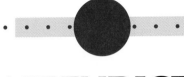

APPENDICES

APPENDIX A: CAPSULAR PATTERN DEFINED

Capsular Pattern

In his classic works (originally published in 1947, with several revisions occurring since that time), Cyriax[1] introduced the concept of the *capsular pattern* as the "pattern of limitation of passive movement of characteristic proportions" that indicates the involvement of the capsule. According to Cyriax,[1] the capsular pattern for each joint varies, with each joint having a characteristic pattern of proportional limitation (when examined using passive range of motion) that indicates that the joint capsule is involved. In the classic "little book" (originally published in 1974) on mobilization of the extremity joints, Kaltenborn[2] agreed with Cyriax[1] that when the whole capsule is shortened, "we will find what Cyriax calls a capsular pattern," which "manifests itself as a characteristic pattern of decreased movements at a joint."[2]

Each joint has a unique capsular pattern. Textbooks vary as to the specific capsular patterns presented for each joint, but most (if not all) references to capsular pattern can be traced to the work of Cyriax[1] and Kaltenborn.[2] Therefore, Table A-1 presents the capsular pattern of the extremities presented by Cyriax[1] and Kaltenborn.[2] Cyriax[1] and Kaltenborn[2] disagree on only one joint: the hip. In the case of the hip joint, the opinions of both Cyriax[1] and Kaltenborn[2] are presented.

One additional note about the capsular pattern specifically relates to the joints of the spine (cervical, thoracic, lumbar, and sacroiliac). Kaltenborn[2] avoids describing the capsular pattern for these joints, hence the name for his text *(Mobilization of the Extremity Joints)*. Cyriax[1] is vague, stating that for the thoracic and lumbar joints, it is difficult to "determine, except in gross arthritis, whether the range is limited or not, taking into account the patient's age and habits." Magee[3] suggests that "only joints that are controlled by muscles have a capsular pattern; joints such as the sacroiliac do not exhibit a capsular pattern." Therefore, this text does not address the capsular pattern of the spine.

Kaltenborn[2] agrees with Cyriax[1] that when the entire capsule is involved, the capsular pattern is always present. However, Kaltenborn[2] does suggest that "limitation of capsular shortening does not necessarily follow a typical pattern. For example, only one part of a capsule may be shortened due to trauma or some other localized lesion of the capsule. In these cases, limitation of movement will be evident only with movements that stretch the affected part of the capsule." In other words, according to Kaltenborn,[2] if the entire capsule is involved, the capsular pattern as described by Cyriax[1] is consistently present. But situations occur where only a part of the capsule is involved, and then the specific capsular pattern is not present.

In these circumstances, Magee[3] suggests that "an analysis of the end feel" will assist in indicating the type of joint involvement present. The end-feel of

Table A–1. CAPSULAR PATTERNS OF EXTREMITY JOINTS

JOINT	ROM RESTRICTION
Upper Extremity	
Shoulder	Lateral rotation is most limited, followed by limitation in abduction; medial rotation is least limited.
Elbow	Flexion is more limited than extension.
Wrist	Flexion and extension are equally limited.
Metacarpophalangeal	Flexion is more limited than extension.
Distal interphalangeal (DIP)	Flexion is more limited than extension.
Proximal interphalangeal (PIP)	Flexion is more limited than extension.
Lower Extremity	
Hip	Flexion, abduction, and medial rotation are grossly limited; extension is slightly limited; lateral rotation is not limited (Cyriax[1]).
	Medial rotation is most limited, followed by extension from zero, then abduction and flexion. Lateral rotation is least limited (Kaltenborn[2]).
Knee	Flexion is more limited than extension.
Ankle (talocrural joint)	Plantarflexion is more limited than dorsiflexion.
Subtalar joint	Inversion (varus) is more limited than eversion (valgus).
Metatarsophalangeal (2nd–5th)	Flexion is more limited than extension.
Metatarsophalangeal (1st)	Extension is more limited than flexion.

a joint motion is examined by applying gentle overpressure at the end of the range of motion and determining the quality of how the joint feels at that end point. Several types of end-feels exist in the body, including muscle, bone-to-bone, springy block, empty, and capsular. If the end-feel is similar to the feel of stretched leather, the capsule is involved. This involvement of the capsule, as determined by examination of passive range of motion indicating a capsular pattern, in conjunction with the end-feel, does have ramifications for treatment. The appropriate treatment of a joint that has been diagnosed as having capsular involvement is manual therapy, including mobilization and manipulation of the joint. For information related to treatment of loss of range of motion due to capsular involvement, the reader is referred to classic texts by the authors Maitland,[4, 5] Kaltenborn,[2] and Cyriax.[1]

References

1. Cyriax J: Textbook of Orthopaedic Medicine, 8th ed. London, Baillière Tindall, 1982.
2. Kaltenborn, FM: Mobilization of the Extremity Joints, 3rd ed. Oslo, Olaf Norlis Bokhandel, 1980.
3. Magee DJ: Orthopedic Physical Assessment, 2nd ed. Philadelphia, WB Saunders, 1992.
4. Maitland GD: Perpheral Manipulation, 2nd ed. London, Butterworths, 1977.
5. Maitland GD: Vertebral Manipulation, 4th ed. London, Butterworths, 1977.

APPENDIX B: SAMPLE DATA RECORDING FORMS

JOINT RANGE OF MOTION			Patient:_____ Age:_____ Indicate: AROM _____ PROM _____			
LEFT				**RIGHT**		
			Date/Examiner's Initials			
			Shoulder			
			Flexion			
			Extension			
			Abduction			
			Medial Rotation			
			Lateral Rotation			
			Elbow/Forearm			
			Flexion			
			Extension			
			Supination			
			Pronation			
			Wrist/Fingers			
			Wrist Flexion			
			Wrist Extension			
			Wrist Abduction			
			Wrist Adduction			
			CMC Flexion			
			CMC Extension			
			CMC Abduction			
			MCP Flexion			
			MCP Extension			
			IP Flexion (indicate digit and whether IP, PIP, or DIP)			

JOINT RANGE OF MOTION

Patient:_____
Age:_____
Indicate:
AROM _____
PROM _____

	LEFT				RIGHT	
			Date/Examiner's Initials			
			Hip			
			Flexion			
			Extension			
			Abduction			
			Adduction			
			Medial Rotation			
			Lateral Rotation			
			Knee			
			Flexion			
			Extension			
			Foot/Ankle			
			Dorsiflexion			
			Plantarflexion			
			Inversion			
			Eversion			
			1st MTP Flexion			
			1st MTP Extension			
			MTP Flexion: Digits 2–5			
			MTP Extension: Digits 2–5			
			IP Flexion (indicate digit and whether IP, PIP, or DIP)			
			IP Extension (indicate digit and whether IP, PIP, or DIP)			

Fig. B–2.

JOINT RANGE OF MOTION

Patient:_____

Age:_____

Measurement Device Used:
_____

Date/Examiner's Initials			
Lumbar			
Flexion			
Extension			
Lateral Flexion - Right			
Lateral Flexion - Left			
Rotation - Right			
Rotation - Left			
Thoracolumbar			
Flexion			
Extension			
Lateral Flexion - Right			
Lateral Flexion - Left			
Rotation - Right			
Rotation - Left			

Fig. B-3.

Fig. B-4.

JOINT RANGE OF MOTION	Patient:_____ Age:_____ Measurement Device Used: _____		
Date/Examiner's Initials			
Cervical			
Flexion			
Extension			
Lateral Flexion - Right			
Lateral Flexion - Left			
Rotation - Right			
Rotation - Left			
Temporomandibular Joint			
Mandibular depression (opening)			
Protrusion			
Lateral Deviation - Right			
Lateral Deviation - Left			

Fig. B-5.

MUSCLE LENGTH			Patient:_____ Age:_____ Indicate: AROM _____ PROM _____

			LEFT			RIGHT		
			Date/Examiner's Initials					
			Latissimus Dorsi					
			Pectoralis Major - General					
			Pectoralis Major - Clavicular					
			Pectoralis Minor					
			Triceps					
			Biceps					
			Forearm Flexor Muscles					
			Forearm Extensor Muscles					

			Date/Examiner's Initials			
			Iliopsoas (indicate test used)			
			Rectus Femoris			
			Quadriceps			
			Hamstrings (indicate test used)			
			Iliotibial Band (indicate test used)			
			Gastrocnemius			
			Soleus (indicate position)			

JOINT RANGE OF MOTION

Patient:_____
Age:_____
Indicate:
  AROM_____
  PROM_____

LEFT   **RIGHT**

Fig. B–6.

C

APPENDIX C: NORMATIVE RANGE of MOTION for the EXTREMITIES and SPINE in ADULTS

While providing normative data for joint range of motion would appear to be a relatively simple task, quite the opposite is true. For many decades, values published by groups such as the American Academy of Orthopaedic Surgeons (AAOS) and the American Medical Association (AMA) have been accepted and used by examiners measuring range of motion (see Tables C–2, C–4, C–5, and C–7).[3–5, 24] However, these "norms" were published without explanation regarding the source of the data. Establishment of normal values for a population must be based on data derived from sufficiently large samples of subjects who are randomly selected from the population in question.[36, 41] That the values published by the AAOS and AMA were derived from such samples is highly doubtful.

Many studies have been published which report data for joint range of motion. Tables C–8 through C–23 provide a comprehensive summary of published data for range of motion of selected joints of the extremities and spine. Tables that provide this same type of information for *all* the major joints of the extremities and the spine are available at www.wbsaunders.com/SIMON/Reese/joint/. In some of the cited studies, researchers have provided information about the population from which range of motion data were derived and about the techniques of data collection, but problems with the sample existed. In the majority of studies, either the sample sizes used were not large enough,* or, if large samples were used, they were not randomized.[15, 20, 23, 25, 29, 33, 40, 53]

In a few studies, large ($n > 100$), randomized samples were used to obtain range of motion data.[26, 30, 34, 38, 47] However, only one study in which large, randomized samples were used also investigated the reliability of the examiner(s), either before, or as part of, the study.[34] The single study that used a large, randomized sample to obtain data, and that examined tester reliability, was a sub-study of the National Health and Nutrition Examination Survey (NHANES I). Goniometric data regarding hip and knee range of motion measurements were gathered in 1891 subjects, aged 25 to 74 years, who were a subset of the total randomized sample of 20,749 U.S. citizens from which data were taken.[34, 48] From the goniometric data obtained on the subset of 1891 subjects, Roach and Miles[48] extracted and analyzed data from 1683 subjects, who were classified as either "black" or "white." These 1683 subjects were then divided according to age, with three age groups identified: 25–39 years, 40–59 years, and 60–74 years. The smallest number of subjects in any

---

* See references 1, 2, 9, 11, 12, 16, 18, 27, 31, 35, 43, 44, 51, 54, 57, 59, 61.

group was greater than 400, so sample sizes were sufficient to provide normative data for hip and knee range of motion for these three age groups. However, a problem existed with the reliability of goniometric data gathered in this study. In fact, goniometric measurements were discontinued after slightly more than half of the intended number of subjects were measured, because "a satisfactory level of reproducibility was not being achieved."[34]

Owing to the numerous problems, as previously discussed, with the "normative" range of motion data that exists in the literature, one can do no more than provide an educated theory regarding normal range of motion for the joints of the extremities and the spine. In the following sections, comparisons are made between the traditionally quoted "norms" of the AAOS and the AMA, and data derived from population samples (flawed though they may be) that report mean values for joint range of motion. Whenever possible, the data selected for comparison are taken from studies that used large, randomized samples. In many cases, insufficient data were available from such studies, and in those cases, data from other studies had to be used for comparison with AAOS and AMA values. Detailed information from a wide range of studies reporting range of motion data for the extremities and spine can be found in Tables C–8 through C–23 and in additional tables available at www.wbsaunders.com/SIMON/Reese/joint/.

NORMATIVE RANGE OF MOTION: UPPER EXTREMITIES

Table C–1 provides suggested normative range of motion values for the upper extremities of adults. Many of the values listed in Table C–1 are identical to values listed by either the AAOS or the AMA (Table C–2). These values were retained because they were supported by studies in the literature that upheld the values of either one group or the other (see Tables C–8 through C–10 and additional tables available at www.wbsaunders.com/SIMON/Reese/joint/). When data were not present to support either the AAOS or the AMA values for a particular movement, normative range of motion values that better reflect the published literature were substituted.

Comparison of normative range of motion data from the literature (see Tables C–8 through C–10 and additional tables available at www.wbsaunders.com/SIMON/Reese/joint/) with values published by the AAOS and the AMA for the upper extremity (Table C–2) yielded differences primarily in the following motions: shoulder flexion, shoulder abduction, and flexion of the interphalangeal (IP) joint of the thumb. Boone and Azen[9] reported mean values for shoulder flexion of 165 ± 5 degrees, and Sabari et al.[52] reported mean values for active shoulder flexion taken in the supine position of 160 ± 12 degrees (Table C–8). These values, taken from adult subjects, are lower than the 180 degrees reported by both the AAOS and the AMA (Table C–2). Although the sample sizes in these studies were small, intrarater reliability for measurements taken in the Sabari et al.[52] study was high (ICC = .95). Additionally, no other study in adults reported values for shoulder flexion range of motion higher than 169 degrees. Therefore, support for a lower value for mean range of motion of shoulder flexion, probably in the range of 0 to 165 degrees, was provided.

A similar argument can be made for shoulder abduction range of motion. Both the AAOS and the AMA again reported values of 180 degrees (Table C–2). While Boone and Azen[9] reported values for shoulder abduction that are similar to those of the AAOS and the AMA, others reported lower values (Table C–9). In a study of 1000 adult males,[25] the mean range

Table C–1. SUGGESTED VALUES FOR NORMAL ROM FOR JOINTS OF THE UPPER EXTREMITY IN ADULTS BASED ON ANALYSIS OF EXISTING DATA

JOINT	ROM
Shoulder	
Flexion	0°–165°
Extension	0°–60°
Abduction	0°–165°
Medial Rotation	0°–70°
Lateral Rotation	0°–90°
Elbow	
Flexion	0°–140°
Extension	0°
Forearm	
Pronation	0°–80°
Supination	0°–80°
Wrist	
Flexion	0°–80°
Extension	0°–70°
Abduction (Radial Deviation)	0°–20°
Adduction (Ulnar Deviation)	0°–30°
1st Carpometacarpal Joint	
Flexion	0°–15°
Extension	0°–20°
Abduction	0°–70°
Metacarpophalangeal Joints	
Flexion	
Thumb	0°–50°
Fingers	0°–90°
Extension	
Thumb	0°
Fingers	0°–20°
Interphalangeal Joints	
Flexion	
IP Joint (Thumb)	0°–65°
PIP Joint (Fingers)	0°–100°
DIP Joint (Fingers)	0°–70°
Extension	
IP Joint (Thumb)	0°–10° to 20°
PIP Joint (Fingers)	0°
DIP Joint (Fingers)	0°

IP, interphalangeal; PIP, proximal interphalangeal; DIP, distal interphalangeal.

of shoulder abduction was 167 ± 13 degrees for passive motion, which is usually somewhat greater than active motion (see Chapter 2). Support for a lower mean range of shoulder abduction was provided by Sabari et al.,[52] who reported a mean value for active shoulder abduction measured in the supine position of 162 ± 19 degrees (intrarater reliability: ICC = .99). Therefore, as with flexion, support was provided for a lower value for mean range of motion of shoulder abduction, probably in the range of 0 to 165 degrees.

In a study of 348 males and females aged 16 to 86 years, in which IP flexion of the thumb was measured with a universal goniometer, active IP flexion averaged 65 ± 12 degrees for the left hand and 64 ± 13 degrees for the right hand (Table C–10).[53] Support for the results obtained by Shaw and Morris[53] was demonstrated in a second study measuring IP flexion in 119 males and females.[33] The subjects in this second study had IP flexion of their

Table C–2. TRADITIONALLY QUOTED VALUES FOR NORMAL ROM FOR JOINTS OF THE UPPER EXTREMITY IN ADULTS

JOINT	ROM VALUES	
Shoulder	AAOS, 1965[3]*	AMA, 1993[5]†
Flexion	0°–180°	0°–180°
Extension	0°–60°	0°–50°
Abduction	0°–180°	0°–180°
Medial Rotation	0°–70°	0°–90°
Lateral Rotation	0°–90°	0°–90°
Elbow		
Flexion	0°–150°	0°–140°
Extension	0°	0°
Forearm		
Pronation	0°–80°	0°–80°
Supination	0°–80°	0°–80°
Wrist		
Flexion	0°–80°	0°–60°
Extension	0°–70°	0°–60°
Abduction (Radial Deviation)	0°–20°	0°–20°
Adduction (Ulnar Deviation)	0°–30°	0°–30°
1st Carpometacarpal Joint		
Flexion	0°–15°	
Extension	0°–20°	0°–50°
Abduction	0°–70°	
Metacarpophalangeal Joints		
Flexion		
Thumb	0°–50°	0°–60°
Fingers	0°–90°	0°–90°
Extension		
Thumb	0°	0°
Fingers	0°–45°	0°–20°
Interphalangeal Joints		
Flexion		
IP Joint (Thumb)	0°–80°	0°–80°
PIP Joint (Fingers)	0°–100°	0°–100°
DIP Joint (Fingers)	0°–90°	0°–70°
Extension		
IP Joint (Thumb)	0°–20°	0°–10°
PIP Joint (Fingers)	0°	0°
DIP Joint (Fingers)	0°	0°

* American Academy of Orthopaedic Surgeons.
† American Medical Association.
IP, interphalangeal; PIP, proximal interphalangeal; DIP, distal interphalangeal.

thumbs measured with a computerized goniometer, and the mean value reported for flexion of the IP joint of the thumb was 67 ± 11 degrees. Therefore, evidence exists to support a lower mean range of motion for IP flexion of the thumb than that reported by the AAOS and the AMA. The mean range of motion for IP flexion of the thumb is probably in the range of 0 to 65 degrees.

NORMATIVE RANGE OF MOTION: THORACIC AND LUMBAR SPINE

A variety of instruments have been used to measure thoracic and lumbar spine range of motion, the most frequently used being the tape measure,

Table C–3. TRADITIONALLY QUOTED VALUES FOR NORMAL ROM OF THORACIC AND LUMBAR SPINE IN ADULTS			
MOTION	SCHOBER*	GONIOMETER†	INCLINOMETER‡
Flexion	3–5 cm	90°	60°
Extension	—	30°	25°
Lateral Flexion	—	30°	25°
Rotation	—	—	30°

    * From Rothschild.[50]
    † Measurement of thoracolumbar spine norms provided by the American Medical Association.[4]
    ‡ Measurement of rotation is for thoracic spine; all other measures are lumbar spine. Norms provided by the American Medical Association.[5]

the goniometer, and the inclinometer. Although, as indicated earlier in this Appendix, concern exists with the publication of previous normative data (given that the origin of the norms is not specified, and data collection procedures are not fully explained), these published norms provide a basis with which to compare published reports of normative range of motion based on actual collection of data with defined methods and procedures. Table C–3 presents traditionally quoted values for range of motion of the thoracic and lumbar spine for each measurement technique. The values in Table C–3 then serve as a base against which actual data on range of motion of the thoracic and lumbar spine, collected and reported in the literature, may be compared.

TAPE MEASURE: ADULTS 20–40 YEARS

As indicated in Table C–3, Rothschild[50] reported a range of 3 to 5 cm for the measurement of lumbar flexion with a tape measure using the Schober technique. In a study publishing normative data on the Schober technique in 172 subjects (primarily male) from ages 20 to 82 years, Fitzgerald et al.[21] reported a measurement of 4 ± 1 cm for lumbar flexion for a subcategory of subjects aged 20 to 40 years (Table C–11), which is in agreement with the suggested norms presented by Rothschild.[50]

However, the Schober technique is no longer used in measurement of lumbar flexion, given the modification of the technique by Macrae and Wright[37] in 1969 (described in Chapter 8). Two studies using the modified Schober technique reported similar measurement of lumbar flexion in 20- to 40-year-old subjects, with Moll and Wright[42] reporting 7 ± 7 cm and Einkauf et al.[19] reporting 6.5 ± 1 cm (Table C–11). (Note: The 20- to 40-year-old age groups were subcategories of a larger study for both Moll and Wright[42] and Einkauf et al.[19]) Van Adrichen and van der Korst[58] reported 6 ± 1 cm in a group of 15- to 18-year-old subjects, and Haley et al.[28] reported a range of 6 to 7 cm in a group of children aged 5 to 9 years (Table C–11).

Based on these publications of data, it appears that the normative value of 3 to 5 cm for the Schober technique of measuring lumbar flexion is not appropriate for the measurement of lumbar flexion using the modified Schober. Given that these studies provide consistent information, a more appropriate norm for lumbar flexion using the modified Schober appears to be 6 to 7 cm. (Table C–4).

Table C–4. SUGGESTED VALUES FOR NORMAL ROM OF THORACIC AND LUMBAR SPINE IN ADULTS			
MOTION	MODIFIED SCHOBER	GONIOMETER	INCLINOMETER
Flexion	6–7 cm	90°	60°
Extension	—	30°	30°
Lateral flexion	—	35°	30°
Rotation	—	—	6°

GONIOMETER: ADULTS 20–40 YEARS

Flexion

As indicated in Table C–3, the AMA suggests that normative range of motion for lumbar flexion measured with a goniometer is 90 degrees. However, to date, no data have been collected to confirm or refute this suggested amount of normative lumbar flexion.

Extension

The suggested range of motion for lumbar extension is 30 degrees (Table C–3). Examining the data of the subjects in the 20- to 84-year-old range, Einkauf et al.[19] reported lumbar extension as 32 ± 15 degrees in a subcategory of 20- to 40-year-olds (Table C–12), in agreement with data provided in Table C–3. Normative data provided for the same age category by Fitzgerald et al.[21] indicated a higher average range of motion, at 40 ± 9 degrees (Table C–12). Given that only two studies have been performed on normative range of motion of lumbar extension as measured with a goniometer, and the fact that one of these studies is in agreement with Table C–3, no strong rationale exists to disagree with the normative data presented in Table C–3 for lumbar extension.

Lateral Flexion

Further examination of the data from the 20- to 40-year-old subcategory in the studies performed by Fitzgerald et al.[21] and Einkauf et al.[19] revealed that measurement of thoracolumbar lateral flexion was 33.5 ± 17 degrees and 36.5 ± 6 degrees, respectively (Table C–13; means of right and left lateral flexion for each study). These data suggest that the normative values presented in Table C–3 are slightly low, and that these values should be adjusted to 35 degrees (Table C–4).

INCLINOMETER: ADULTS 20–40 YEARS

Flexion

Table C–3 suggests that normative lumbar flexion range of motion measured using an inclinometer is 60 degrees. Lumbar flexion measured with an inclinometer is less than the amount of flexion measured with a goniometer because the inclinometer procedure allows measurement of lumbar mobility and subtracts any motion in the hips. Review of published investigations as to the amount of lumbar flexion measured with an inclinometer yielded three studies[14, 17, 39] that reported very consistent values ranging from 55 to 63 degrees (Table C–11). Therefore, 60 degrees appears to be an appropriate value for the norm of lumbar flexion measured with an inclinometer (Table C–4).

Extension

Three studies have examined lumbar extension using an inclinometer, with all investigations[14, 17, 39] reporting extension means ranging from 27 to 32 degrees (Table C–12). Based on these data, the normative range of motion of

25 degrees reported in Table C–3 appears low, and the published studies suggest that 30 degrees of lumbar extension might be a more appropriate norm (Table C–4).

Lateral Flexion

Table C–3 presents the norm for range of motion for lateral flexion as 25 degrees. Dillard et al.[17] investigated lateral flexion using the inclinometer and reported 37 degrees of lateral flexion (Table C–13). Therefore, a rationale appears to exist for having a norm of at least 30 degrees for lateral flexion (Table C–4).

Rotation

The AMA suggests that rotation be measured with an inclinometer by having the subject flex to horizontal and then rotate the spine as far as possible. The AMA then suggests that normative rotation using this technique is 30 degrees (Table C–3). However, range of motion determined using this technique reported in the literature comes nowhere close to 30 degrees. Boline et al.[8] reported 6 degrees of motion for both right and left rotation (Table C–14). Based on this study, the 30-degree norm reported in Table C–3 is much too high.

SUMMARY: THORACIC AND LUMBAR SPINE, ADULTS 20–40 YEARS

As indicated previously, Table C–3 was presented to provide a base against which studies that collected data on actual range of motion in the thoracic and lumbar spine could be compared. Based on the review of literature related to normative data, and with knowledge of the limitation dependent on sample size described in Chapter 2, Table C–4 provides recommended normative ranges of motion for tape measure (flexion only), goniometer, and inclinometer measurement of thoracic and lumbar spine range of motion.

NORMATIVE RANGE OF MOTION: CERVICAL SPINE

Table C–5 presents suggested normative ranges of motion for the cervical spine as measured by tape measure, goniometer, inclinometer, and Cervical Range of Motion (CROM) device. These data are presented as a basis for discussion of published reports based on actual data collection.

TAPE MEASURE: ADULTS 20–40 YEARS

No "normative" data have been suggested as being considered normal for measurement of cervical range of motion with a tape measure. In reviewing the only two studies reporting mean data for cervical range of motion as measured with a tape measure, consistent data were reported in the studies by Balogun et al.[6] and Hsieh and Yeung[32] (Tables C–15 through C–18). Therefore, these data are provided in Table C–5 as appropriate until future research refutes this information.

	TABLE			
MOTION	**MEASURE***	**GONIOMETER†**	**INCLINOMETER‡**	**CROM§**
Flexion	1–4 cm	45°	50°	50°
Extension	20 cm	45°	60°	75°
Lateral Flexion	15 cm	45°	45°	45°
Rotation	10 cm	—	80°	70°

Table C–5. SUGGESTED VALUES FOR NORMAL ROM OF CERVICAL SPINE IN ADULTS

* Cervical spine norms derived from data by Balogun et al.[6] and Hsieh and Yeung.[32]
† Cervical spine norms provided by the American Medical Association.[4]
‡ Cervical spine norms provided by the American Medical Association.[5]
§ Cervical spine norms derived from means of male and female data from ages 20–40 years according to study by Youdas et al.[63] CROM, Cervical Range of Motion device.
Note: The American Academy of Orthopedic Surgeons[24] does not provide normative data using a tape measure, inclinometer, or CROM for cervical range of motion.

GONIOMETER AND INCLINOMETER: ADULTS 20–40 YEARS

Although Youdas et al.[62] reported on the reliability of the goniometer, no studies have reported actual range of motion collected in the measurement of the cervical spine using that device. Additionally, no investigations including normative data related to cervical range of motion measured with the inclinometer have been published. Therefore, given that no other data suggest otherwise, the norms provided by the second edition[4] (for measurement with the goniometer) and the fourth edition[5] (for measurement with the inclinometer) of the AMA's *Guides to Physical Impairment and Disability* are provided in Table C–5.

CROM: ADULTS 20–40 YEARS

Information on cervical range of motion measured with the CROM device presented in Table C–5 is derived from the data provided by Youdas et al.[63] by calculating the overall means of the combined data for males and females in the 20- to 40-year-old age brackets. The reasons for using the data supplied by Youdas et al.[63] as the "standard" and not using other studies examining range of motion provided by the CROM device are twofold. The study by Youdas et al.[63] is the only study to examine cervical range of motion across the age span using a large sample size ($n = 337$), and this study is referenced by the manufacturer of the CROM device for providing normal values (Performance Attachment Associates; St. Paul, Minn).

Two studies other than the investigation by Youdas et al.[63] have provided data on cervical flexion and extension as measured by the CROM device. Studies by Ordway et al.[45] and by Capuano-Pucci et al.[13] (Table C–15 and C–16) provide support for the 50-degree range of motion for flexion and the 75-degree range of motion for extension suggested by Youdas et al.[63] (Table C–5). In the only other study providing data using the CROM device to measure lateral flexion and rotation of the cervical spine, Capuano-Pucci et al.[13] (Tables C–17 and C–18) are in agreement with the 45-degree measurement for lateral flexion and the 70-degree measurement for rotation suggested by Youdas et al.[63] (Table C–5). Therefore, support exists for the suggested normative ranges of cervical motion for subjects aged 20 to 40 years presented in Table C–5.

NORMATIVE RANGE OF MOTION: LOWER EXTREMITIES

Table C–6 provides suggested normative range of motion values for the lower extremities of adults. Fewer of the values listed for the lower extremities, than for the upper extremities, are identical to values listed by either the AAOS or the AMA (Table C–7). While the literature supported retaining some AAOS and AMA values (see Tables C–19 through C–23 and additional tables available at www.wbsaunders.com/SIMON/Reese/joint/), many of the original AAOS and AMA values were altered to better reflect published data. Some values, such as those for hip adduction, knee flexion, and ankle dorsiflexion, were altered only slightly from the AAOS or the AMA values, owing to information gleaned from published studies. However, in other cases, data were not present to support either the AAOS or the AMA values, and normative range of motion values for those particular movements were changed to better reflect the published literature. Motions with values more substantially changed from the AAOS or AMA values include hip extension, hip medial rotation, hip lateral rotation, and flexion and extension of the 1st metatarsophalangeal (MTP) joint.

The mean range of hip extension has been lowered from 0 to 30 degrees, as reported by the AAOS and the AMA, to 0 to 20 degrees. This decrease in the mean hip extension range of motion is supported by three studies that investigated hip range of motion in adult subjects (Table C–19). Both Roaas and Anderson[47] and Ahlberg et al.[2] measured hip extension in adult males aged 30 to 40 years. Mean hip extension reported by the two studies was 10 ± 5 degrees for the Roaas and Anderson[47] study ($n = 105$), and 14 ± 6 degrees for the Ahlberg et al.[2] study ($n = 50$). Similarly, Boone and Azen[9]

JOINT	ROM
Table C–6. SUGGESTED VALUES FOR NORMAL ROM FOR JOINTS OF THE LOWER EXTREMITY IN ADULTS BASED ON ANALYSIS OF EXISTING DATA	
Hip	
Flexion	0°–120°
Extension	0°–20°
Abduction	0°–40° to 45°
Adduction	0°–25° to 30°
Medial Rotation	0°–35° to 40°
Lateral Rotation	0°–35° to 40°
Knee	
Flexion	0°–140° to 145°
Extension	0°
Ankle/Foot	
Dorsiflexion*	0°–15° to 20°
Plantarflexion†	0°–40° to 50°
Inversion†	0°–30° to 35°
Eversion*	0°–20°
1st Metatarsophalangeal (MTP) Joint	
Flexion	0°–20°
Extension	0°–80°

* Component of pronation. (ROM values apply to foot, not to isolated subtalar joint, motion.)

† Component of supination. (ROM values apply to foot, not to isolated subtalar joint, motion.)

JOINT	ROM VALUES	
Hip	**AAOS, 1965[3]***	**AMA, 1984[4]†**
Flexion	0°–120°	0°–100°
Extension	0°–30°	0°–30°
Abduction	0°–45°	0°–40°
Adduction	0°–30°	0°–20°
Medial Rotation	0°–45°	0°–50°
Lateral Rotation	0°–45°	0°–40°
Knee		
Flexion	0°–135°	0°–150°
Extension	0°–10°	0°
Ankle/Foot		
Dorsiflexion‡	0°–20°	0°–20°
Plantarflexion§	0°–50°	0°–40°
Inversion§	0°–35°	0°–30°
Eversion‡	0°–15°	0°–20°
1st Metatarsophalangeal (MTP) Joint		
Flexion	0°–45°	0°–30°
Extension	0°–70°	0°–50°

Table C–7. TRADITIONALLY QUOTED VALUES FOR NORMAL ROM FOR JOINTS OF THE LOWER EXTREMITY IN ADULTS

* American Academy of Orthopaedic Surgeons.
† American Medical Association.
‡ Component of pronation.
§ Component of supination.

reported mean hip extension values of 12 ± 6 degrees in a study of 56 males aged 20 to 54 years. Only two studies reported mean hip extension values higher than 15 degrees. Data from the NHANES I, reported by Roach and Miles,[48] yielded a mean value for hip extension of 22 ± 8 degrees, while Svenningsen et al.[56] reported mean values of 24 degrees for hip extension in adults (Table C–19). Since none of the studies that have examined hip extension range of motion in adults reported hip extension values in the 30-degree range, the value for mean hip extension range of motion was lowered to 0 to 20 degrees.

Several studies that have investigated hip rotation provide support for lowered values for hip medial and lateral rotation range of motion (Tables C–20 and C–21). Four groups of investigators measured active hip rotation range of motion in adult subjects while the subjects were seated with their hips and knees flexed to 90 degrees.[27, 47, 48, 54] Mean values for hip medial rotation from the four studies ranged from a low of 33 ± 6 degrees to a high of 37 ± 7 degrees. For hip lateral rotation, the mean values reported ranged from a low of 33 ± 5 degrees to a high of 36 ± 8 degrees. With the exception of a study by Boone and Azen,[9] the only reports of active hip rotation in adults exceeding 40 degrees come from studies in which the sample population is from a culture in which increased hip motion has been identified.[2, 23, 30]

In adult subjects younger than 45 years of age, extension of the 1st MTP joint appears to exceed the norms of 0 to 50 degrees or 0 to 70 degrees, as published by the AMA and the AAOS, respectively. Data gathered from male[35] or from male and female[12, 31] adult subjects demonstrates 1st MTP extension in the 75- to 95-degree range, when the subject is younger than 45 years of age (Table C–22). Conversely, mean flexion of the 1st MTP joint appears to be less than reported by either the AMA or the AAOS (Table C–7). Mean values reported for 1st MTP flexion did not exceed 20 degrees when a universal goniometer was used to measure the motion,[12] and values did not exceed 25 degrees when motion was measured using radiographic techniques (Table C–23).[35]

Table C–8. INVESTIGATIONS REPORTING DATA FOR SHOULDER FLEXION ROM

STUDY	SAMPLE	AGES	METHOD USED	NUMBER OF EXAMINERS	TYPE OF MOTION	RELIABILITY COEFFICIENT CALCULATED?	ROM
Boone & Azen[9]	53 M	1–19 years	AAOS	1	AROM	No	168° ± 4°
Boone & Azen[9]	56 M	20–54 years	AAOS	1	AROM	No	165° ± 5°
Sabari et al.[52]	30 (# M & F not stated)	17–92 years	Supine	1	AROM	ICC .95	160° ± 12°
Sabari et al.[52]	30 (# M & F not stated)	17–92 years	Sitting	1	AROM	ICC .97	158° ± 15°
Sabari et al.[52]	30 (# M & F not stated)	17–92 years	Supine	1	PROM	ICC .94	163° ± 13°
Sabari et al.[52]	30 (# M & F not stated)	17–92 years	Sitting	1	PROM	ICC .95	160° ± 15°
Walker et al.[59]	60 (30 M, 30 F)	60–84 years	AAOS	1	AROM	Pearson's r > .81	165° ± 10°
Watanabe et al.[60]	339/Japanese	Birth to 2 years	Not stated	Not stated	PROM	Unknown	172° – 180°

M, males; F, females; AAOS, American Academy of Orthopaedic Surgeons; AROM, active range of motion; ICC, intraclass correlation; PROM, passive range of motion.

Table C–9. INVESTIGATIONS REPORTING DATA FOR SHOULDER ABDUCTION ROM

STUDY	SAMPLE	AGES	METHOD USED	NUMBER OF EXAMINERS	TYPE OF MOTION	RELIABILITY COEFFICIENT CALCULATED?	ROM
Boone & Azen[9]	53 M	1–19 years	AAOS	1	AROM	No	185° ± 4°
Boone & Azen[9]	56 M	20–54 years	AAOS	1	AROM	No	183° ± 9°
Gunal et al.[25]	1000 M/ Turkish	18–22 years	AAOS	2	PROM	No	166° ± 6° (R) 168° ± 19° (L)
Sabari et al.[52]	30 (# M & F not stated)	17–92 years	Supine	1	AROM	ICC .99	162° ± 19°
Sabari et al.[52]	30 (# M & F not stated)	17–92 years	Sitting	1	AROM	ICC .97	156° ± 17°
Sabari et al.[52]	30 (# M & F not stated)	17–92 years	Supine	1	PROM	ICC .98	163° ± 17°
Sabari et al.[52]	30 (# M & F not stated)	17–92 years	Sitting	1	PROM	ICC .95	158° ± 16°
Walker et al.[59]	60 (30 M, 30 F)	60–84 years	AAOS	1	AROM	Pearson's r > .81	165° ± 19°
Watanabe et al.[60]	339/Japanese	Birth to 2 years	Not stated	Not stated	PROM	Unknown	177°–187°

M, males; F, females; AAOS, American Academy of Orthopaedic Surgeons; AROM, active range of motion; ICC, intraclass correlation; PROM, passive range of motion; R, right; L, left.

Table C–10. INVESTIGATIONS REPORTING DATA FOR INTERPHALANGEAL FLEXION (THUMB) ROM

STUDY	SAMPLE	AGES	METHOD USED	NUMBER OF EXAMINERS	TYPE OF MOTION	RELIABILITY COEFFICIENT CALCULATED?	ROM
Jenkins et al.[33]	119 (50 M, 69 F)	16–72 years	Elbow flexed to 90°; wrist/forearm neutral	1	AROM	No	67° ± 11°
Shaw & Morris[53]	348 (199 M, 149 F)	16–86 years	Not stated	Not stated	AROM	No	64° ± 13° (R) 65° ± 12° (L)

M, males; F, females; AROM, active range of motion; R, right; L, left.

Table C–11. INVESTIGATIONS REPORTING DATA FOR THORACIC AND LUMBAR FLEXION ROM

STUDY	SAMPLE SIZE	AGES (YEARS)	INSTRUMENTATION	METHOD USED	NUMBER OF EXAMINERS	ROM	RELIABILITY ESTABLISHED?
Haley et al.[28]	282 (140 M, 142 F)	5–9	Tape Measure	Modified Schober	1	6–7 cm ± 1 cm	ICC* .83
Einkauf et al.[19]	109 F	20–84	Tape Measure	Modified Schober	2	5–7 cm ± 1 cm	Unknown correlation (inter) .98
Fitzgerald et al.[21]	172 (168 M, 4 F)	20–82	Tape Measure	Schober	Not reported	2–4 cm ± 1 cm	Pearson's *r* (inter) 1.0
Moll and Wright[42]	237 (119 M, 118 F)	15–75	Tape Measure	Modified Schober	Not reported	5–7 cm ± 1 cm	No
van Adrichem & van der Korst[58]	66 (34 M, 32 F)	15–18	Tape Measure	Modified Schober	Not reported	6 cm ± 1 cm	No
Mayer et al.[39]	13	$\bar{x}$ = 31	Double Inclinometer	—	1	55° ± 9°	No
Chiarello & Savidge[14]	12 (4 M, 8 F)	23–35	Double Inclinometer	—	3	59° ± 5°	ICC (inter) .74
Dillard et al.[17]	20 (10 M, 10 F)	20–40	Double Inclinometer	—	1	63° ± 11°	Pearson's *r* .79
Breum et al.[10]	47 (27 M, 20 F)	18–38	BROM†	—	1	56° ± 10°	ICC .63

M, males; F, females.
* Intraclass correlation.
† Back Range of Motion device.

Table C–12. INVESTIGATIONS REPORTING DATA FOR THORACIC AND LUMBAR EXTENSION ROM

STUDY	SAMPLE SIZE	AGES (YEARS)	INSTRUMENTATION	NUMBER OF EXAMINERS	ROM	RELIABILITY ESTABLISHED?
Beattie et al.[7]	100 (63 M, 37 F)	20–76	Tape Measure Modified Schober	1	.58–2.0 cm ± 0–1 cm	ICC* .93
Einkauf et al.[19]	109 F	20–84	Goniometer	2	18°–36°	Unknown correlation (inter) .93
Fitzgerald et al.[21]	172 (168 M, 4 F)	20–82	Goniometer	Not reported	16°–41°	Pearson's *r* (inter) .88
Mayer et al.[39]	13	$\bar{x}$ = 31	Double Inclinometer	1	27° ± 13°	No
Chiarello & Savidge[14]	12 (4 M, 8 F)	23–35	Double Inclinometer	3	32° ± 10°	ICC (inter) .65
Dillard et al.[17]	20 (10 M, 10 F)	20–40	Double Inclinometer	Not reported	29° ± 8°	Pearson's *r* .28
Breum et al.[10]	47 (27 M, 20 F)	18–38	BROM†	1	22° ± 8°	ICC .35

M, males; F, females.
* Intraclass correlation.
† Back Range of Motion device.

Table C–13. INVESTIGATIONS REPORTING DATA FOR THORACIC AND LUMBAR LATERAL FLEXION ROM

STUDY	SAMPLE SIZE	AGES (YEARS)	INSTRUMENTATION	METHOD USED	NUMBER OF EXAMINERS	ROM	RELIABILITY ESTABLISHED?
Rose[49]	18 (15 M, 3 F)	$\bar{x}$ = 19.5 ± 4.6	Tape Measure	Marks at lateral thigh	1	23 cm ± 3 cm (R) 23 cm ± 3 cm (L)	Pearson's r .89 (R), .78 (L)
Einkauf et al.[19]	109 F	20–84	Goniometer	Thoracolumbar	2	24°–36° (R) 20°–33° (L)	Pearson's r (intra) .89 (R), .78 (L)
Fitzgerald et al.[21]	172 (168 M, 4 F)	20–82	Goniometer	Thoracolumbar	Not reported	18°–38° (R) 19°–39° (L)	Pearson's r (inter) .76 (R), .91 (L)
Dillard et al.[17]	20 (10 M, 10 F)	20–40	Single Inclinometer	Lumbar	1	37° ± 8° (R) 37° ± 8° (L)	Pearson's r .59 (R), .62 (L)
Breum et al.[10]	47 (27 M, 20 F)	18–38	BROM*	Lumbar	1	33° ± 6° (R) 34° ± 6° (L)	ICC† .89 (R), .92 (L)

M, males, F, females; R, right; L, left.
* Back Range of Motion device.
† Intraclass correlation.

Table C–14. INVESTIGATIONS REPORTING DATA FOR THORACIC AND LUMBAR ROTATION ROM

STUDY	SAMPLE SIZE	AGES (YEARS)	INSTRUMENTATION	METHOD USED	NUMBER OF EXAMINERS	ROM	RELIABILITY ESTABLISHED?
Dillard et al.[17]	20 (10 M, 10 F)	20–40	Double Inclinometer	"Standing at edge of table"	1	28° ± 5° (R) 29° ± 8° (L)	Pearson's r .64 (R), .40 (L)
Boline et al.[8]	25 (17 M, 8 F)	$\bar{x}$ = 33 ± 4.1	Single Inclinometer	Flexed to horizontal and rotate	2	6° ± 3° (R) 6° ± 3° (L)	ICC† (inter) .73
Breum et al.[10]	47 (27 M, 20 F)	18–38	BROM*	Sitting	Not reported	8° ± 6° (R) 7° ± 4° (L)	ICC .57 (R), .56 (L)

M, males; F, females; R, right; L, left.
* Back Range of Motion device.
† Intraclass correlation.

Table C–15. INVESTIGATIONS REPORTING DATA FOR CERVICAL FLEXION ROM

STUDY	SAMPLE SIZE	AGES (YEARS)	INSTRUMENTATION	NUMBER OF EXAMINERS	ROM	RELIABILITY ESTABLISHED?
Ordway et al.[45]	20 (9 M, 11 F)	20–49	CROM*	Not reported	48° ± 13°	No
Youdas et al.[63]	337 (166 M, 177 F)	11–97	CROM	5	36°–64° ± 8°–11°	ICC† (intra) .23–.88
Capuano-Pucci et al.[13]	20 (4 M, 16 F)	$\bar{x}$ = 23.5 ± 3	CROM	2	50° ± 9°	Pearson's r (intra) .63, .91
Balogun et al.[6]	21 (15 M, 6 F)	18–26	Tape Measure	3	4 cm ± 2 cm	Pearson's r (intra) .26, .49, .48
Hsieh & Yeung[32]	34 (27 M, 7 F)	14–31	Tape Measure	2	1 cm ± 2 cm	Pearson's r (intra) .86, .95

M, males; F, females.
* Cervical Range of Motion device.
† Intraclass correlation.

Table C–16. INVESTIGATIONS REPORTING DATA FOR CERVICAL EXTENSION ROM

STUDY	SAMPLE SIZE	AGES (YEARS)	INSTRUMENTATION	NUMBER OF EXAMINERS	ROM	RELIABILITY ESTABLISHED?
Ordway et al.[45]	20 (9 M, 11 F)	20–49	CROM*	Not reported	79° ± 18°	No
Youdas et al.[63]	337 (166 M, 177 F)	11–97	CROM	5	52°–86° ± 10°–18°	ICC† (intra) .89–.96
Capuano-Pucci et al.[13]	20 (4 M, 16 F)	x̄ = 23.5 ± 3	CROM	2	71° ± 9°	Pearson's r (intra) .90, .82
Balogun et al.[6]	21 (15 M, 6 F)	18–26	Tape Measure	3	19 cm ± 2 cm	Pearson's r (intra) .72, .87, .88
Hsieh & Yeung[32]	34 (27 M, 7 F)	14–31	Tape Measure	2	22 cm ± 2 cm	Pearson's r (intra) .79, .94

M, males; F, females.
* Cervical Range of Motion device.
† Intraclass correlation.

Table C–17. INVESTIGATIONS REPORTING DATA FOR CERVICAL LATERAL FLEXION ROM

STUDY	SAMPLE SIZE	AGES (YEARS)	INSTRUMENTATION	NUMBER OF EXAMINERS	ROM	RELIABILITY ESTABLISHED?
Youdas et al.[63]	337 (166 M, 177 F)	11–97	CROM*	5	22°–49° (R) 22°–47° (L)	ICC† (intra) .60–.94
Capuano-Pucci et al.[13]	20 (4 M, 16 F)	x̄ = 23.5 ± 3	CROM	2	43° ± 7° (R) 44° ± 8° (L)	Pearson's r (intra) .79, .90
Balogun et al.[6]	21 (15 M, 6 F)	18–26	Tape Measure	3	13 cm ± 2 cm(R) 13 cm ± 2 cm(L)	Pearson's r (intra) .53–.77
Hsieh & Yeung[32]	34 (27 M, 7 F)	14–31	Tape Measure	2	12 cm ± 2 cm(R) 12 cm ± 2 cm(L)	Pearson's r (intra) .86, .91

M, males; F, females; R, right; L, left.
* Cervical Range of Motion device.
† Intraclass correlation.

Table C–18. INVESTIGATIONS REPORTING DATA FOR CERVICAL ROTATION ROM

STUDY	SAMPLE SIZE	AGES (YEARS)	INSTRUMENTATION	NUMBER OF EXAMINERS	ROM	RELIABILITY ESTABLISHED?
Youdas et al.[63]	337 (166 M, 177 F)	11–97	CROM*	5	44°–75° (R) 45°–72° (L)	ICC† (intra) .58–.99
Capuano-Pucci et al.[13]	20 (4 M, 16 F)	x̄ = 23.5 ± 3	CROM	2	70° ± 7° (R) 69° ± 7° (L)	Pearson's r (intra) .62, .89
Balogun et al.[6]	21 (15 M, 6 F)	18–26	Tape Measure	3	11 cm ± 3 cm(R) 11 cm ± 2 cm(L)	Pearson's r (intra) .59–.86
Hsieh & Yeung[32]	34 (27 M, 7 F)	14–31	Tape Measure	2	11 cm ± 2 cm(R) 11 cm ± 2 cm(L)	Pearson's r (intra) .78, .88

M, males; F, females; R, right; L, left.
* Cervical Range of Motion device.
† Intraclass correlation.

Table C–19. INVESTIGATIONS REPORTING DATA FOR HIP EXTENSION ROM

STUDY	SAMPLE	AGES	METHOD USED	NUMBER OF EXAMINERS	TYPE OF MOTION	RELIABILITY COEFFICIENT CALCULATED?	ROM
Ahlberg et al.[2]	50 M/Saudi Arabian	30–40 years	AAOS	1	PROM	No	$14° \pm 6°$
Boone & Azen[9]	53 M	1–19 years	AAOS	1	AROM	No	$7° \pm 7°$
Boone & Azen[9]	56 M	20–54 years	AAOS	1	AROM	No	$12° \pm 6°$
Broughton et al.[11]	57 (# M & F not stated)	Neonates; 1–7 days	Not sufficiently described	1	PROM	No	$-34° \pm 6°$
Broughton et al.[11]	57 (# M & F not stated)	3 months	Not sufficiently described	1	PROM	No	$-19° \pm 6°$
Broughton et al.[11]	57 (# M & F not stated)	6 months	Not sufficiently described	1	PROM	No	$-8° \pm 6°$
Coon et al.[16]	44 (25 M, 19 F)	6 weeks	Supine, contralateral hip flexed	1	PROM	No	$-19° \pm 6°$
Coon et al.[16]	44 (25 M, 19 F)	3 months	Supine, contralateral hip flexed	1	PROM	No	$-7° \pm 4°$
Coon et al.[16]	40 (19 M, 21 F)	6 months	Supine, contralateral hip flexed	1	PROM	No	$-7° \pm 4°$
Drews et al.[18]	54 (26 M, 28 F)	12 hours–6 days	Sidelying, contralateral hip flexed	2	PROM	Pearson's *r* (inter) .56 (L) .74 (R)	$-28° \pm 6°$
Forero et al.[22]	60 (34 M, 26 F)/ (42 Hispanic, 15 white, 3 black)	1–3 days	Supine, contralateral hip flexed	1	PROM	Pearson's *r* .99	$-30° \pm 4°$
Haas et al.[26]	400 (192 M, 208 F)/(200 white, 200 black)	1 hour–3 days	Supine, contralateral hip flexed	2	PROM	No	$-30° \pm 8°$
Mundale et al.[43]	36 (16 M, 20 F)	20–30 years	Mundale technique	Not stated	PROM	95% within ± 4°	$-11°$
Phelps et al.[46]	25 (# M & F per group not stated)	9 months	Prone, both hips flexed over end of table	1	PROM	No	$-10° \pm 3°$
Phelps et al.[46]	25 (# M & F per group not stated)	12 months	Prone, both hips flexed over end of table	1	PROM	No	$-9° \pm 5°$
Phelps et al.[46]	18 (# M & F per group not stated)	18 months	Prone, both hips flexed over end of table	1	PROM	No	$-4° \pm 3°$
Phelps et al.[46]	18 (# M & F per group not stated)	24 months	Prone, both hips flexed over end of table	1	PROM	No	$-3° \pm 3°$
Roaas & Anderson[47]	105 M (210 hips)/Swedish	30–40 years	AAOS, 1965; contralateral hip flexed	1	PROM	No	$9° \pm 5°$ (R) $10° \pm 5°$ (L)
Roach & Miles[48]	433 (200 M, 233 F)/(346 white, 87 black)	25–39 years	Prone, with knee extended	1	AROM	"Satisfactory level of reproducibility not achieved."	$22° \pm 8°$

(Table continued on following page)

Table C–19. (Cont.)

STUDY	SAMPLE	AGES	METHOD USED	NUMBER OF EXAMINERS	TYPE OF MOTION	RELIABILITY COEFFICIENT CALCULATED?	ROM
Roach & Miles[48]	727 (368 M, 359 F)/(565 white, 162 black)	40–59 years	Prone, with knee extended	1	AROM	"Satisfactory level of reproducibility not achieved."	18° ± 7°
Roach & Miles[48]	523 (253 M, 270 F)/(402 white, 121 black)	60–74 years	Prone, with knee extended	1	AROM	"Satisfactory level of reproducibility not achieved."	17° ± 8°
Svenningsen et al.[56]	103 (51 M, 52 F)	4 years	AAOS	1	PROM	No	29°
Svenningsen et al.[56]	102 (50 M, 52 F)	6 years	AAOS	1	PROM	No	26°
Svenningsen et al.[56]	104 (52 M, 52 F)	8 years	AAOS	1	PROM	No	27°
Svenningsen et al.[56]	134 (65 M, 69 F)	11 years	AAOS	1	PROM	No	25°
Svenningsen et al.[56]	114 (57 M, 57 F)	15 years	AAOS	1	PROM	No	26°
Svenningsen et al.[56]	206 (102 M, 104 F)	Adult; $\bar{x}$ = 23 years	AAOS	1	PROM	No	24°
Walker et al.[59]	60 (30 M, 30 F)	60–84 years	AAOS	1	AROM	Pearson's r >.81	−11° ± 4°
Watanabe et al.[60]	62/Japanese	Neonates	Not stated	Not stated	PROM	Unknown	−25°
Watanabe et al.[60]	62/Japanese	4 weeks	Not stated	Not stated	PROM	Unknown	−12°
Watanabe et al.[60]	54/Japanese	4–8 months	Not stated	Not stated	PROM	Unknown	−4°
Watanabe et al.[60]	45/Japanese	8–12 months	Not stated	Not stated	PROM	Unknown	3°
Watanabe et al.[60]	64/Japanese	1 year	Not stated	Not stated	PROM	Unknown	15°
Watanabe et al.[60]	64/Japanese	2 years	Not stated	Not stated	PROM	Unknown	21°
Waugh et al.[61]	40 (18 M, 22 F)	9 months	Prone, both hips flexed over end of table	1	PROM	No	−10° ± 3°

M, males; F, females; AROM, active range of motion; PROM, passive range of motion; AAOS, American Academy of Orthopaedic Surgeons.

Table C–20. INVESTIGATIONS REPORTING DATA FOR HIP LATERAL ROTATION ROM

STUDY	SAMPLE	AGES	METHOD USED	NUMBER OF EXAMINERS	TYPE OF MOTION	RELIABILITY COEFFICIENT CALCULATED?	ROM
Ahlberg et al.[2]	50 M/Saudi Arabian	30–40 years	AAOS	1	PROM	No	73° ± 11°
Boone & Azen[9]	53 M	1–19 years	AAOS–seated	1	AROM	No	51° ± 6°
Boone & Azen[9]	56 M	20–54 years	AAOS–seated	1	AROM	No	44° ± 5°
Coon et al.[16]	44 (25 M, 19 F)	6 weeks	Prone, hip extended, knee flexed to 90°	1	PROM	No	48° ± 11°
Coon et al.[16]	44 (25 M, 19 F)	3 months	Prone, hip extended, knee flexed to 90°	1	PROM	No	45° ± 5°
Coon et al.[16]	40 (19 M, 21 F)	6 months	Prone, hip extended, knee flexed to 90°	1	PROM	No	46° ± 5°
Drews et al.[18]	54 (26 M, 28 F)	12 hours–6 days	Supine, hip and knee flexed to 90°; contralateral hip and knee extended; stationary arm—parallel anterior midline of trunk; moving arm—tibial crest axis—midpatella	2	PROM	Pearson's *r* (inter) .63 (L) .79 (R)	114° ± 10°
Ellison et al.[20]	100 (25 M, 75 F)	20–41 years	Prone, knee flexed to 90°	1	PROM	ICC .96	36° ± 8° (L) 35° ± 7° (R)
Forero et al.[22]	60 (34 M, 26 F) (42 Hispanic, 15 white, 3 black)	1–3 days	Supine, hip/knee flexed to 90°	1	PROM	Pearson's *r* .99	92° ± 3°
Giladi et al.[23]	295 males	18–20 years	AAOS, hip flexed to 90°	Not stated	Not stated	No	57° ± 9°
Haas et al.[26]	400 (192 M, 208 F)/(200 white, 200 black)	1 hour–3 days	Supine, hips and knees flexed to 90°	2	PROM	No	89° ± 14°
Haley[27]	50 F	21–50 years	Seated, hip and knee flexed to 90°	1	AROM	No	33° ± 5°
Haley[27]	50 F	21–50 years	Seated, hip and knee flexed to 90°	1	PROM	No	45° ± 5°
Haley[27]	50 F	21–50 years	Supine, hip extended	1	AROM	No	31° ± 6°
Haley[27]	50 F	21–50 years	Supine, hip extended	1	PROM	No	43° ± 5°
Hoaglund et al.[30]	211 (112 M, 99 F)/Chinese	55–85+ years	Hip flexed to 90°	1	PROM (according to photo; not stated)	No	62° ± 13°
Hoaglund et al.[30]	211 (112 M, 99 F)/Chinese	55–85+ years	Hip neutral flexion/ extension	1	PROM (according to photo; not stated)	No	53° ± 9°
Phelps et al.[46]	25 (# M & F per group not stated)	9 months	Prone, hip extended, knee flexed to 90°	1	PROM	No	56° ± 7°

(Table continued on following page)

Table C–20. (Cont.)

STUDY	SAMPLE	AGES	METHOD USED	NUMBER OF EXAMINERS	TYPE OF MOTION	RELIABILITY COEFFICIENT CALCULATED?	ROM
Phelps et al.[46]	25 (# M & F per group not stated)	12 months	Prone, hip extended, knee flexed to 90°	1	PROM	No	58° ± 9°
Phelps et al.[46]	18 (# M & F per group not stated)	18 months	Prone, hip extended, knee flexed to 90°	1	PROM	No	52° ± 9°
Phelps et al.[46]	18 (# M & F per group not stated)	24 months	Prone, hip extended, knee flexed to 90°	1	PROM	No	47° ± 9°
Roaas & Anderson[47]	105 M (210 hips)/Swedish	30–40 years	AAOS	1	PROM	No	34° ± 7°
Roach & Miles[48]	433 (200 M, 233 F)/(346 white, 87 black)	25–39 years	Seated, hip and knee flexed to 90°	1	AROM	"Satisfactory level of reproducibility not achieved"	34° ± 8°
Roach & Miles[48]	727 (368 M, 359 F)/(565 white, 162 black)	40–59 years	Seated, hip and knee flexed to 90°	1	AROM	"Satisfactory level of reproducibility not achieved"	32° ± 8°
Roach & Miles[48]	523 (253 M, 270 F)/(402 white, 121 black)	60–74 years	Seated, hip and knee flexed to 90°	1	AROM	"Satisfactory level of reproducibility not achieved"	29°
Simoneau et al.[54]	60 (21 M, 39 F)	18–27 years	Seated, hip and knee flexed to 90°	6	AROM	ICC (inter) .90	36° ± 8°
Simoneau et al.[54]	60 (21 M, 39 F)	18–27 years	Prone, hip extended, knee flexed to 90°	6	AROM	ICC (inter) .93	45° ± 11°
Svenningsen et al.[56]	103 (51 M, 52 F)	4 years	AAOS	1	PROM	No	46°
Svenningsen et al.[56]	102 (50 M, 52 F)	6 years	AAOS	1	PROM	No	45°
Svenningsen et al.[56]	104 (52 M, 52 F)	8 years	AAOS	1	PROM	No	43°
Svenningsen et al.[56]	134 (65 M, 69 F)	11 years	AAOS	1	PROM	No	42°
Svenningsen et al.[56]	114 (57 M, 57 F)	15 years	AAOS	1	PROM	No	43°
Svenningsen et al.[56]	206 (102 M, 104 F)	Adult; $\bar{x}$ = 23 years	AAOS	1	PROM	No	42°
Walker et al.[59]	60 (30 M, 30 F)	60–84 years	AAOS—seated	1	AROM	Pearson's r >.81	32° ± 6°
Watanabe et al.[60]	62/Japanese	Birth	Not stated	Not stated	PROM	Unknown	77°
Watanabe et al.[60]	62/Japanese	4 weeks	Not stated	Not stated	PROM	Unknown	66°
Watanabe et al.[60]	54/Japanese	4–8 months	Not stated	Not stated	PROM	Unknown	66°
Watanabe et al.[60]	45/Japanese	8–12 months	Not stated	Not stated	PROM	Unknown	79°
Watanabe et al.[60]	64/Japanese	1 year	Not stated	Not stated	PROM	Unknown	74°
Watanabe et al.[60]	57/Japanese	2 years	Not stated	Not stated	PROM	Unknown	58°

M, males; F, females; AAOS, American Academy of Orthopaedic Surgeons; AROM, active range of motion; PROM, passive range of motion; ICC, intraclass correlation.

Table C–21. INVESTIGATIONS REPORTING DATA FOR HIP MEDIAL ROTATION ROM

STUDY	SAMPLE	AGES	METHOD USED	NUMBER OF EXAMINERS	TYPE OF MOTION	RELIABILITY COEFFICIENT CALCULATED?	ROM
Ahlberg et al.[2]	50 M/Saudi Arabian	30–40 years	AAOS	1	PROM	No	37° ± 12°
Boone & Azen[9]	53 M	1–19 years	AAOS; seated	1	AROM	No	50° ± 6°
Boone & Azen[9]	56 M	20–54 years	AAOS; seated	1	AROM	No	44° ± 4°
Coon et al.[16]	44 (25 M, 19 F)	6 weeks	Prone, hip extended, knee flexed to 90°	1	PROM	No	24° ± 5°
Coon et al.[16]	44 (25 M, 19 F)	3 months	Prone, hip extended, knee flexed to 90°	1	PROM	No	26° ± 3°
Coon et al.[16]	40 (19 M, 21 F)	6 months	Prone, hip extended, knee flexed to 90°	1	PROM	No	21° ± 4°
Drews et al.[18]	54 (26 M, 28 F)	12 hours–6 days	Supine, hip and knee flexed to 90°; contral hip and knee extended; stat arm—parallel ant midline of trunk; moving arm—tibial crest; axis—midpatella	2	PROM	Pearson's r (inter) .91 (L) .78 (R)	80° ± 9°
Ellison (L) et al.[20] (R)	100 (25 M, 75 F)	20–41 years	Prone, knee flexed to 90°	1	PROM	ICC .98/.99	38° ± 11° 38° ± 11°
Forero et al.[22]	60 (26 F, 34 M) (42 Hispanic/ 15 white/ 3 black)	1–3 days	Supine, hip and knee flexed to 90°	1	PROM	Pearson's r .99	76° ± 6°
Giladi et al.[23]	295 M/Israeli	18–20 years	AAOS, hip flexed to 90°	Not stated	Not stated	No	53° ± 11°
Haley[27]	50 F	21–50 years	Seated, hip and knee flexed to 90°	1	AROM	No	37° ± 7°
Haley[27]	50 F	21–50 years	Seated, hip and knee flexed to 90°	1	PROM	No	45° ± 5°
Haley[27]	50 F	21–50 years	Supine, hip extended	1	AROM	No	26° ± 5°
Haley[27]	50 F	21–50 years	Supine, hip extended	1	PROM	No	38° ± 6°
Hoaglund et al.[30]	112 M	55–85+ years	Hip flexed to 90°	1	PROM (according to photo; not stated)	No	22° ± 8°
Hoaglund et al.[30]	99 F	55–85+ years	Hip flexed to 90°	1	PROM (according to photo; not stated)	No	31° ± 10°
Hoaglund et al.[30]	112 M	55–85+ years	Hip neutral, flex/extension	1	PROM (according to photo; not stated)	No	29° ± 11°

(Table continued on following page)

Table C-21. (Cont.)

STUDY	SAMPLE	AGES	METHOD USED	NUMBER OF EXAMINERS	TYPE OF MOTION	RELIABILITY COEFFICIENT CALCULATED?	ROM
Hoaglund et al.[30]	99 F	55–85+ years	Hip neutral, flex/extension	1	PROM (according to photo; not stated)	No	37° ± 8°
Haas et al.[26]	400 (192 M, 208 F)/(200 black/ 200 white)	1 hour–3 days	Supine, hips and knees flexed to 90°	2	PROM	No	62° ± 13°
Phelps et al.[46]	25 (# M & F per group not stated)	9 months	Prone, hip extended, knee flexed to 90°	1	PROM	No	41° ± 8°
Phelps et al.[46]	25 (# M & F per group not stated)	12 months	Prone, hip extended, knee flexed to 90°	1	PROM	No	44° ± 9°
Phelps et al.[46]	18 (# M & F per group not stated)	18 months	Prone, hip extended, knee flexed to 90°	1	PROM	No	45° ± 8°
Phelps et al.[46]	18 (# M & F per group not stated)	24 months	Prone, hip extended, knee flexed to 90°	1	PROM	No	52° ± 10°
Roaas & Anderson[47]	105 M/ Swedish	30–40 years	AAOS	1	PROM	No	33° ± 8°
Roach & Miles[48]	433 (200 M, 233 F)/(87 black/ 346 white)	25–39 years	Seated, hip and knee flexed to 90°	1	AROM	"Satisfactory" level of reproducibility not achieved.	33° ± 7°
Roach & Miles[48]	727 (368 M, 359 F)/(162 black/ 565 white)	40–59 years	Seated, hip and knee flexed to 90°	1	AROM	"Satisfactory" level of reproducibility not achieved.	31° ± 8°
Roach & Miles[48]	523 (253 M, 270 F)/(121 black/ 402 white)	60–74 years	Seated, hip and knee flexed to 90°	1	AROM	"Satisfactory" level of reproducibility not achieved.	30° ± 7°
Simoneau, et al.[54]	39 F	18–27 years	Seated, hip and knee flexed to 90°	6	AROM	ICC (inter) .91	35° ± 6°
Simoneau, et al.[54]	21 M	18–27 years	Seated, hip and knee flexed to 90°	6	AROM	ICC (inter) .91	30° ± 7°
Simoneau, et al.[54]	39 F	18–27 years	Prone, hip extended, knee flexed to 90°	6	AROM	ICC (inter) .94	38° ± 9°
Simoneau, et al.[54]	21 M	18–27 years	Prone, hip extended, knee flexed to 90°	6	AROM	ICC (inter) .94	32° ± 9°
Svenningsen et al.[56]	103 (51 M, 52 F)	4 years	AAOS	1	PROM	No	56°
Svenningsen et al.[56]	102 (50 M, 52 F)	6 years	AAOS	1	PROM	No	55°
Svenningsen et al.[56]	104 (52 M, 52 F)	8 years	AAOS	1	PROM	No	54°
Svenningsen et al.[56]	134 (65 M, 69 F)	11 years	AAOS	1	PROM	No	48°
Svenningsen et al.[56]	114 (57 M, 57 F)	15 years	AAOS	1	PROM	No	45°
Svenningsen et al.[56]	206 (102 M, 104 F)	Adult; $\bar{x}$ = 23 years	AAOS	1	PROM	No	45°
Walker et al.[59]	30 M	60–84 years	AAOS	1	AROM	Pearson's r >.81	22° ± 6°
Walker et al.[59]	30 F	60–84 years	AAOS	1	AROM	Pearson's r >.81	36° ± 7°

Table C–21. (Cont.)

STUDY	SAMPLE	AGES	METHOD USED	NUMBER OF EXAMINERS	TYPE OF MOTION	RELIABILITY COEFFICIENT CALCULATED?	ROM
Watanabe et al.[60]	62 Japanese	Birth	Not stated	Not stated	PROM	Unknown	21°
Watanabe et al.[60]	62 Japanese	4 weeks	Not stated	Not stated	PROM	Unknown	24°
Watanabe et al.[60]	54 Japanese	4–8 months	Not stated	Not stated	PROM	Unknown	39°
Watanabe et al.[60]	45 Japanese	8–12 months	Not stated	Not stated	PROM	Unknown	38°
Watanabe et al.[60]	64 Japanese	1 year	Not stated	Not stated	PROM	Unknown	49°
Watanabe et al.[60]	57 Japanese	2 years	Not stated	Not stated	PROM	Unknown	59°

M, males; F, females; AAOS, American Academy of Orthopaedic Surgeons; AROM, active range of motion; PROM, passive range of motion; ICC, intraclass correlation.

Table C–22.	INVESTIGATIONS REPORTING DATA FOR FIRST MTP EXTENSION						
STUDY	SAMPLE	AGES	METHOD USED	NUMBER OF EXAMINERS	TYPE OF MOTION	RELIABILITY COEFFICIENT CALCULATED?	ROM
Buell et al.[12]	15 (# M & F not stated)	19–30 years	STJN; midtarsal joint fully pronated, medial alignment	Not stated	AROM	No	88°
Buell et al.[12]	24 (# M & F not stated)	30–45 years	STJN; midtarsal joint fully pronated, medial alignment	Not stated	AROM	No	77°
Buell et al.[12]	11 (# M & F not stated)	Older than 45 years	STJN; midtarsal joint fully pronated, medial alignment	Not stated	AROM	No	62°
Buell et al.[12]	15 (# M & F not stated)	19–30 years	STJN; midtarsal joint fully pronated, medial alignment	Not stated	PROM	No	95°
Buell et al.[12]	24 (# M & F not stated)	30–45 years	STJN; midtarsal joint fully pronated, medial alignment	Not stated	PROM	No	82°
Buell et al.[12]	11 (# M & F not stated)	Older than 45 years	STJN; midtarsal joint fully pronated, medial alignment	Not stated	PROM	No	65°
Hopson et al.[31]	20 (10 M, 10 F)	21–43 years	Supine, medial alignment of UG	1	PROM	ICC .95	96° ± 10°
Hopson et al.[31]	20 (10 M, 10 F)	21–43 years	Supine, dorsal alignment of UG	1	PROM	ICC .91	85° ± 11°
Hopson et al.[31]	20 (10 M, 10 F)	21–43 years	Seated, partial weight bearing, medial alignment	1	PROM	ICC .95	100° ± 6°
Hopson et al.[31]	20 (10 M, 10 F)	21–43 years	Standing, full weight bearing, medial alignment	1	PROM	ICC .98	110° ± 11°
Joseph[35]	17 M	Younger than 30 years	Angles measured from lateral radiographs	Not stated	AROM	No	54° (R) 56° (L)
Joseph[35]	17 M	30–45 years	Angles measured from lateral radiographs	Not stated	AROM	No	52° (R) 52° (L)
Joseph[35]	16 M	Older than 45 years	Angles measured from lateral radiographs	Not stated	AROM	No	46° (R) 44° (L)

(Table continued on following page)

Table C–22.	(Cont.)						
STUDY	SAMPLE	AGES	METHOD USED	NUMBER OF EXAMINERS	TYPE OF MOTION	RELIABILITY COEFFICIENT CALCULATED?	ROM
Joseph[35]	16 M	Younger than 30 years	Angles measured from lateral radiographs	Not stated	PROM	No	78° (R) 77° (L)
Joseph[35]	17 M	30–45 years	Angles measured from lateral radiographs	Not stated	PROM	No	76° (R) 75° (L)
Joseph[35]	16 M	45 and under	Angles measured from lateral radiographs	Not stated	PROM	No	71° (R) 63° (L)
Walker et al.[59]	60 (30 M, 30 F)	60–84 years	AAOS	1	AROM	Pearson's r >.81	61° ± 13°

M, males; F, females; AAOS, American Academy of Orthopaedic Surgeons; MTP, metatarsophalangeal; AROM, active range of motion; PROM, passive range of motion; STJN, subtalar joint neutral; R, right; L, left; UG, universal goniometer; ICC, intraclass correlation.

Table C–23.	INVESTIGATIONS REPORTING DATA FOR FIRST MTP FLEXION ROM						
STUDY	SAMPLE	AGES	METHOD USED	NUMBER OF EXAMINERS	TYPE OF MOTION	RELIABILITY COEFFICIENT CALCULATED?	ROM
Buell et al.[12]	15 (# M & F not stated)	19–30 years	STJN; midtarsal joint fully pronated, medial alignment	Not stated	PROM	No	20°
Buell et al.[12]	24 (# M & F not stated)	30–45 years	STJN; midtarsal joint fully pronated, medial alignment	Not stated	PROM	No	17°
Buell et al.[12]	11 (# M & F not stated)	45 years and under	STJN; midtarsal joint fully pronated, medial alignment	Not stated	PROM	No	14°
Joseph[35]	17 M	Younger than 30 years	Angles measured from lateral radiographs	Not stated	AROM	No	26° ± 2° (R) 25° ± 2° (L)
Joseph[35]	17 M	30–45 years	Angles measured from lateral radiographs	Not stated	AROM	No	24° ± 2° (R) 23° ± 2° (L)
Joseph[35]	16 M	Older than 45 years	Angles measured from lateral radiographs	Not stated	AROM	No	18° ± 2° (R) 21° ± 2° (L)
Walker et al.[59]	60 (30 M, 30 F)	60–84 years	AAOS	2	AROM	Pearson's r >.81	7° ± 12°

M, males; F, females; AAOS, American Academy of Orthopaedic Surgeons; MTP, metatarsophalangeal; AROM, active range of motion; PROM, passive range of motion; STJN, subtalar joint neutral; R, right; L, left.

References

1. Ahlbäck SO, Lindahl O: Sagittal mobility of the hip-joint. Acta Orthop Scand 1964;34: 310–322.
2. Ahlberg A, Moussa M, Al-Nahdi M: On geographical variations in the normal range of joint motion. Clin Orthop 1988;234:229–231.
3. American Academy of Orthopaedic Surgeons: Joint Motion: Method of Measuring and Recording. Chicago, American Academy of Orthopaedic Surgeons, 1965.
4. American Medical Association: Guides to the Evaluation of Permanent Impairment, 2nd ed. Chicago, 1984.
5. American Medical Association: Guides to the Evaluation of Permanent Impairment, 4th ed. Chicago, 1993.
6. Balogun JA, Abereoje OK, Olaogun MO, Obajuluwa VA: Inter- and intratester reliability of measuring neck motions with tape measure and Myrin gravity-reference goniometer. J Orthop Sports Phys Ther 1989;10:248–253.
7. Beattie P, Rothstein JM, Lamb RL: Reliability of the attraction method for measuring lumbar spine backward bending. Phys Ther 1987;67:364–369.
8. Boline PD, Keating JC, Haas M, Anderson AV: Inter examiner reliability and discriminant validity of inclinometric measurement of lumbar rotation in chronic low-back pain patients and subjects without low-back pain. Spine 1992;17:335–338.
9. Boone DC, Azen SP: Normal range of motion of joints in male subjects. J Bone Joint Surg 1979;61:756–759.
10. Breum J, Wiberg J, Bolton JE: Reliability and concurrent validity of the BROM II for measuring lumbar mobility. J Manipulative Physiol Ther 1995;18:497–502.
11. Broughton NS, Wright J, Menelaus MB: Range of knee motion in normal neonates. J Pediatr Orthop 1993;13:263–264.
12. Buell T, Green DR, Risser J: Measurement of the first metatarsophalangeal joint range of motion. J Am Podiatr Med Assoc 1988;78:439–448.
13. Capuano-Pucci D, Rheault W, Aukai J, et al.: Intratester and intertester reliability of the cervical range of motion device. Arch Phys Med Rehabil 1991;72:338–340.
14. Chiarello CM, Savidge R: Interrater reliability of the Cybex EDI-320 and fluid goniometer in normals and patients with low back pain. Arch Phys Med Rehabil 1993;74:32–37.
15. Cobe HM: The range of active motion at the wrist of white adults. J Bone Joint Surg 1928;10:763–774.
16. Coon V, Donato G, Honser C, et al.: Normal ranges of hip motion in infants six weeks, three months, and six months of age. Clin Orthop 1975;110:256–260.
17. Dillard J, Trafimow J, Andersson GBJ, Cronin K: Motion of the lumbar spine: Reliability of two measurement techniques. Spine 1991;16:321–324.
18. Drews JE, Vraciu JK, Pellino G: Range of motion of the joints of the lower extremities of newborns. Phys Occup Ther Pediatr 1984;4:49–62.
19. Einkauf DK, Gohdes ML, Jensen GM, Jewell MJ: Changes in spinal mobility with increasing age in women. Phys Ther 1987;67:370–375.
20. Ellison JB, Rose SJ, Sahrmann SA: Patterns of hip rotation range of motion: A comparison between healthy subjects and patients with low back pain. Phys Ther 1990;70:537–541.
21. Fitzgerald GK, Wynveen KJ, Rheault W, Rothschild B: Objective assessment with establishment of normal values for lumbar spinal range of motion. Phys Ther 1983;63:1776–1781.
22. Forero N, Okamura LA, Larson MA: Normal ranges of hip motion in neonates. J Pediatr Orthop 1989;9:391–395.
23. Giladi M, Milgrom C, Stein M et al.: External rotation of the hip. Clin Orthop 1987;216:131–134.
24. Greene WB, Heckman JD: The Clinical Measurement of Joint Motion. Rosemont, Ill, American Academy of Orthopaedic Surgeons, 1994.
25. Gunal I, Kose N, Erdogan O: Normal range of motion of the joints of the upper extremity in male subjects, with special reference to side. J Bone Joint Surg Am 1996;78:1401–1404.
26. Haas SS, Epps CH, Adams JP: Normal ranges of hip motion in the newborn. Clin Orthop 1973;19:114–118.
27. Haley ET: Range of hip rotation and torque of hip rotator muscle groups. Am J Phys Med 1953;32:261–270.
28. Haley SM, Tada WL, Carmichael EM: Spinal mobility in young children. Phys Ther 1986;66:1697–1703.
29. Hewitt D: The range of active motion at the wrist of women. J Bone Joint Surg 1928;10:775–787.
30. Hoaglund FT, Yau A, Wong WL: Osteoarthritis of the hip and other joints in southern Chinese in Hong Kong. J Bone Joint Surg 1973;55A:545–557.
31. Hopson MM, McPoil TG, Cornwall MW: Motion of the first metatarsophalangeal joint: Reliability and validity of four measurement techniques. J Am Podiatr Med Assoc 1995;85:198–204.

32. Hsieh C, Yeung B: Active neck motion measurements with a tape measure. J Orthop Sports Phys Ther 1986;8:88–92.

33. Jenkins M, Bamberger HB, Black L, Nowinski R: Thumb joint flexion. What is normal? J Hand Surg [Br] 1998;23:796–797.

34. Johnson CL, Fulwood R, Abraham S, et al.: Basic data on anthropometric measurements and angular measurements of the hip and knee joints for selected age groups 1–74 years of age, United States, 1971–75. Hyattsville, Md: National Center for Health Statistics (National Health Survey Series 11, No. 219); 1981. US Dept of Health and Human Services publication (PHS) 81–1669.

35. Joseph J: Range of movement of the great toe in men. J Bone Joint Surg 1954;36B:450–457.

36. Krejcie, RV, Morgan DW: Determining sample size for research activities. Educ Psychol Measurement 1970;30:607–610.

37. Macrae IF, Wright V: Measurement of back movement. Ann Rheum Dis 1969;28:584–589.

38. Mallon WJ, Brown HR, Nunley JA: Digital ranges of motion: Normal values in young adults. J Hand Surg 1991;16A:882–887.

39. Mayer TG, Tencer AF, Kristoferson S, Mooney V: Use of noninvasive techniques for quantification of spinal range-of-motion in normal subjects and chronic low-back dysfunction patients. Spine 1984;9:588–595.

40. Milgrom C, Giladi M, Simkin A, et al.: The normal range of subtalar inversion and eversion in young males as measured by three different techniques. Foot Ankle Int 1985;6:143–145.

41. Minium EW: Statistical Reasoning in Psychology and Education. New York, John Wiley & Sons, 1978.

42. Moll JMV, Wright V: Normal range of motion: An objective clinical study. Ann Rheum Dis 1971;30:381–386.

43. Mundale MO, Hislop HJ, Babideau RJ, et al.: Evaluation of extension of the hip. Arch Phys Med Rehabil 1956;37:75–80.

44. Nigg BM, Fisher V, Allinger TL, et al.: Range of motion of the foot as a function of age. Foot Ankle Int 1992;13:336–343.

45. Ordway NR, Seymour R, Donelson RG, et al.: Cervical sagittal range-of-motion analysis using three methods. Spine 1997;22:501–508.

46. Phelps E, Smith LJ, Hallum A: Normal ranges of hip motion of infants between nine and 24 months of age. Dev Med Child Neurol 1985;27:785–792.

47. Roaas A, Anderson G: Normal range of motion of the hip, knee and ankle joints in male subjects, 30–40 years of age. Acta Orthop Scand 1982;53:205–208.

48. Roach KE, Miles TP: Normal hip and knee active range of motion: The relationship to age. Phys Ther 1991;71:656–665.

49. Rose MJ: The statistical analysis of the intra-observer repeatability of four clinical measurement techniques. Physiotherapy 1991;77:89–91.

50. Rothschild BM: Rhematology: A Primary Care Approach. Brooklyn, NY, Yorke Medical Books, 1982.

51. Ryu J, Cooney WP, Askew LJ, et al.: Functional ranges of motion of the wrist joint. J Hand Surg 1991;16A:409–419.

52. Sabari JS, Maltzev I, Lubarsky D, et al: Goniometric assessment of shoulder range of motion: Comparison of testing in supine and sitting positions. Arch Phys Med Rehabil 1998;79:647–651.

53. Shaw SJ, Morris MA: The range of motion of the metacarpophalangeal joint of the thumb and its relationship to injury. J Hand Surg 1992;17B:164–166.

54. Simoneau CC, Hoenig KJ, Lepley JE, Papanek PE: Influence of hip position and gender on active hip internal and external rotation. J Orthop Sports Phys Ther 1998;28:158–164.

55. Smith JR, Walker JM: Knee and elbow range of motion in healthy older individuals. Phys Occup Ther Geriatr 1983;2:31–38.

56. Svenningsen S, Terjesen T, Auflem M, Berg V: Hip motion related to age and sex. Acta Orthop Scand 1989;60:97–100.

57. Tiberio D, Bohannon RW, Zito MA: Effect of subtalar joint position on the measurement of maximum ankle dorsiflexion. Clin Biomech (Bristol, Avon) 1989;4:189–191.

58. Van Adrichem JAM, van der Korst JK: Assessment of the flexibility of the lumbar spine. Scand J Rheumatol 1973;2:87–91.

59. Walker JM, Sue D, Miles-Elkousy N, et al.: Active mobility of the extremities in older subjects. Phys Ther 1984;64:919–923.

60. Watanabe H, et al.: The range of joint motions of the extremities in healthy Japanese people: The difference according to age. Cited in Walker, JM: Musculoskeletal development: A review. Phys Ther 1991;71:878.

61. Waugh KG, Minkel JL, Parker R, Coon VA: Measurement of selected hip, knee, and ankle joint motions in newborns. Phys Ther 1983;63:1616–1621.

62. Youdas JW, Carey TR, Garrett TR: Reliability of measurement of cervical spine range of motion—Comparison of three methods. Phys Ther 1991;71:98–104.

63. Youdas JW, Garrett TR, Suman VJ, et al.: Normal range of motion of the cervical spine: An initial goniometric study. Phys Ther 1992;72:770–780.

INDEX

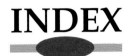

Note: Page numbers followed by the letter f refer to figures. Page numbers followed by the letter b refer to boxed material and those followed by t refer to tables.